ALLE ZEIT WACH 1842

G. Gasbarrini S. Pretolani (Eds.)

Basic and Clinical Aspects of Helicobacter pylori Infection

With 76 Figures

Springer-Verlag
Berlin Heidelberg New York
London Paris Tokyo
Hong Kong Barcelona
Budapest

Professor G. Gasbarrini
I. Patologia Medica
Policlinico S. Orsola
Via Massarenti 9
I-40138 Bologna
Italy

Dr. S. Pretolani
I. Patologia Medica
Policlinico S. Orsola
Via Massarenti 9
I-40138 Bologna
Italy

ISBN 3-540-56720-8 Springer-Verlag Berlin Heidelberg New York
ISBN 0-387-56720-8 Springer-Verlag New York Berlin Heidelberg

Library of Congress Cataloging-in-Publication Data. Basic and Clinical Aspects of Helicobacter pylori infection / G. Gasbarrini, S. Pretolani (eds.). p. cm. Proceedings of the Fourth Workshop of the European Helicobacter Pylori Study Group, held in Bologna, Italy, Nov. 1991. Includes bibliographical references and index. ISBN 3-540-56720-8 (alk. paper). – ISBN 0-387-56720-8 (alk. paper). 1. Helicobacter pylori infections – Congresses. I. Gasbarrini, G. II. Pretolani, S. (Stefano), 1956– . III. European Helicobacter Pylori Study Group, Workshop (4th; 1991; Bologna, Italy) [DNLM: 1. Helicobacter Infections – pathology – congresses. 2. Helicobacter Infections – drug therapy – congresses. 3. Helicobacter pylori – pathogenicity – congresses. 4. Peptic Ulcer-parasitology – congresses. 5. Gastritis – parasitology – congresses. WC 200 8311 1991] – QR201.H44B37 1993 616.9'31 – dc20 DNLM/DLC 93-43056

Printed in Germany

Typesetting: Thomson Press (India) Ltd., New Delhi

23/3130/SPS – 543210 – Printed on acid-free paper

Preface

A century ago the Italian pathologist Bizzozero described the relationships between spiral bacteria and the mammalian gastrointestinal tract. Since 1982, when *Helicobacter pylori* was discovered, gastroduodenal disease have been completely revised as a consequence of the results of basic and clinical research in this field.

Progress in understanding the pathogenesis of this bacterium has been made by studying *H. pylori* infection in animal models. More specific diagnostic tools have been developed using new molecular biology techniques. Future trends are directed towards preparing a specific *H. pylori* vaccine.

A new classification for gastritis, the Sydney System, including *H. pylori* gastritis, was proposed in 1990. As concerns the clinical approach to peptic ulcer disease in the 1990's, the majority of authors agree on the importance of *H. pylori* eradication. Moreover, recent clinical studies suggest that *H. pylori* infection can be associated with other gastroduodenal diseases, such as nonulcer dyspepsia and gastric cancer. Multicenter trials to standardize serological methods and evaluate the efficacy of new antimicrobial therapy schedules are planned throughout different European countries.

The fourth Workshop of the European *Helicobacter Pylori* Study Group was held in Bologna, Italy, in November 1991. Two years before Bologna University celebrated its ninth centennial, giving evidence of being the oldest University in the modern world. Thus the *H. pylori* story that has continued for more than a century has been discussed once again at the University with the oldest tradition in the world.

The papers presented at the fourth Workshop in Bologna were selected out of 363 original contributions sent to the organizing committee from 30 different countries and five continents. Of those 363 papers 49 were selected; these were presented orally and discussed in the plenary sessions at the workshop, and they have been compiled in extended form together with the lectures in this book. The opportunity of this choice is confirmed by the fact that 2 years after their presentation, the majority of these studies are surprisingly up to date and represent a fundamental advance in the knowledge of *H. pylori* infection.

The reader will find in this volume several topics on current problems related to gastroduodenal pathology and *H. pylori* infection:

symptoms and histology of nonulcerous dyspepsia, the role of surgical infections in geriatric age, pathogenic mechanisms associated with structural factors of the bacterium (toxins, adhesions, agglutinins) as well with the host immune response, the role of serology in the diagnosis of the infection, some aspects of molecular biology of the bacterium, and the newest therapeutic approaches.

We think that this book will be useful not only to researchers, looking for the most recent data on those topics, but also to the general practitioner who needs a comprehensive overview of the impact of this bacterium on gastroduodenal pathology and information about the therapeutic options.

This volume represents a continuation of the books already published as proceedings of the previous meetings of the EHPSG, also in its editorial and typographic features. Publishing these proceedings, within an acceptable time, is an important activity of the EHPGS and should be maintained in the future. It is with pleasure that we present this most recent collection of papers.

Stefano Pretolani
(Secretary of
IV Workshop of EHPSG)

Giovanni Gasbarrini
(President of
IV Workshop of EHPSG)

Contents

Nonulcer Dyspepsia

Nonulcer Dyspepsia
C. O'Morain and M. Buckley 3

Nonulcer Dyspepsia: Psychological Considerations
M. Farnè 8

Nonulcer Dyspepsia and *Helicobacter pylori*: Effect of Eradication on Symptoms and Gastritis
S. Pretolani, F. Bonvicini, E. Brocchi, M. Baraldini, D. Cilla, S. Baldinelli, E. Bazzocchi, P. Pasini, and G. Gasbarrini (With 4 Figures) 11

Upper Gastrointestinal Endoscopy and the Prevalence of *Helicobacter pylori* Infection in Recurrent Abdominal Pain of Childhood
M. Ashorn, R. Karikoski-Leo, T. Ruuska, A. Miettinen, and M. Mäki 19

The Value of Serodiagnosis of *Helicobacter pylori* in Predicting Negative Gastroscopy
P.R. Hawtin, D. Sharpstone, S. Vyas, J. Treasure, D. Fine, and D.G. Newell (With 1 Figure) 23

The Icelandic Nonulcer Dyspepsia/*Helicobacter pylori* Study: Symptomatic Response and Eradication Rate with De-Nol or De-Nol Plus Metronidazol in Treatment of *Helicobacter*-Positive Patients with Nonulcer Dyspepsia
E. Oddsson, H. Guðjónsson, A. Theodors, S. Björnsson, O. Gunnlaugsson, M. Gormsen, O. Steingrímsson, J.J. Jóhannsson, and B. Thjodleifsson (With 1 Figure) 26

Long-Term Follow-up of Children with *Helicobacter pylori*-Associated Nonulcer Dyspepsia After Eradication of the Infection
C. De Giacomo, P. Perotti, E. Giacobone, R. Daturi, L. Villani, and R. Fiocca 29

Helicobacter pylori, Surgery, and Aging

The Role of Ulcer Surgery Today
R. Bittner 35

Effect of Single-Shot Antibiotic Treatment on *Helicobacter pylori* in Patients Undergoing Ulcer Operation
M. Büchler, H. Frieß, F. Flock, A. Stanescu, K. Baczako, and P. Malfertheiner 41

The Aging Stomach
J.H. Baron 48

Pathogenic Mechanisms of *Helcobacter pylori* Infection: Virulence

Construction of a Molecular Population Genetic Framework for the Characterization of *Helicobacter pylori* Pathogenesis by Multilocus Enzyme Electrophoresis
M.F. Go, D.Y. Graham, and J.M. Musser 57

The Flagella of *Helicobacter pylori*: Molecular Analysis and Potential in Pathogenesis
C.W. Penn and C.J. Luke 60

Identification of Potential S Layer Proteins of *Helicobacter pylori*
B. Eschweiler, B. Gerstenecker, T. Moriki, B. Bohrmann, and M. Kist (With 6 Figures) 65

Urease as a Colonisation Factor in *Helicobacter*
A.A. McColm, J. Bagshaw, C. O'Malley, and A. McLaren (With 4 Figures) 74

Affinity and Ion Exchange Chromatography in the Purification and Characterization of *Helicobacter pylori* Cytotoxin-Associated Proteins
I. Luzzi, M. Bugnoli, C. Pezzella, N. Figura, I. Benedetti, D. Armellini, and A. Rossolini 79

Neutralization of the Vacuolating Toxin from *Helicobacter pylori* by Antisera from Patients with Duodenal or Gastric Ulcer
H. Goossens, Y. Glupczynski, J.P. Lambert, A. Burette, L. Vlaes, and J.P. Butzler 82

Helicobacter pylori: Phospholipase C and Haemolysis
M.A. Daw, H.X. Xia, and C. O'Morain 85

Haemaglutinins of *Helicobacter pylori* and Adherence to HEp-2 Cells
C.S. Goodwin 90

Partial Purification and Characterization of Sialic Acid Specific Soluble Haemagglutinin(s) of *Helicobacter pylori* Strain NCTC 11637
J. Lelwala-Guruge, A.S. Kreger, W. Shen, and T. Wadström (With 1 Figure) 92

Pathogenic Mechanisms of *Helicobacter pylori* Infection: Host Response

The Role of *Helicobacter pylori* Gastritis in Ulcerogenesis and Carcinogenesis
E. Solcia, R. Fiocca, L. Villani, O. Luinetti, A. Gianatti, E. Trespi, G. Stella, M. Cornaggia, A. Chiaravalli, and C. Capella (With 5 Figures) 101

Isolation and Phenotypical Characterization of T-Lymphocytes Isolated from the Gastric Mucosa of Patients With and Without *Helicobacter pylori*
W.P. Brooks, G. Meimarakis, R.A. Hatz, E. Bayerdörffer, G. Enders, and H.J. Krämling (With 4 Figures) 113

Demonstration of the Major Cytotoxin-Association Protein of *Helicobacter pylori* in Gastric Biopsies by Western Blotting
N. Figura, M. Bugnoli, S. Quaranta, M. Corsetti, D. Armellini, M. Matergi, L. Di Gregorio, L. Abate, E. Esposito, and P.F. Bayeli (With 1 Figure) 119

Gastric Functions and *Helicobacter pylori* Infection in Patients with Fundic Atrophic Gastritis
R. Corinaldesi, A. Tucci, V. Stanghellini, C. Tosetti, S. Gasperoni, G.F. Paparo, G. Biasco, S. Siringo, and L. Barbara 122

Peptic Ulcer in the Elderly: Not a *Helicobacter*-Related Condition?
J.I. Wyatt, T.M. Shallcross, and R.V. Heatley 125

Serology of *Helicobacter pylori* Infection

Introduction
L.P. Andersen and D.G. Newell 131

The Use of *Helicobacter pylori* Serology in Diagnosis and Treatment Monitoring
L.P. Andersen 133

The Use of Serological Detection of *Helicobacter pylori* in Epidemiology
D. Forman 136

Helicobacter pylori Serology: Kit Evaluation and Comparison
E. De Koster, P. Denis, H. Goossens, J.F. Nyst, and M. Deltenre 139

Standards for Serologic Study of Infection with *Helicobacter pylori*
R. Feldman, S.J.W. Evans, J. Deeks, B. Rathbone, and The *Helicobacter pylori* Serology Study Group (With 5 Figures) 145

Helicobacter pylori Antigenic Preparations
A.R. Stacey 154

The Value of Class and Subclass ELISAs and Antibody Specificity in Monitoring Treatment of *Helicobacter pylori*
A.R. Stacey, G.D. Bell, and D.G. Newell (With 2 Figures) 159

Future Prospects for *Helicobacter pylori* Serology
D.G. Newell 164

The *Helicobacter pylori* San Marino Study: Seroepidemiology of *Helicobacter pylori* Infection in the Republic of San Marino
G. Gasbarrini, S. Pretolani, G.C. Ghironzi, G. Giulianelli, E. Tonelli, M.R.A. Gatto, S. Ferrari, F. Mégraud, M. Baraldini, D. Cilla, S. Baldinelli, E. Bazzocchi, and F. Bonvicini (With 5 Figures) 168

Molecular Biology of *Helicobacter pylori*

Construction of Isogenic Mutants of *Helicobacter pylori* Deficient in Urease Activity
R.L. Ferrero, V. Cussac, P. Courcoux, and A. Labigne (With 1 Figure) 179

Cloning of a *Helicobacter pylori* Flagellin Gene and Construction of a Nonflagellated Mutant by Transformation-Mediated Allelic Exchange
R. Haas, H. Leying, J.P.M. Van Putten, T.F. Meyer, G. Geis, S. Suerbaum, and W. Opferkuch (With 2 Figures) 183

Identification and Characterization of an Adhesion Gene of *Helicobacter pylori* by Cloning
D.G. Evans, T.K. Karjalainen, D.J. Evans Jr., D.Y. Graham, and C.H. Lee 189

Molecular Cloning and Nucleotide Sequence Determination of *htr*A, a Gene Encoding a 48-kDa Stress Protein of *Helicobacter pylori*
H. Kleanthous, C.L. Clayton, D.D. Morgan, M.J. Pallen, and S. Tabaqchali (With 5 Figures) 195

Diagnosis of *Helicobacter pylori* in Gastric Juice Aspirates Using Polymerase Chain Reaction
T.U. Westblom, S. Phadnis, S. Normark, and S.J. Czinn . . 203

Molecular Fingerprinting of *Helicobacter pylori*: An Evaluation of Methods
D.D. Morgan, C. Clayton, H. Kleanthous, C. McNulty, and S. Tabaqchali (with 5 Figures) 206

Developments in Ribotyping of *Helicobacter pylori*
R.J. Owen (With 2 Figures) 213

The 130-kDa Vacuolating Cytotoxin-Associated Protein Is a Component of Cytotoxic *Helicobacter pylori* Organisms
M. Bugnoli, D. Armellini, R. Rappuoli, A. Rossolini, Z.Y. Xiang, and N. Figura (With 1 Figure) 219

The Cloning and Partial Sequence Analysis of the Catalase Gene of *Helicobacter pylori*
D.G. Newell, P.J.M. Nuijten, A.R. Stacey, and S.L. Hazell 223

Binding of *Helicobacter pylori* to Extracellular Matrix Proteins
A.P. Moran, P. Kuusela, and T.U. Kosunen (With 2 Figures) 227

Therapeutic Approaches

Helicobacter pylori: Clinical Aspects
J.J. Misiewicz 237

H_2 Receptor Antagonists: Is There a Place in the Treatment of *Helicobacter pylori* Infection?
C. Scarpignato, M. Felder, and G. Dobrilla
(With 4 Figures) 241

Proton Pump Inhibitors in the Management of *Helicobacter pylori*-Related Diseases
M. Deltenre, E. De Koster, and J.F. Nyst 251

Pharmacology of Bismuth-Containing Medicines Used to Treat *Helicobacter pylori* Infections
D.W.R. Hall 258

Bismuth and *Helicobacter pylori*
P. Malfertheiner, M. Nilius, and U. Kreusel
(With 5 Figures) 266

Antibiotics in *Helicobacter pylori* Treatment
C.S. Goodwin 280

Clinical Application of Antibiotics in Eradicating *Helicobacter pylori*
C. O'Morain, H.X Xia, and M.A. Daw 283

Cytoprotective Drugs and *Helicobacter pylori* Infection
M. Del Tacca, G. Natale, and C. Blandizzi
(With 4 Figures) 290

Approaches to the Treatment of *Helicobacter pylori* Infection
G. Bianchi Porro and M. Lazzaroni (With 3 Figures) 298

Subject Index 307

List of First Authors

Addresses are given at the beginning of the respective contribution

Andersen, L.P. 131, 133
Ashorn, M. 19

Baron, J.H. 48
Bianchi Porro, G. 298
Bittner, R. 35
Brooks, W.P. 113
Büchler, M. 41

Corinaldesi, R. 122

Daw, M.A. 85
De Giacomo, C. 29
De Koster, E. 139
Del Tacca, M. 290
Deltenre, M. 251

Eschweiler, B. 65
Evans, D.G. 189

Farné, M. 8
Feldman, R. 145
Ferrero, R.L. 179
Figura, N. 119, 219
Forman, D. 136

Gasbarrini, G. 168
Go, M.F. 57
Goodwin, C.S. 90, 280
Goossens, H. 82

Haas, R. 183
Hall, D.W.R. 258
Hawtin, P.R. 23

Kleanthous, H. 195

Lelwala-Guruge, J. 92
Luzzi, I. 79

Malfertheiner, P. 266
Mc Laren, A. 74
Misiewicz, J.J. 237
Moran, A.P. 227
Morgan, D.D. 206

Newell, D.G. 164, 223

O'Morain, C. 3, 283
Oddsson, E. 26
Owen, R.J. 213

Penn, C.W. 60
Pretolani, S. 11

Scarpignato, C. 241
Solcia, E. 101
Stacey, A.R. 154, 159

Westblom, T.U. 203
Wyatt, J.I. 125

Nonulcer Dyspepsia

Nonulcer Dyspepsia

C. O'Morain and M. Buckley

Introduction

Dyspepsia is a term widely used in clinical practice. Physicians describe patients as having dyspepsia when the patients themselves say that they have indigestion. Dyspepsia derives from the Greek words *dys* (bad) and *peptein* (to digest). Indigestion is derived from Latin, but the two words otherwise have the same construction and the same meaning. Dyspepsia and indigestion have been used to describe symptoms presumed to have originated in the gut anywhere from the oesophagus to the colon.

Definition and Classification

Non-ulcer dyspepsia is usually used to describe patients who have dyspeptic symptoms for more than 3 months, and who have a normal endoscopy, normal biochemistry and no evidence of gall bladder disease [1]. Symptoms ranging from abdominal pain and discomfort, post-prandial fullness, abdominal bloating, belching, early satiety, anorexia, nausea, vomiting, heartburn and regurgitation have been grouped together under the term non-ulcer dyspepsia. For research and clinical purposes symptoms should be grouped into reflux, ulcer, mortility and non-specific dyspepsia:

Reflux-like dyspepsia
- Heartburn
- Acid regurgitation

Ulcer-like dyspepsia
- Epigastric pain
- Night pain causing the patient to awaken
- Pain relieved by food or antacids
- Pain with a pattern of remission and relapses

Motility-like dyspepsia
- Nausea or vomitting
- Early satiety/anorexia
- Post prandial bloating

Department of Gastroenterology, Meath/Adelaide Hospitals, Trinity College, Dublin, Ireland

Gasbarrini/Pretolani (Eds.)
Basic and Clinical Aspects of H. pylori Infection

Excessive belching
Upper abdominal discomfort
Non-specific dyspepsia
Symptoms which do not fit into any of the above categories

An organic aetiology is suggested by this classification. Patients who have predominantly reflux symptoms have macroscopically normal-appearing oesophagus, but biopsies from the oesophagus may reveal changes of reflux. Furthermore, 24-h ambulatory pH probe may also reveal abnormalities. A 24-h ambulatory pH recording is particularly useful in patients who have non-cardiac chest pain [2]. If a definite diagnosis is made of gastro-oesophageal reflux with a normal endoscopy, H_2 antagonist treatment is usually successful.

Non-specific dyspepsia may be due to an abnormality of motility affecting the antrum [3]. Patients with non-specific dyspepsia may well have some psychological overlay [4]. Patients who have *Helicobacter pylori* infection and a macroscopically normal endoscopy often have ulcer-like dyspepsia symptoms [5].

Prevalence

Non-ulcer dyspepsia is a common condition. A recent review in which previous studies were pooled covered 3667 patients who underwent endoscopy; 33.6% had normal findings, 23% gastric oesophageal reflux, 20% gastritis, 19% ulcers, and 2% cancer [6]. The prevalence of non-ulcer dyspepsia is greater in patients aged under 25 years, where a normal endoscopy is found in 38% of patients and cancer is rarely found [7]. However, it is still significant in patients aged over 60 in that 20% of patients with dyspepsia have a normal endoscoy [8]. This would suggest that it is a life-long condition. In a prospective study of 77 patients with non-ulcer dyspepsia, 68% continued to have pain at 5 years, although fewer than half had pain that interfered with their capacity to work [9]. Early studies reported a high rate of peptic ulcers developing in patients originally diagnosed as having X-ray negative dyspepsia [10]. This was also supportive of a role for *H. pylori*. *H. pylori* causes gastritis which later results in a duodenal ulcer. *H. pylori* raises the local pH in the vicinity of antral cells, causing gastrin to be secreted which in turn acts systemically on the parietal cells to secrete acid. The resulting hyperacidity gives rise to the formation of gastric metaplasia in the duodenum, a response to any injurous condition. That part of the duodenum with gastric metaplasia then becomes infected by *H. pylori*, resulting in ulceration.

Aetiology

The aetiology of non-ulcer dyspepsia remains unknown. The disease probably includes a spectrum of causes. Gastric acid secretion, upper gastrointestinal tract motility abnormalities, evnironmental and psychological factors have all been suggested. There is no significant difference in basal or peak acid secretion between patients with non-ulcer dyspepsia and controls [11]. In a small study of patients with non-ulcer dyspepsia injection of pentagastrin was associated with pain. Inhibiting acid secretion with H_2 antagonists did not significantly reduce pain [2]. Thus the role that acid plays in non-ulcer dyspepsia is uncertain, and it is likely to be small.

Studies of the upper gastrointestinal tract motility in patients with non-ulcer dyspepsia who have symptoms suggestive of gastroparesis have antral hypomotility after meals. Abnormal gastric myoelectric activity has also been documented in some patients. Delayed gastric emptying for solids and liquids has been reported in 25%–50% [13].

It is frequently assumed that diet plays an important role in dyspepsia although food intolerance, as established by double-blind challenge testing, appears to be rare [14]. There is no evidence that smoking, alcohol or coffee are associated with non-ulcer dyspepsia. Analgesic drugs, however, may be an important cause of dyspepsia in selected patients [15]. Psychological stress can also be the cause of gastrointestinal symptoms. Major life-events stress is not more common in patients with non-ulcer dyspepsia [16]. Patients with non-ulcer dyspepsia reportedly have more somatic complaints than do ulcer patients and controls, suggesting that personality may be important in the pathogenesis of non-ulcer dyspepsia [17].

Recently Dinan and Keeling suggested that non-ulcer dyspepsia is characterised by a neurochemical dysfunction in the central nervous system [18]. Buspirone stimulates 5-hydroxytryptamine (5-HT) receptors and brings about the release of prolactin, and there is evidence to suggest that the extent of prolactin release after a challenge with buspirone is an indicator of the sensitivity to central 5-HT receptors. In a study of 17 patients with a diagnosis of non-ulcer dyspepsia, 8 normal healthy controls and 6 patients with peptic ulcer disease were given a challenge of 60 mg buspirone orally, and prolactin release over a 3-h period was monitored. The mean prolactin response was significantly greater in patients with non-ulcer dyspepsia than in healthy controls and in those with peptic ulcer disease. The results suggest the central 5-HT receptors may be supersensitive in non-ulcer dyspepsia.

A preliminary study of the efficacy of a 5-HT blocker in over 30 patients with the syndrome lends support to the above finding.

Helicobacter pylori

This workshop highlights the role of *H. pylori* in non-ulcer dyspepsia particularly in those patients whose predominant symptom is pain.

Bismuth subcitrate and bismuth subsalicylate, besides having effectcs on the gastric mucosa, suppress but usually do not eradicate *H. pylori* infection [19]. The role of *H. pylori* in non-ulcer dyspepsia may be in patients who have ulcer type dyspepsia. However it is important to remember that there is a high placebo response (30%–60%) to all drug treatments in dyspepsia. However, most trials do suggest that bismuth is effective, and statistically significant symptom improvement over placebo has been demonstrated in several trials, but not all [20, 21].

All these investigations have several shortcomings, and particularly study blinding was difficult as bismuth usually causes reversible black discolouration of stools. More importantly, all the studies used symptom measures that were not validated and may be inadequate. Despite this bismuth may be a useful drug for a small sub-group of patients with non-ulcer dyspepsia who have associated *H. pylori* gastritis.

In a recent study we randomised patients who had non-ulcer dyspepsia and had *H. pylori* gastritis to either of three treatment regimes, colloidal bismuth subcitrate 1 q.i.d.; amoxycillin 500 mg t.d.s., and metronidazole 400 mg t.d.s. for 1 week; colloidal bismuth subcitrate plus amoxycillin plus metronidazole [22]. Eradication rates were 37%, 56% and 55%, respectively, for these treatment regimes. Although gastritis scores improved significantly only in patients in whom *H. pylori* had been eradicated, mean symptom scores after treatment were similar in patients who had or had not been eradicated. Similarly the mean symptom score improved whether or not gastritis improved. The observations were similar for treatment groups analysed individually. However, in the long term after 1 year follow-up there was a significant improvement in these patients who had *H. pylori* eradicated in that they needed fewer treatment courses during that year and had at review significantly fewer symptoms.

Conclusion

Non-ulcer dyspepsia is a costly condition resulting in extensive investigation with the use of empiric treatment.

The present workshop has revealed some very interesting data in clarifying the role of *H. pylori* in the sub-group of patients with non-ulcer dyspepsia with symptoms that are ulcer in type. It has also highlighted the debate of recurrent abdominal pain in childhood. It is possible that *H. pylori* may play a role in this condition. However, we await long-term studies to see whether eradication of *H. pylori* alters the natural history of the disease.

A confident diagnosis is important since unnecessary investigation results in considerable expense and anxiety. Serological testing may reduce endoscopy workload. In the terms of treatment the strong placebo response is observed. Long-term studies should be initiated to determine whether eradication of *H. pylori* alters the natural history of the disease.

References

1. Talley NJ (1991) Non-ulcer dyspepsia: myths and realities. Ailment Pharmacol Ther 5 [Suppl]: 145–162
2. Klauser AG, Schindbeck NE, Muller-Lissner SA (1990) Symptoms of gastroesophageal reflux disease. Lancet 335: 205–208

3. Kerlin P (1989) Postprandial antral hypomotility in patients with idiopathic nausea and vomiting. Gut 30: 54–59
4. Richter JE (1991) Stress and psychologic and environmental factors in functional dyspepsia. Scand J Gastroenterol 26 [Suppl 182]: 40–46
5. Rokkas T, Pursey C, Uzoeching E et al. (1987) *Campylobacter pylori* and non-ulcer dyspepsia. Am J Gastroenterol 82: 1149–1152
6. Richter JE (1991) Dyspepsia: organic causes and differential characteristics from functional dyspepsia. Scand J Gastroenterol 26 [Suppl 182]: 11–16
7. Forbut LN, Gribble RJ, Baron JH (1987) Gastrointestinal endoscopy in the young. BJ 295: 365
8. Lockhart SP, Schofield PM, Gribble RJ, Baron JH (1985) Upper gastrointestinal endoscopy in the elderly. BJ 290: 283
9. Bonnevie O (1982) Outcome of non-ulcer dyspepsia. Scand J Gastroenterol 17 [Suppl 79]: 135–138
10. Krag E (1969) The pseudo-ulcer syndrome: a clinical radiographic and statistical follow-up study of patients with ulcer symptoms but no demonstrable ulcer in the stomach or duodenum. Dan Med Bull 16: 6–9
11. Nyren O (1991) Secretory abnormalities in functional dyspepsia. Scand J Gastroenterol 26 [Suppl 182]: 29–32
12. Bates S, Sjoden PO, Fellenius J, Nyren O (1989) Blocked and non-blocked acid secretion and reported pain in ulcer, non-ulcer dyspepsia and normal subjects. Gastroenterology 97: 376–383
13. Malagelada JR (1991) Gastrointestinal motor disturbances in functional dyspepsia. Scand J Gastroeterol 26 [Suppl 182]: 29–32
14. Farrah DA, Culder I, Benson L et al. (1985) Specific food intolerance: its place as a cause of gastrointestinal symptoms. Gut 26: 164–168
15. Talley NJ, McNeil D, Piper DW (1988) Environmental factors and chronic unexplained dyspepsia: association with acetominopher but no other analgesies, alcohol, coffee, tea or smoking. Dig Dis Sci 33: 641–648
16. Talley NJ, Piper DW (1986) Major life event stress and dyspepsia of unknown cause: a case control study. Gut 27: 127–134
17. Talley NJ (1991) Non-ulcer dyspepsia: myths and realities. Ailment Pharmacol Ther 5 [Suppl 1]: 145–162
18. Dixon TG, Yatham LN, Barry S, Chua A, Keeling PWN (1990) Serotoxin supersensitivity: the pathophysiologic basis of non-ulcer dyspepsia? A preliminary report of buspironel prolactin responses. Scand J Gastroenterol 25: 541–544
19. Ormond JE, Talley NJ (1990) *Helicobacter pylori*: controversies and an approach to management. May Clin Proc 65: 414–426
20. Borody T, Hennessy W, Daskalopoulos G et al. (1987) Double-blind trial of De-Nol in non-ulcer dyspepsia associated with *Campylobacter pyloridis* gastritis. Gastroenterology 92: 1324 (abstract)
21. McNulty CZM, Gearty JC, Crump B et al. (1986) *Campylobacter pyloridis* and associated gastritis: investigator blind placebo-controlled trial of bismuth and erythromycin ethylsuccinate. Br Med J 293: 645–649
22. Patchett S, Beattie S, Leen E, Keane C, O'Morain C (1991) Eradicating *Helicobacter pylori* and symptoms of non-ulcer dyspepsia. Br Med J 303: 1238–1240

Nonulcer Dyspepsia: Psychological Considerations

M. Farnè

It is commonly recognized that emotional factors affect the gastric mucosa. As early as 1833 William Beaumont made some most important findings on emotions and digestion [1]. However, it is surprising that few formal studies have so far investigated the psychological aspects of nonulcer dyspepsia [11]. Over the years, I have made some observations on patients who, according to data in the literature, could be diagnosed as nonulcer dyspeptics [10–12]. The patients numbered 26 (16 women and 10 men; mean age 37.4 years), but since at the time I did not know of the present workshop, I did not organize the observations into a precise experimental design. At any rate, from them it is possible to infer that in the nonulcer dyspepsia problem there are two psychological components: (a) stress and emotional factors, and (b) personality variables.

Stress and Emotional Factors

Emotional factors and stress-producing situations have long been recognized as influential in the pathogenesis of various disorders of the gut [11]; in fact, stress alters secretion, motility, and vascularity, and many of what Selye [9] called "signs of danger" of distress involve the gastro-intestinal tract. As far as nonulcer dyspepsia is concerned, I think there is an indirect demonstration of the influence of stress in the observations that I have made. I frequently use autogenic training, a method inducing a relaxation response (the opposite of the stress response), which has been applied in a large number of medical disorders [7]. Changes induced by autogenic training correspond largely to similar changes induced by parasympathomimetic medications.

The 26 nonulcer dyspeptic patients were in the early phase of their illness (which was between 6 and 12 months old), referred to me by their general practitioner, and were treated singly with autogenic training only (i.e., without either specific drugs or psychotherapy). After 10 months of the training, the patients were subjected to a structured interview, and the outcome was discussed with the family physician in each case.

One must keep in mind that there is a natural tendency for nonulcer dyspepsia to improve, and that a large placebo response makes evaluation of different treatments difficult [2]. In my cases, after 10 months of autogenic therapy

Dipartimento di Psicologia, Università degli Studi, Bologna, Italy

Gasbarrini/Pretolani (Eds.)
Basic and Clinical Aspects of H. pylori Infection

there was complete disappearance or a clear improvement of the disorder in 20 subjects, while the effects remained limited in the other 6. This discounts the hypothesis of a placebo effect; also, this closely reproduces the general results obtained with autogenic training in patients with distress symptoms [3].

Personality Variables

Examining the psychological aspects of specific illnesses requires great care to avoid the so-called psychosomatic fallacy. This consists partly in the belief that there are personality characteristics going hand-in-hand with certain specific somatic disorders. In reality, experimental research has never substantiated this belief. Even the well-known type A behavior pattern, generally considered a specific coronary risk factor, is now being shown to be rather a nonspecific disease vulnerability condition (see, e.g., [8]).

At the moment, it is only possible to say that there are general groups of illnesses associated with general groups of personality traits. In this context, the studies of Fisher are relevant [6]. This author has described a special kind of personality called "barrier" (B).
The low-B person is characterized by:

1. Low level of goal setting
2. Inability to persist at tasks
3. Fear of the consequences of being aggressive
4. Suggestibility, dependence on group interactions
5. Difficulty in permitting himself a direct course of self-gratification
6. Vulnerability to stress
7. Psychosomatic symptoms in the body interior (e.g., asthma, nonulcer dyspepsia, accelerated heartbeat).

According to Fisher's results, high B subjects manifest more psychosomatic symptoms in the outer body sectors (skin, muscles, e.g., rheumatoid artritis) while low B subjects have a predisposition to psychosomatic symptoms in the inner body sectors (heart, stomach, lungs, e.g., asthma). Analyzing the scores obtained by the 26 nonulcer dyspeptic patients on the B-MMPI scale [4, 5], the B trait turned out very low in 13 of them (50%), relatively low in 9, and relatively high in the remaining 4.

The result may confirm Fisher's opinion on the association between low B characteristics and psychosomatic symptoms in the inner body.

In conclusion, as a psychologist with a medical background I am convinced that some things are too important to be left only to psychologists. However, I am even more convinced of the fact that in our life, in our health, and in our illness the psychological element plays a fundamental role.

References

1. Beaumont W (1833) Experiments and observations on the gastric juice and the physiology of digestion. Allen, Plattsburg
2. Colin-Jones DG (1988) Management of dyspepsia: report of a working party. Lancet 12: 576–579
3. Farnè M, Corallo A (1992) Signs of distress and autogenic training: an experimental study. Boll Soc Ital Biol Sper (in press)
4. Farnè M, Sebellico A, Gnugnoli D (1986) An objective measure of the Barrier personality trait: results of an inquiry. Boll Soc Ital Biol Sper 62: 1165–1169
5. Farnè M, Cutajar R, Sebellico A (1990) The Barrier inventory: a validity study. Boll Soc Ital Biol Sper 66: 387–390
6. Fisher S (1986) Development and structure of the body image. Lawrence Erlbaum, Hillsdale
7. Luthe W, Shultz JH (1969) Autogenic therapy. Grune and Stratton, New York
8. Rimè B et al. (1989) Type A behaviour pattern: specific coronary risk factor or general disease-prone condition? Br J Med Psychol 62: 229–238
9. Selye H (1976) The stress of life, 2nd edn. McGraw-Hill, New York
10. Svedlund J, Sjodin I, Dotevall G (1988) GSRS: clinical rating scale for gastrointestinal symptoms in patients with irritable bowel syndrome and pepetic ulcer disease. Dig Dis Sci 33: 129–134
11. Talley N, Phillips SF (1988) Non-ulcer dyspepsia: potential causes and pathophysiology. Ann Intern Med 108: 865–879
12. Talley N et al. (1988) A patient questionnaire to identify bowel disease. Ann Intern Med 111: 671–674

Nonulcer Dyspepsia and *Helicobacter pylori*: Effect of Eradication on Symptoms and Gastritis

S. Pretolani, F. Bonvicini, E. Brocchi, M. Baraldini, D. Cilla, S. Baldinelli, E. Bazzocchi, P. Pasini, and G. Gasbarrini

Introduction

It is now well established that *Helicobacter pylori* is the principal cause of chronic gastritis [1] and it is also considered the main permissive factor for the recurrence of peptic ulcer disease [2, 3].

As *H. pylori* infection is also demonstrated in 50% of patients presenting with dyspepsia [4, 5], it has been suggested that *H. pylori* gastric colonization and associated gastritis may contribute to the developing of symptoms in patients with nonulcer dyspepsia (NUD) [6].

NUD is a common clinical entity with a prevalence of 30% in the general population and diffused all over the world [7]. However, there is a wide spectrum of clinical presentation of subjects with NUD, suggesting that different subgroups of patients have different underlying pathophysiologic mechanisms. The definition of NUD as proposed in 1988 by an international working party was addressed to the presence of symptoms referable to the proximal alimentary tract (upper abdominal pain or discomfort, heartburn, nausea or vomiting) lasting for more than 1 month [8]. Recently a working team report has proposed a revised classification of dyspepsia using positive symptoms-based criteria in order to develop consensus guidelines for diagnosis and management [9]. In this classification *H. pylori* has been considered as one of the possible pathophysiological mechanisms of the subgroup ulcer-like functional dyspepsia. However, some studies have found an association between *H. pylori* and ulcer-like symptoms [10, 11] while others have failed to confirm any significant difference in symptom pattern between those dyspeptic patients with and without the infection [12, 113].

Therefore we undertook a prospective study to assess the role of *H. pylori* in the pathogenesis of NUD (or ulcer-like functional dyspepsia) evaluating: (a) the symptom pattern, the presence of environmental factors (smoking, alcohol and H_2-antagonist use) and gastric histopathology according to the *H. pylori* status in a population of NUD patients and (b) the effect of *H. pylori* eradication on symptoms and histological appearance in a selected group of *H. pylori*-positive NUD patients.

1st Department of Internal Medicine, University of Bologna, Policlinico S. Orsola, Via Massarenti 9, 40138 Bologna, Italy

Gasbarrini/Pretolani (Eds.)
Basic and Clinical Aspects of H. pylori Infection

Patients and Methods

All patients referred to our department of medicine over 8 months with a history of dyspepsia lasting for more than 1 month were admitted to the study. After biochemical, ultrasonographic and endoscopic examinations, we excluded patients with evidence of gastroesophageal reflux disease, peptic ulcer (active or inactive), pancreatic or hepatobiliary diseases, gastrointestinal surgery, and other major organic diseases. We also excluded subjects who were receiving nonsteroidal anti-inflammatory drugs as well those who had taken antibiotics or bismuth up to 1 month before the study. In a total of 174 patients with NUD (93 females, 81 males, age 18–84 years, mean 49) we evaluated the presence and severity of symptoms by a standardized questionnaire. Five symptoms of NUD (heartburn, epigastric pain, burping, bloating, nausea and vomiting) were separately assessed by a visual analogue scale (VAS): on a nongraded scale from 0 (absent) to 100 (severe and incapacitating symptom) the patient marked the actual level of the symptom. This scale seems to be superior to other rating scales and has been previously validated [14]. Smoking, alcohol use, and previous H_2-antagonist treatment were also recorded.

Multiple gastric biopsies were taken during endoscopy for *H. pylori* detection and histopathologic examination. A modified microtiter urease test [15] was used to evaluate the presence of urease activity on fresh biopsies from both antrum and corpus. Two other biopsy specimens from antrum and corpus were fixed in 10% buffered formalin, embedded in paraffin and sectioned. A modified Giemsa stain was used to detect *H. pylori* on sections [16]. Patients were considered positive for *H. pylori* when both methods yielded positive results. Hematoxilin and eosin stain was used to diagnose histological gastritis according to the Sydney System for gastritis [17].

Treatment Study

Fifty-four of 174 NUD patients agreed to undergo a treatment for the eradication of *H. pylori* infection. Informed consent was obtained from all patients. They were randomly assigned to receive either colloidal bismuth subcitrate (CBS), 120 mg four times daily, plus metronidazole (METRO), 250 mg three times daily, for 2 weeks, or amoxicillin (AMO) 500 mg three times daily plus METRO, 250 mg three times daily, for 2 weeks. The two groups were similar as regards sex, age, and symptom scores. Endoscopy and multiple gastric biopsies were repeated at 4 weeks and 8 months after the cessation of the treatment. Interviews with VAS scale compilation were performed at 2 and 8 months after the cessation of the treatment.

Statistical Analysis

Statistical analysis was carried out with χ^2 test with Yate's correction, Fischer's exact test, and *t*-test of significance when appropriate. A p value of $<.05$ was considered significant.

Results

H. pylori was present in 107 (61.5%) of 174 NUD patients. Prevalence rates of infection according to sex, age, smoking, alcohol and H_2 antagonists are reported in Fig. 1. No difference in prevalence of *H. pylori* was detected between males and females (47/107 = 43.9% vs 60/107 = 56.1%, p = n.s.). There were also no differences with respect to smoking (39/107 = 36.4% vs 15/67 = 22.4%, p = n.s.) and to alcohol consumption (26/107 = 24.3% vs 14/67 = 20.9%, p = n.s.). In contrast, a significantly higher prevalence of the infection was found according to age (35/107 = 32.7% in the age group 18–39 years vs 34/67 = 50.7% in the age group 40–65 years, $\chi^2 = 8.02$, $p < .005$) and to previous H_2 antagonist treatment (32/107 = 29.9% vs 6/67 = 9%, $\chi^2 = 9.4$, $p < .005$).

The presence of NUD symptoms (heartburn, epigastric pain, burping, nausea and vomiting, bloating) as well the presence of endoscopic antritis and histological gastritis according to the *H. pylori* status are reported in Fig. 2. No differences were found between *H. pylori*-positive and negative patients as regards pain, vomiting, and endoscopic antritis. Heartburn (43/107 = 40% vs 14/67 = 20.9%, $\chi^2 = 6.1$, $p < .02$) and burping (54/107 = 50.5% vs 16/67% = 23.9%, $\chi^2 = 11.3$, $p < .001$) were significantly associated with *H. pylori* presence. There was a higher prevalence of bloating in *H. pylori*-negative patients (31/67 = 46.2% vs 29/107 = 27%, $\chi^2 = 5.8$, $p < .02$). Histological gastritis was nearly always associated with *H. pylori* infection (104/107 = 97% vs 10/67 = 14.9%, $\chi^2 = 21.5$, $p < .0005$).

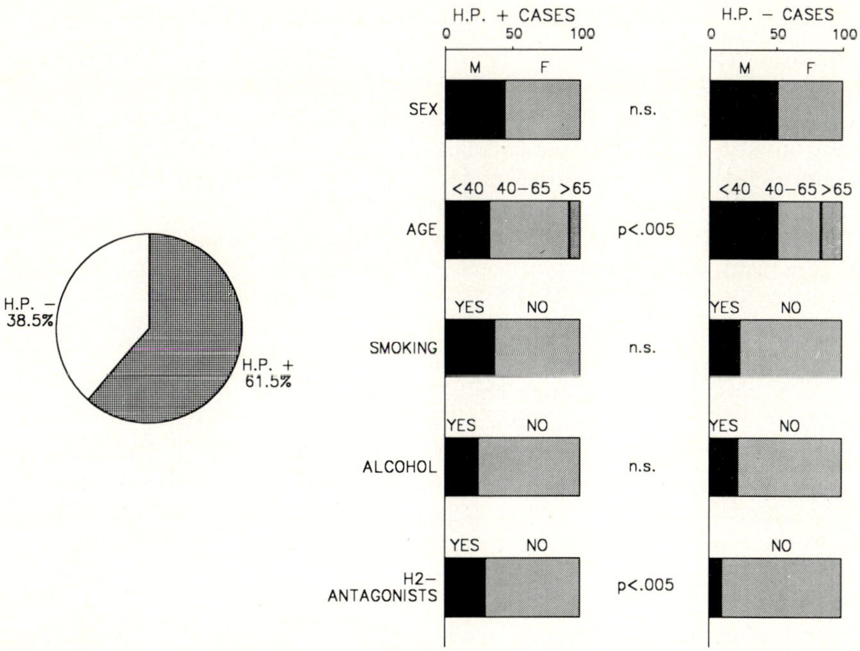

Fig. 1. Prevalence of *Helicobacter pylori* (*H.P.*) infection according to sex, age, smoking, alcohol consumption and H_2 antagonist use in 174 nonulcer dyspepsia patients

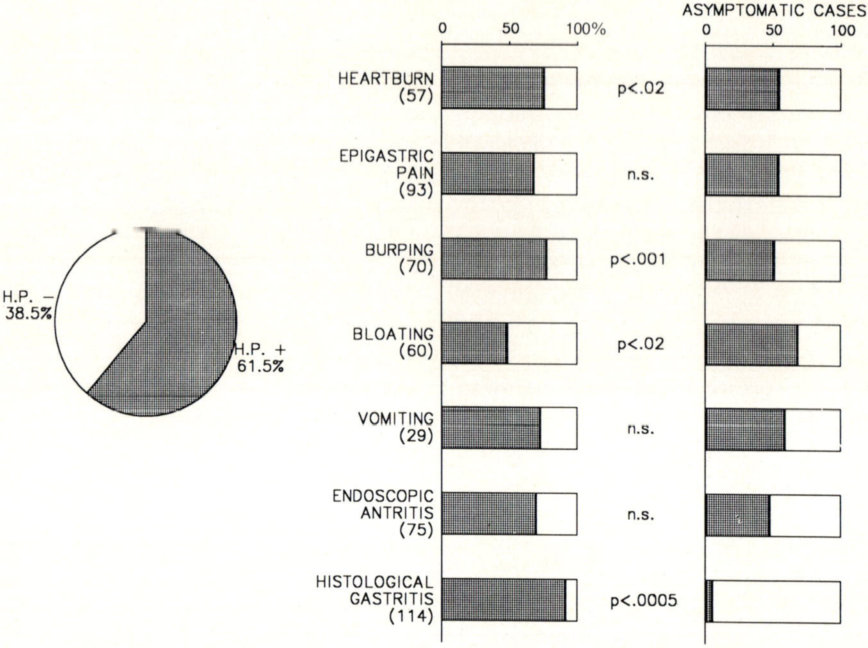

Fig. 2. Association of symptoms, endoscopic antritis and histologic gastritis with *Helicobacter pylori* (*H.P.*) infection in 174 NUD patients

Treatment Study

Forty-eight of the 54 selected patients completed the treatment and the scheduled follow-up at 8 months. Six patients failed to complete the study: two were lost to control and four (three in AMO/METRO group and one in CBS/METRO group) reported gastric intolerance to the drugs.

Eradication of *H. pylori* infection was obtained in a total of 31/48 (64.5%) NUD patients, with no difference between the two treatment groups (16/25 = 64% in CBS/METRO and 15/23 = 65% in AMO/METRO, p = n.s.). Histological gastritis improved in 29/31 (93.5%) of the patients in whom symptoms were eradicated as compared with 1/17 (5.9%) in the noneradicated group, $p < .0005$.

As regards the symptom scores, a significant reduction at 2 months after treatment was shown for heartburn (mean 6.51 before vs 1.95 after, $p < .001$) and burping (7.45 before vs 3.4 after, $p < .002$) in the patients with successful eradication. Also patients in whom *H. pylori* was not eradicated displayed a similar trend in reduction of these scores, and the differences between the two groups were not significant. However, when the patients were examined at 8 months after the treatment, those in whom the infection was eradicated maintained low scores (mean 2.15 for heartburn, $p < 0.001$ and 3.8 for burping, $p < .002$) while those in which *H. pylori* was still present showed an increase to pretreatment levels in mean symptom score (mean 5.42 for heartburn, p = n.s., 5.87 for burping, p = n.s.; Figs. 3 and 4). No differences were found at 8 months

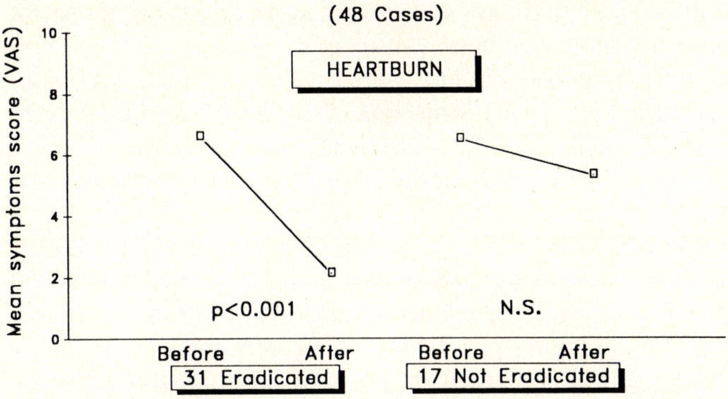

Fig. 3. Effect of *Helicobacter pylori* eradication on heartburn mean score 8 months after cessation of treatment in 48 NUD patients

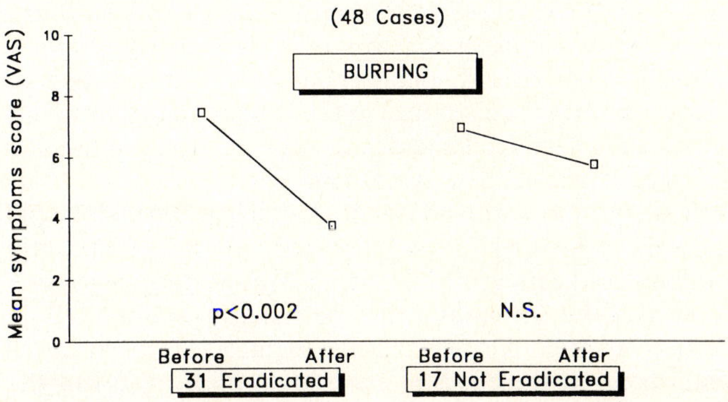

Fig. 4. Effect of *Helicobacter pylori* eradication on burping mean score 8 months after cessation of treatment in 48 NUD patients

with respect to 4 weeks after the cessation of the treatment in the two groups as concerns the presence of histological gastritis (5/31 in eradicated vs 16/17 in noneradicated).

Discussion

Previous studies have clearly demonstrated that *H. pylori* is one of the main causative agents of gastric inflammation. There is also evidence from volunteer and treatment studies that *H. pylori* infection can induce acute dyspeptic symptoms [18, 19]. However, the relationship between chronic nonulcer dyspepsia and *H. pylori* remains to be clarified. Several reports have demonstrated that the eradication of *H. pylori* infection leads to improvement in gastritis histologically [20, 21]. Some studies have reported a correlation between improvement of symptoms with clearance of bacteria [6, 11], whereas others have not [21–23].

It is conceivable that differences in diagnostic criteria and evaluation of specific symptoms may account for these conflicting results.

In this study non-ulcer dyspepsia patients were carefully selected, according to the most recent classification [8, 9] with special attention to identify the subset of patients with ulcer-like NUD. Moreover, each symptom received a VAS score, either in the general NUD population or in the treatment study population.

We found *H. pylori* infection in 61.5% of NUD patients, with a higher prevalence in older subjects. These results are similar to those reported in previous works [4–6, 20, 24]. The slight higher prevalence of infection in our study population could be explained by the higher proportion of subjects aged 40–65. It has been shown that in this age group the prevalence of *H. pylori* infection increases, probably due to a cohort effect [25]. No differences in the prevalence of *H. pylori* were detected according to sex, smoking and alcohol consumption, which was also consistent with previous data.

In contrast, *H. pylori* positive-NUD patients have been more frequently treated with H_2 antagonists (30% vs 9% of those *H. pylori* negative). Heartburn and burping were two symptoms significantly associated to *H. pylori* infection. A possible explanation and link for these findings could be that in a subset of NUD patients. *H. pylori* infection can induce specific ulcer-like symptoms: the antisecretory treatment in such patients could be considered as a symptomatic relief for the long-term persistence of these symptoms.

As other works have shown, too, we found no correlation between endoscopic findings and presence of *H. pylori* [6]. Histological gastritis was significantly associated to *H. pylori*, and eradicating the infection led to the disappearing of gastritis which persisted over the 8-months follow-up time. In contrast, NUD patients in whom infection is not eradicated continue to have gastritis at histological level. These data confirm the effect of eradication of *H. pylori* in the elimination of chronic gastritis independently of the drugs used [6, 20, 26].

Our data give further evidence that *H. pylori* gastritis might be responsible for some symptoms of ulcer-like NUD. A significant improvement in mean symptom scores for heartburn and burping was shown at the end of the treatment when eradication was obtained. As an other researcher found [27] even patients in whom infection was not eradicated had an improvement in mean symptom scores short term after treatment. However, at 8 months after treatment this score reduction has disappeared in *H. pylori* infected patients while remaining in those in whom infection was eradicated. Therefore, it is possible that a placebo effect could account for the short-term symptom improvement in patients in whom infection persists. In contrast, the persistence of improved symptom scores in the infection-free NUD population might suggest the real effect of a mechanism acting through the elimination of *H. pylori* infection and recovery from the associated acute and chronic inflammatory infiltrate of the stomach.

In conclusion, our study shows that *H. pylori* might play a role in the pathogenesis of symptoms in a subset of patients with NUD (ulcer-like type). Double-blind placebo-controlled studies could confirm the real effect of the eradication of infection in the long term in these patients.

References

1. Peterson WL (1991) *Helicobacter pylori* and peptic ulcer disease. N Engl J Med 324: 1043–1048
2. Rauws EAJ, Tytgat GNJ (1990) Cure of duodenal ulcer associated with eradication of *Helicobacter pylori*. Lancet 335: 1233–1235
3. Graham DY, Lew GM, Klein PD, Evans DG, Evans DJ, Saeed ZA, Malaty HM (1992) Effect of treatment of *Helicobacter pylori* infection on the long term recurrence of gastric or duodenal ulcer. Ann Intern Med 116: 705–708
4. Rokkas T, Pursey C, Uzoechina E, Dorrington L, Simmons NA, Filipe MI, Sladen GE (1987) *Campylobacter pylori* and non-ulcer dyspepsia. Am J Gastroenterol 82: 1149–1152
5. Loffeld RJLF, Potters HVOJ, Arends JW, Stobbering E, Flendrig JA, Van Spreeuwel JP (1988) *Campylobacter* associated gastritis in patients with non-ulcer dyspepsia. J Clin Pathol 41: 85–88
6. Kang JY, Tay HH, Wee A, Guan R, Math MV, Yap I (1991) Effect of colloidal bismuth subcitrate on symptoms and gastric histology in non-ulcer dyspepsia. A double blind placebo controlled study. Gut 31: 476–480
7. Tibblin G (1985) Introduction to the epidemiology of dyspepsia. Scand J Gastroenterol 20 [Suppl 109]: 29–33
8. Colin-Jones DG, Bloom B, Bodemar G, Cream G, Freston J, Gugler R, Malagelada J, Nyrén O, Petersen H, Piper D (1988) Management of dyspepsia: report of a working party. Lancet 1: 576–579
9. Talley NJ, Colin-Jones DG, Koch KL, Nyrén O, Stanghellini V (1991) Functional dyspepsia: a classification with guidelines for diagnosis and management. Gastroenterol Int 4: 145–160
10. Deltenre M, Nyst JF, Jonas C, Glupczynsky Y, Deprez C, Burette A (1989) Données cliniques, endoscopiques et histologiques chez 1100 patients dont 574 colonisés par *Campylobacter pylori*. Gastroenterol Clin Biol 13: 89B–95B
11. Rokkas T, Pursey C, Uzoechina E, Dorrington L, Simmons NA, Filipe MI, Sladen GE (1988) Non-ulcer dyspepsia and short term De-nol therapy: a placebo controlled trial with particular reference to the role of *Helicobacter pylori*. Gut 29: 1386–1391
12. Sobala GM, Dixon MF, Axon ATR (1990) Symptomatology of *Campylobacter pylori*-associated dyspepsia. Eur J Gastroenterol Hepatol 2: 445–449
13. Börsch G, Schmidt G, Wegener M, Sandmann M, Adamek R, Leverkus F, Reytemeyer E (1988) *Campylobacter pylori*: prospective analysis of clinical and histological factors associated with colonization of the upper gastrointestinal tract. Eur J Clin Invest 18: 133–138
14. Jørgensen LS, Bønløkke L, Wamberg P (1985) Non-ulcer upper dyspepsia. Aspects of pain. Scand J Gastroenterol 20: 46–50
15. Pretolani S, Bonvicini F, Baraldini M, Micaletti E, Brocchi E, Caletti GC, Gasbarrini G (1988) The value of microtiter urease test in grading of *Campylobacter* gastric colonization anf associated gastritis. In: Gasbarrini G, Stefanini GF, Desideri D (eds) Attualità gastroenterologia. Editrice Compositori, Bologna, pp 503–506
16. Gray SF, Wyatt JI, Rathbone BJ (1986) Simplified techniques for identifying *Campylobacter pyloridis*. J Clin Pathol 39: 1279
17. Price AB (1991) They Sydney system: histological division. J Gastroenterol Hepatol 6: 209–222
18. Marshall BJ, Armstrong J, McGreiche G, Glancy R (1985) Attempts to fulfil Koch's postulates for pyloric *Campylobacter*. Med J Aust 142: 436–439
19. Morris A, Nicholson G (1987) Ingestion of *Campylobacter pyloridis* causes gastritis and raises fasting pH. Am J gastroenterol 82: 192–199
20. Rauws EAJ, Langenberg W, Houthoff HJ, Zanen HC, Tytgat GNJ (1988) *Campylobacter pyloridis*-associated chronic active antral gastritis: a prospective study of its prevalence and the effects of antibacterial and antiulcer treatment. Gastroenterology 94: 33–40
21. Goh KL, Parasakhti N, Peh SC, Wong NW, Lo YL, Puthucheary SD (1991) Helicobacter pylori infection and non-ulcer dyspepsia: the effect of treatment with colloidal bismuth subcitrate. Scand J Gastroenterol 26: 1123–1131
22. Morgan D, Kraft W, Bender M, Pearson A (1988) Nitrofurans in the treatment of gastritis associated with Campylobacter pylori. Gastroenterology 95: 1178–1184
23. Glupczynski Y, Burette A, Labbe M, Deprez C, De Reuck M, Deltenre M (1988) Campylobacter pylori-associated gastritis: a double blind placebo controlled trial with amoxycillin. Am J Gastroenterol 83: 365–372

24. Rathbone BJ, Wyatt JI, Worsley BW (1986) Systemic and local antibodies responses to gastric *Campylobacter pyloridis* in non-ulcer dyspepsia. Gut 27: 642–647
25. Mendall MA, Goggin PM, Molineaux M, Levy J, Toosy T, Strachan D, Northfield TC (1992) Childhood living conditions and *Helicobacter pylori* seropositivity in adult life. Lancet 339: 896–897
26. Oderda G, Dellolio D, Morra I, Ansaldi N (1989) *Campylobacter pylori* gastritis long term results of treatment with amoxycillin. Arch Dis Child 64: 326–329
27. Patchett S, Beattie S, Leen E, Keane K, O'Morain C (1991) Eradicating *Helicobacter pylori* and symptoms of non-ulcer dyspepsia. BMJ 303: 1238–1240

Upper Gastrointestinal Endoscopy and the Prevalence of *Helicobacter pylori* Infection in Recurrent Abdominal Pain of Childhood

M. Ashorn, R. Karikoski-Leo, T. Ruuska, A. Miettinen, and M. Mäki

Introduction

Recurrent abdominal pain (RAP) is probably the most common complaint among children. It is characterized as a minimum of three episodes of pain occurring over a period longer than 3 months [1]. In different studies the prevalence of RAP has varied from 9% to 15%; however, new epidemiological studies are rare [7]. The etiology of RAP has remained for the most part obscure. Only about 10% of children with RAP have been diagnosed as having an organic background for their pain, whereas the rest have been explained by psychosomatic symptoms [10, 11]. It has even been suggested that diagnostic studies should therefore be limited. Endoscopy has usually been avoided because of the minimal information it would bring to the etiology of RAP [3].

The recent interest in *Helicobacter pylori* infections, gastritis, and duodenal ulcer has given a new perspective and brought a more invasive diagnostic approach to children with abdominal pain and dyspepsia [4, 8]. To clarify the possible organic pathology of RAP by endoscopic methods, we report the findings of 82 consecutive children complaining of recurrent abdominal pain.

Subjects and Methods

Over 2.5 years 82 consecutive children referred to the outpatient clinic with recurrent complaints of gastrointestinal pain and associated symptoms such as diarrhea, nausea, vomiting, and regurgitation underwent upper gastrointestinal endoscopy. The children had symptoms for at least 3 months. The median age was 11.5 years, with a range from 3 to 16 years. The upper gastrointestinal endoscopy was performed using Olympus GIF XP 10 and XP 20 endoscopes. Biopsies were taken for routine histology and for identification of *H. pylori* by culture. Esophageal long-term pH recordings were performed on selected patients. *H. pylori* antibodies were determined by an enzyme immunoassay using acid glycine extract antigen, derived from *H. pylori* strain ATCC 43504 (= NCTC 11637). Serological evaluation was performed in 59 children with RAP.

Department of Pediatrics, Tampere University Hospital, 33520 Tampere, Finland

Gasbarrini/Pretolani (Eds.)
Basic and Clinical Aspects of H. pylori Infection

Results

Gastroscopy revealed macroscopic changes and histological evaluation microscopic ones in 48 out of 82 children (58.2%) with RAP. Four children had other diseases: lactose malabsorption ($n = 2$), hydronephrosis ($n = 1$), and yersinosis ($n = 1$). Altogether 30 of the children (36.6%) retained the initial diagnosis of RAP. Patients with endoscopically verified mucosal damage had similar clinical characteristics to those without pathological findings (Table 1). Of the symptoms associated with RAP none correlated significantly to the endoscopic damage.

H. pylori infection was demonstrated in 18 (22%) of the children with RAP, and gastritis was found in 48 (58.5%) of the children (Table 2). The diagnosis of gastritis was based on histology alone in 16 patients. Positivity for *H. pylori* was based on positive histology and culture in 11 out of 18 cases, on histology in only 6 cases, and on positive culture alone in one case. Of the 16 *H. pylori* positive children examined 12 (75%) were also positive for serum IgG class

Table 1. Patient characteristics and associated symptoms of 82 consecutive children complaining of recurrent abdominal pain (RAP): the children are divided into two groups, those with organic pathology and those retaining the initial diagnosis RAP

	Organic pathology ($n = 52$)	RAP ($n = 30$)	p
Sex (M/F)	27/25	14/16	
Age (years)			
Median	11.5	11.0	NS
Range	3–16	4–16	
Duration of abdominal pains (months)			
Mean	21.8	17.2	NS
SD	15.6	19.2	
Range	3–72	3–72	
Diarrhea	16 (30.8%)	8 (26.7%)	NS
Nausea	8 (15.4%)	5 (16.7%)	NS
Vomiting	13 (25%)	8 (26.7%)	NS
Regurgitation	9 (17.3%)	2 (6.7%)	NS

Table 2. Findings and characteristics of 48 children with recurrent abdominal pain syndrome associated with gastric inflammation: those positive versus those negative for *H. pylori*

	Positive	Negative	p
Gastritis	18 (37.5%)	30 (62.5%)	
Duodenal ulcer	3	0	.047
Esophagitis	0	8	.016
Age (years)			
Median	12	11	NS
Range	3–16	5–16	
Duration of symptoms (months)			
Mean	26.1	16.2	NS
Range	3–72	3–36	

antibodies to *H. pylori*. Antibodies were also determined in 43 otherwise *H. pylori* negative patients, in whom no positive response in IgG class was seen.

Children positive for *H. pylori* had, in general, a longer history of abdominal pain compared to those without *H. pylori* infection; the difference, however was not significant (Table 2). We did not notice any difference in the character of pain (intensity, location) between the groups with or without *H. pylori* infection.

All the children with esophagitis also had gastroesophageal reflux disease, and their antral biopsies were negative for *H. pylori* despite clear inflammation in the gastric mucosa.

Discussion

This study shows that abnormal endoscopic finding is more common than previously thought in children with typical "psychosomatic" RAP syndrome. Our material is selected, however, because children with a positive history of obvious lactose intolerance did not undergo upper gastrointestinal endoscopy. Moreover, many children with RAP are not referred to the outpatient clinic. We therefore conclude that the present finding of 3.7% of duodenal ulcer disease and 22% of *H. pylori* gastritis in children with RAP is an overestimate of this infection, at least in Finland.

We do not know the exact prevalence of *H. pylori* infection in pediatric age groups in Finland, but according to studies in adult blood donors *H. pylori* colonization correlates with increasing age, and the prevalence is in young adults 10% in our country [6]. Even so, our figures are in agreement with those of Glassman et al. [5]. In a more selected material the frequency was even as high as 63% [8].

In the present study all children with *H. pylori* infection had gastritis or duodenal ulcer disease. Without treatment and bacterial eradication, *H. pylori* infection and ulcer disease is known to cause long-term morbidity and ulcer relapses. It has also recently been shown that chronic gastritis precedes the formation of peptic ulcer [12]. Thus it would also seem clinically relevant to treat children with *H. pylori* infection and RAP. In dyspeptic children both symptoms and gastritis are resolved in a parallel way with the eradication of the etiologic agent [2, 9]. It remains to be seen, however, whether treatment of *H. pylori* affects the symptoms in children with psychosomatic RAP.

In our material, only 7% of the pathological findings could have been diagnosed by means other than endoscopy. Histology can also clarify the diagnosis in a high number of cases so that biopsies should always be taken, even on a normal-appearing mucosa. Endoscopically diagnosed esophagitis was the organic pathology associated with RAP in 10% of the children in the present series. According to this study there does not seem to be any specific set of symptoms which could differentiate nonorganic from organic background in children complaining of recurrent abdominal pain.

If all children with RAP cannot be studied endoscopically for the presence of *H. pylori* infection, the measurement of serum antibodies to *H. pylori* promises to be the method of choice in determining which children should be investigated more invasively. In our study a sensitivity of 75% was reached by using the determination of IgG antibodies by an enzyme immunoassay in detecting *H. pylori* infection. It is possible that the sensitivity of this assay could be further increased by the determination of IgA antibodies in addition to IgG or by using a lower cutoff level for seropositivity.

We conclude that organic pathology is more common than is now presumed in children with typical psychosomatic, recurrent, even mild abdominal pain syndrome. So far the role of gastritis with or without *H. pylori* infection in causing pain has not been clearly demonstrated.

References

1. Apley J, Naish N (1958) Recurrent abdominal pain: a field survey of 1000 school children. Arch Dis Child 33: 165–170
2. Drumm B, Sherman P, Chiasson D, Karmali M, Cutz E (1988) Treatment of *Campylobacter pylori*-associated antral gastritis in children with bismuth subsalicylate and ampicillin. J Pediatr 113: 908–912
3. Galler JR, Neustein S, Walker WA (1980) Clinical aspects of recurrent abdominal pain in children. In Oski FA, Stockman JA (eds) Year book of pediatrics, Year Book Medical Publishers, Chicago
4. Galssman MS, Schwarz SM, Medow MS et al. (1989) *Campylobacter pylori*-related gastrointestinal disease in children: incidence and clinical findings. Dig Dis Sci 34: 1501–1504
5. Glassman MS, Dallal S, Berzin SH et al. (1990) *Helicobacter pylori*-related gastroduodenal disease in children: diagnostic uitlity of enzyme linked immunosorbent assay. Dig Dis Sci 35: 993–997
6. Kosunen TU, Höök J, Rautelin HI, Myllylä G (1989) Age-dependent increase of *Campylobacter pylori* antibodies in blood donors. Scand J Gastroenterol 24: 110–114
7. Lundby L, Sandbaek A, Juul S (1990) Recurrent abdominal pain in schoolchildren aged 9–12 years. Ugeskr Laeger 152: 2851–2854
8. Oderda G, Vaira D, Holton J, Dowsett JF, Ansaldi N (1989) Serum pepsinogen I and IgG antibody to *Campylobacter pylori* in non-specific abdominal pain in childhood. Gut 30: 912–916
9. Oderda G, Holton J, Altare F, Vaira D, Ainley C, Ansaldi N (1989) Amoxycillin plus tinidazole for *Campylobacter pylori* gastritis in children: assessment by serum IgG antibody, pepsinogen I, and gastrin levels. Lancet I: 690–692
10. Rappaport L (1989) Recurrent abdominal pain: theories and pragmatics. Pediatrician 16: 78–84
11. Recurrent abdominal pain in childhood. Leading article (1980) BMJ 1: 1096–1097
12. Sipponen P, Varis K, Fräki O, Korri UM, Seppälä K, Siurala M (1990) Cumulative 10-year risk of symptomatic duodenal and gastric ulcer in patients with or without chronic gastritis: a clinical follow-up study of 454 outpatients. Scand J Gastroenterol 25: 966–973

The Value of Serodiagnosis of *Helicobacter pylori* in Predicting Negative Gastroscopy

P.R. Hawtin[1], D. Sharpstone[2], S. Vyas[3], J. Treasure[4], D. Fine[2], and D.G. Newell[5]

Introduction

Increasing constraints with escalating demands on endoscopy resources have prompted interest in evaluating ways of predicting clinically non-significant endoscopies. Previous systems have attempted to identify high-risk patients by collating known predisposing factors to ulcer disease. These have largely proved unsatisfactory due to their poor specificity and sensitivity. The main potential for reducing endoscopic workload lies in serodiagnosis of *Helicobacter pylori*. Screening by serology is now possible with a high sensitivity and specificity and has been suggested as an alternative. However, for serology to be adopted routinely further prospective studies are needed to establish the role of such a screening protocol. A prospective study was therefore undertaken with the following aims: (a) to validate an enzyme-linked immunosorbent assay (ELISA) against antral biopsy culture and histology and (b), to evaluate the predictive values of an ELISA result against endocopic findings.

Methods

An indirect ELISA was adopted as described by Newell et al. [1] which used an acid extract of a single strain of *H. pylori* and a conjugate that labels all classes of immunoglobulin. The ELISA was validated against antral culture and/or histology in 154 patients attending routine upper gastro-intestinal (GI) endoscopy. *H. pylori* culture was by direct plating antral biopsies onto blood agar and Skirrow's medium and incubated for up to 5 days under microaerophilic conditions. Histological examination included a modified Giemsa stain to increase the sensitivity of *H. pylori* detection and to identify any other non-culturable spiral bacteria. Serodiagnosis only was then performed on a further 301 patients attending an open-access upper GI endoscopy list. All 456 patients

[1] Public Health Laboratory, Southampton General Hospital, Tremona Road, Southampton, SO9 4XY, UK
[2] Medical Unit, Southampton General Hospital, Tremona Road, Southampton, SO9 4XY, UK
[3] Medical Unit, Bournemouth General Hospital, Tremona Road, Southampton SO9 4XY, UK
[4] Histopathology, Southampton General Hospital, Tremona Road, Southampton, SO9 4XY, UK
[5] Central Veterinary Laboratory, Weybridge, UK

Gasbarrini/Pretolani (Eds.)
Basic and Clinical Aspects of H. pylori Infection

completed a questionnaire about risk factors for peptic ulceration such as drug history, alcohol and smoking. Results were analysed by the Mann-Whitney *U* test and multi-variate regression. At endoscopy pathological findings were scored on a 4-point scale as follows: 0 = normal, 1 = mild inflammation, 2 = moderate inflammation, 3 = ulceration.

Results

For all ages, the sensitivity of the ELISA against culture and histology was 90% with a specificity of 83%. The negative predictive value was 89%. However, we found that when the negative predictive value was calculated for specified age groups (Fig. 1), it was 100% up to the age of 45 ($n = 43$); above 45 years the negative predictive value fell to 76% ($n = 111$). The reason for this is not clear at present. When the ELISA was compared with significant endoscopic findings alone, i.e. a break in the mucosa such as erosions or ulceration, the negative predictive value (93%) was significant only in those aged under 45 years. If a screening strategy of the under 45 year group by serology were adopted, the endoscopic saving would be 66%. However, 7% of significant pathology would have been missed. In our study these were: (a) three cases of moderate oesophagitis and (b) two cases of moderate gastritis; (one patient had undergone gastric surgery for leiomyoma). There were no cases of frank peptic ulceration missed.

The statistical analysis of the questionnaire identified risk factors for peptic ulceration. Significance was reached for a history of smoking and alcohol in patients with oesophagitis. Gastritis correlated with a past history of ulceration and with male sex with duodentitis. The ELISA correlated strongly with upper GI disease, including oesophagitis.

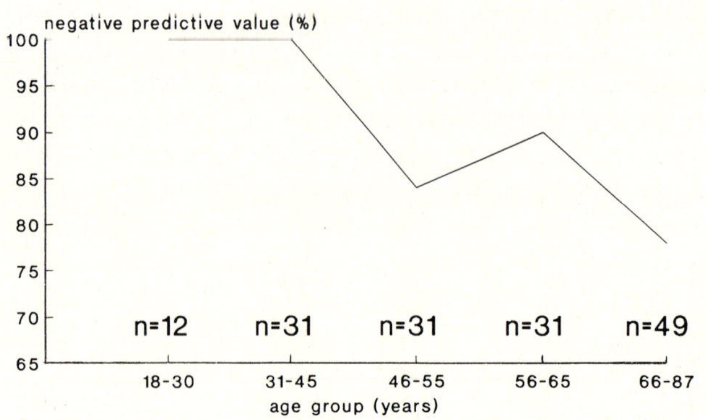

Fig. 1. Negative predictive value of ELISA in the different age groups

Conclusions

1. For subjects aged under 45 years, a negative ELISA result predicts the absence of *H. pylori* infection (negative predictive value of 100%).
2. For subjects aged under 45 years, a negative ELISA result also predicts the absence of serious pathological findings at endoscopy (negative predictive value of 93%).
3. If patients aged under 45 years who have a negative ELISA result were not endoscoped, the workload would be reduced by 15%.

Thus a negative ELISA finding in the under 45 year age group could be used as a screening test and patients reassured that it is unlikely that significant upper GI pathology has been missed.

Reference

1. Newell DG, Johnston BJ, Ali MH, Reed PI (1988) An enzymelinked immunosorbent assay for the serodiagnosis of *Campylobacter pylori*-associated gastritis. Scand J Gastroenterol 23 [Suppl 142]: 53–57

The Icelandic Nonulcer Dyspepsia/*Helicobacter pylori* Study: Symptomatic Response and Eradication Rate with De-Nol or De-Nol Plus Metronidazol in Treatment of *Helicobacter*-positive Patients with Nonulcer Dyspepsia

E. Oddsson, H. Guðjónsson, A. Theodors, S. Björnsson, O. Gunnlaugsson, M. Gormsen, O. Steingrímsson, J.J. Jóhannsson, and B. Thjodleifsson

Nonulcer dyspepsia is a common condition. From earlier studies we know that the incidence of *Helicobactor pylori* in dyspeptic patients in Iceland is 78% [1]. Until recently no therapy proven effective for these patients [5]. A Finnish study of sucralfate has shown some effect [2], but in a similar study recently concluded we found no difference between sucralfate and placebo. Short-term studies with bismuth subcitrate (De-Nol) and metronidazol have shown some effect [3, 4]. It therefore seemed pertinent to do a study with longer follow-up of these drugs. The Icelandic nonulcer dyspepsia *Helicobactor pylori* study was a collaborative study done at three hospitals in Reykjavík.

The aim of this study was to evaluate the effect of De-Nol [colloidal bismuth subcitrate] with placebo and compare the efficacy of this treatment with De-Nol and metronidazol on eradication of *Helicobactor pylori* and the symptomatic response in a group of *Helicobactor*-positive patients with nonulcer dyspepsia.

Methods

A total of 69 patients were randomized in to two groups. All patients had chronic upper dyspeptic symptoms of at least 4 weeks' duration, with endoscopic gastritis but without endoscopic gastric or duodenal ulceration. All had a positive quick urease test (CLO test). The two treatment groups were clinically comparable, except for previous history of peptic ulcer that was registered in 15 patients in the metronidazol group but in only 5 in the placebo group.

There were 34 patients in each group (Fig. 1). Both groups were treated with De-Nol 240 mg twice daily for 28 days, the patients in the metronidazol group receiving metronidazol 400 mg three times daily for the first 10 days of the treatment period and the patients in the placebo group receiving placebo tablets for the same length of time. At inclusion, and after 4, 12, and 26 weeks the patients were checked for symptoms and diary cards collected. All patients were endoscoped prior to inclusion and at 12 weeks. If they were *Helicobacter* negative

Reykjavík Hospitals, Reykjavík, Iceland

Gasbarrini/Pretolani (Eds.)
Basic and Clinical Aspects of H. pylori Infection

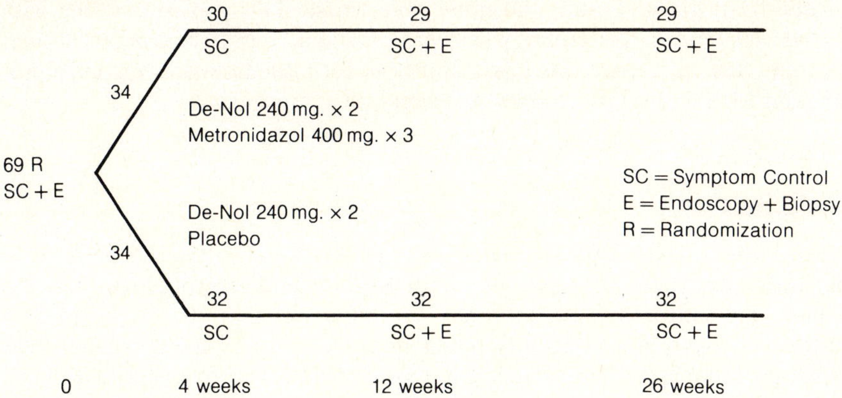

Fig. 1. Set-up of the study

at 12 weeks they also had an endoscopy at 26 weeks. At each endoscopy biopsies were obtained for CLO and Jatrox urease tests, culture, and histology.

Results

The success at eradicating *Helicobacter pylori* was not impressive in this study. In the De-Nol/metronidazol group 11 patients were *Helicobacter* negative at 12 weeks (37%) and 9 patients (28%) at 26 weeks. The corresponding numbers were 2 and 1 in the De-Nol and placebo groups, or 6% and 3%. The eradication rate was significantly better in the patients treated with De-Nol/metronidazol, both at 12 and at 26 weeks ($p < 0.05$).

Patients in both groups had good symptomatic response, 90% and 67% in the De-Nol/metronidazol group and 75% and 59% in the De-Nol/placebo group. This is statistically not significant.

The symptomatic response in this study, however, seemed to correlate better with the eradication of *Helicobacter* than it did with the two treatments (Table 1). The difference was small at 12 weeks with two patients symptom free in each group, two and ten patients reporting their symptoms being worse. At 26 weeks the difference was evident; more patients had become symptom free in the

Table 1. Symptomatic response at 12 and 26 weeks

	12 Weeks			26 Weeks		
	Healed	Improved	Worse	Healed	Improved	Worse
Helicobacter negative	2	9	2	7	3	0
Helicobacter positive	2	36	10	1	32	18

Differences at 26 weeks statistically significant ($p < 0.05$).

Helicobacter-negative group, and none were worse. This was in contrast with the *Helicobacter*-positive group, where more patients report worsening of their symptoms. The difference was significant both for patients who were asymptomatic and for those who reported worsening of symptoms.

Conclusions

This study compared De-Nol alone with De-Nol and metronidazol and the patients were followed for 6 months. We found: (a) that the eradication of *Helicobacter pylori* is significantly better with De-Nol and metronidazol than with De-Nol alone; (b) that there is good symptomatic improvement with both treatments at 12 and 26 weeks; and (c) that symptomatic improvement is significanly better sustained in *Helicobacter*-negative patients at 26 weeks.

References

1. Jóhannsson JH, Hardardóttir H, Sigvaldadóttir E, Kristjánsdóttir S, Thjodleifsson B, Oddsson E, Steingrimsson O (1989) *Camphylobacter pylori* in the stomach mucosa. Iceland Med J. 75: 191–196
2. Kairaluoma MI, Hentilae R, Alavaikko M et al. (1987) Sucralfate versus placebo in treatment of non-ulcer dyspepsia. Am J Med 83 [S 3B]: 51–55
3. Kang JY, Tay HH, Wee A, Guan R, Math MV, Yap I (1990) Effect of colloidal bismuth subcitrate on symptoms and gastric histology in non-ulcer dyspepsia. A double blind placebo study. Gut 31: 476–480
4. Patchett S, Beattie S, Leen E, Keane C, O'Morain C (1991) Eradicating *Helicobacter pylori* and symptoms of non-ulcer dyspepsia. BMJ 303: 1238–1240
5. Veldhuyzen van Zanten SJO, Tytgat KMAJ, Jalali S, Goodacre RL, Hunt RH (1989) Can gastritis symptoms be evaluated in clinical trials? An overview of treatment of gastritis, nonulcer dyspepsia and *Campylobacter*-associated gastritis. J Clin Gastroenterol 1(5): 496–501

Long-Term Follow-up of Children with *Helicobacter pylori*-Associated Nonulcer Dyspepsia After Eradication of the Infection

C. De Giacomo[1], P. Perotti[1], E. Giacobone[2], R. Daturi[2], L. Villani[3], and R. Fiocca[3]

Introduction

Helicobacter pylori infection has been described in children with peptic ulcer disease and chronic type B gastritis. In all reported pediatric series the most frequent symptom associated with the infection was recurrent epigastric or abdominal pain. Combination of amoxycillin with colloidal bismuth subcitrate [2] or with tinidazole [4] eradicated the infection and improved symptoms and gastritis in approximately 70% of infected children. Follow-up of these patients was generally limited to a few months after discontinuation of therapy. To study the outcome of the disease after successful treatment we prospectively followed-up children and adolescents with *H. pylori*-associated nonulcer dyspepsia for a mean period of 3 years after eradication of the infection.

Patients and Methods

Nineteen children and adolescents (age range 4–19 years) were evaluated endoscopically for recurrent epigastric or abdominal pain and upper digestive complaints. As children are usually not able to give detailed information about abdominal pain (location, severity, relationship to meals, etc), symptoms were recorded but not scored. Histologic and microbiologic examination of antral specimens showed evidence of *H. pylori*-associated chronic gastritis in all patients. Histologic classification and grading of chronic gastritis were based on evaluation of mononuclear cell infiltration of the lamina propria, intraepithelial granulocytes, epithelial lesions, and mucin depletion, as previously published [2]. Fully informed written consent was obtained before endoscopy and biopsics.

At diagnosis serum samples were collected from each patient to measure *H. pylori*-specific IgG and IgA by means of enzyme-linked immunosorbent assay [3]. This method allowed us to identify infected children with 95% sensitivity and 84% specificity. IgG and IgA seropositivity showed 100% positive predictive-

[1] Clinica Pediatrica, IRCCS Policlinico S. Matteo, 27100 Pavia, Italy
[2] Servizio di Analisi Microbiologiche, IRCCS Policlinico San Matteo, 27100 Pavia, Italy
[3] Istituto di Anatomia Patologica, IRCCS Policlinico San Matteo, 27100 Pavia, Italy

Gasbarrini/Pretolani (Eds.)
Basic and Clinical Aspects of H. pylori Infection

ness; absence of IgG or IgA seropositivity gave 95% negative predictiveness [3]. Of 19 patients 17 were seropositive for IgG and/or IgA.

All these children were treated with amoxycillin (70 mg/kg per day in two divided doses for 2 weeks) and colloidal bismuth subcitrate (480 mg/1.7 m^2 body surface per day in three or four divided doses for 4 weeks). Such treatment resulted in eradication of the infection and significant improvement of gastritis in up to 70% of children treated [2]. *H. pylori* eradication was evaluated by follow-up endoscopy and antral biopsy at least 1 month after discontinuating treatment (mean 6 months for all patients).

These 19 patients entered a follow-up study with periodic examinations and recording of symptoms at 3, 6, and 12 months. After the first year patients were evaluated once a year or in the case of recurrence of symptoms. In addition, *H. pylori* specific IgG and IgA titers were measured. Further endoscopies with antral biopsies were proposed to patients with recurrence of symptoms.

Results

The follow-up period of these 19 patients ranged from 1 year to 4 years and 11 months (mean 3 years). Symptoms improved in all patients during treatment. At the time of endoscopic reevaluation all 19 patients revealed improvement or disappearance of abdominal pain and digestive complaints. Seven patients had subsequent recurrence of symptoms, suggesting relapse of the infection. Symptoms were similar to those experienced before starting treatment and usually developed 8–12 months later.

After treatment serum titers of *H. pylori* specific antibodies decreased progressively in all patients. Values below the cutoff points of seropositivity were achieved within 1 year in all but two patients with borderline values for IgG.

During follow-up one symptomatic patient had IgG and IgA increase, while one without symptoms had IgG increase. Seven children (five symtomatics and two asymptomatics) had further endoscopic reevaluation. Two of six symptomatic seronegative children and the child without symptoms but with IgG seropositivity refused further endoscopy.

H. pylori relapse was seen only in the child with recurrence of symptoms and seropositivity for both IgG and IgA. The remaining six were persistently negative and histologically healed.

Discussion

H. pylori infection is strongly associated with peptic ulcer disease and chronic gastritis in man. It has been found in approximately half of adults with nonulcer dyspepsia. Although definition of nonulcer dyspepsia is relative to adult patients [1], recurrent abdominal pain is the main symptom in children with *H. pylori* infection. The ability of children to define their symptoms depends on age.

Children younger than 10 years usually locate their pain in the periumbilical region and are not able to define other characteristics. Nonetheless, recurrent abdominal pain is usually associated with upper digestive complaints (regurgitation, vomiting, eruttation, disconfort after meals, etc.) similar to those referred by dyspeptic adults. Thus the association of recurrent abdominal pain and upper digestive symptoms may reasonably be considered as the pediatric equivalent of nonulcer dyspepsia in adults.

In children *H. pylori* infection has been shown in association with chronic gastritis and, less frequently than in adults, with peptic ulcers. Eradication of the infection with double therapy was associated with improvement in clinical picture and histologic lesions. Although eradication of the infection has been described [2, 4], no data are currently available about long-term follow-up of these children.

We studied the outcome of 19 children and adolescents in whom *H. pylori* infection was eradicated and chronic gastritis significantly improved. Due to the high rate of relapse, which generally occurs within 4 weeks after stopping treatment, we evaluated children at least 1 month after discontinuation of drugs. Further follow-up was based on clinical and serologic surveillance. Symptoms recurred in 7 of 19 patients, but *H. pylori* relapse was evident only in 1 of 5 reevaluated. The lack of scoring symptoms could be the reason of the poor correlation of symptoms with *H. pylori* relapse. Development of a specific clinical score of dyspepsia for children could be an important help in the management of dyspeptic children.

Serology indentified correctly the symptomatic child who relapse by an increase of both specific IgG and IgA; in addition, all seronegative children who had a repeat endoscopy remained *H. pylori* negative in spite of recurrence of dyspepsia. All but one of the remaining asymptomatic patients were seronegative, suggesting that it is possible to obtain a long-term eradication in the majority of children. It seems reasonable to maintain that only two of 19 children relapsed (one confirmed), independently of the recurrence of symptoms. Serology represents a reliable method of follow-up of children treated for *H. pylori* infection.

References

1. Anonymous (1988) Management of dyspepsia: report of a working party. Lancet 1: 576–579
2. De Giacomo C, Fiocca R, Villani L, Lisato L, Licardi G, Diegoli N, Donadini A, Maggiore G (1990) *Helicobacter pylori* infection and chronic gastritis: clinical, serological, and histologic correlations in children treated with amoxicillin and colloidal bismuth subcitrate. J Pediatr Gastroenterol Nutr 11: 310–316
3. De Giacomo C, Lisato L, Negrini R, Licardi G, Maggiore G (1991) Serum immune response to *Helicobacter pylori* in children: epidemiologic and clinical applications. J Pediatr 119: 205–210
4. Oderda G, Vaira D, Holton J, Ainley C, Altare F, Ansaldi N (1989) Amoxycillin plus tinidazole for *Campylobacter pylori* gastritis in children: assessment by serum IgG antibody, pepsinogen I, and gastrin levels.

Helicobacter pylori, Surgery, and Aging

The Role of Ulcer Surgery Today

R. Bittner

Surgical therapy of gastroduodenal ulcers has again reached a turning point. The development of new, more potent drugs such as omeprazol and the discovery of *Helicobacter pylori* as a possible etiological factor in the pathogenesis of ulcer disease call for a revision of established therapeutic strategies. Today, partial gastric resection has its place in peptic ulcer treatment only in a few selected indications: (a) suspicion of malignancy, (b) recurrent ulcer following, highly selective vagotomy (HSV), refractory to conservative therapy, and (c) complicated large ulcer. In gastric ulcer the indication for resection should be set rather liberally because a chronic benign ulcer often cannot be distinguished macroscopically from a malignant one, and biopsies can yield false negative results. Even definite healing tendencies under conservative therapy are not reliable criteria for benign status. However, partial gastrectomy should no longer be used electively for duodenal ulcer. It is too dangerous and may produce troublesome side effects such as dumping and bile reflux; long-term sequelae include loss of weight, bone disease, and anemia and increase the chance of eventual death from gastric cancer.

Vagotomy is thus the mainstay of surgical treatment especially for duodenal ulcer since the 1970s. However, should vagotomy be truncal, selective, or highly selective, combined with antrectomy or with drainage-procedure, or should the pylorus be kept intact? Is a single operative method suitable for all patients, or should the operation be tailored to the patient's individual requirements? If the case of the latter, what criteria govern the choice of operation? The questions are endless and certainly cannot all be answered here. According to all published literature, highly selective vagotomy is still the safest procedure because of the absence of any breach in the continuity of the gastrointestinal tract or a suture line that might leak or bleed and of any stoma or blind loop. Moreover, in comparison to truncal vagotomy and selective gastric vagotomy with pyloroplasty the unwanted late postoperative side effects are far fewer after HSV. Therefore the HSV, in which the antropyloric pump unit remains in its inervation and stomach and duodenum are not be opened, was the operative method of choice (the "gold standard") of surgical therapy in peptic ulcer disease over the past two decades.

Since the introduction of the H_2-receptor blocking agents in clinical practice in 1977 the therapeutic strategy as well as the role of the surgeon in peptic ulcer therapy at all is more challenged. Worldwide the number of operations

Department of General Surgery, Marienhospital, Böheimstr. 37, 70178 Stuttgart, Germany

Gasbarrini/Pretolani (Eds.)
Basic and Clinical Aspects of H. pylori Infection

has fallen drastically. Medical therapy is replacing surgical interventions. The maxim "A tablet a day keeps the surgeon away" is becoming for surgeons a bitter reality. In this context one can understand the title of the recent published article of Sir J. Alexander-Williams in the *British Medical Journal*: "A requiem for vagotomy" [1]. Although the essay represents modern thinking, in my opinion it does not withstand critical scrutiny. For example, if the role of the surgeon is reduced to the treatment of ulcer complications, the question arises of how he is to gain his experience and technical know-how to treat and cure severe complications if an elective surgical ulcer therapy no longer exists. In our hospital over the past 27 months we performed emergency operations in 39 patients suffering from a bleeding or perforated peptic ulcer. Mortality in these complicated ulcer cases was below 10%. One must ask this percentage will not likely rise drastically if the surgeon lacks the experience gained in elective ulcer surgery?

The aims of ulcer therapy should be (a) to relieve pain, (b) to heal the ulcer, and (c) to keep the ulcer healed. Despite all euphoria concerning the success of drug therapy, nearly all ulcers can be initially healed medically although the *disease* as such remains. Even under long-term drug therapy the recurrence rate is about 30% in 1 year, not to mention the long-term side effects, which cannot as yet be assessed. We must therefore consider antiandrogenic effects, mental confusion, and interference with liver enzymes – and since the introduction of omeprazol, with its nearly complete acid blockade, the bacterial overgrowth in the stomach and upper intestine, possible food poisoning, high circulating gastrin level, and development of carcinoid tumors or gastric carcinomas. Comparing therapeutic regimes, we must also consider the costs of therapy. HSV cures the ulcer at once. The initial cost of hospital care, surgery, and anesthesia is high, but thereafter medical costs are minimal unless the patient develops recurrent ulceration.

Medical treatment with H_2 receptor antagonists is much cheaper than HSV in the short term. However, the need for continuous treatment and assessment over many years, repeat endoscopies, and loss of time from work means that in Europe medical treatment is more expensive than surgical in the long term. In the Federal Republic of Germany the costs of the two strategies are equal after 6 years, after which HSV is the cheaper option. In Great Britain this period of time is even shorter, 4–5 years. In addition, in poor countries, containing most of the world's population, patients with peptic ulcer are unlikely to be able to affort the costs of treatment with H_2 blockers (about U.S. $400 per year), and if ulcer symptoms are severe, surgery remains the only hope there. Furthermore, the immense psychological advantage for the patient following a successful operation should not be neglected. The psychological advantage means freedom from disease, pills, physicians, endoscopy, hospitals, and the need for compliance. Many patients do not want to change life-style, go to bed early, avoid stress, take pills regularly, and do what wives, mothers, or physicians tell them to do.

With a HSV all three aims of ulcer therapy can be achieved. No other operative approach has been examined so closely regarding hazards and benefits. Multiple studies have scrutinized risks, side effects, and long-term results, which today can be followed up for more than 20 years. Considering risks, a literature

Table 1. Duodenal ulcer: reported mortality

Author	Year	n	Mortality: n(%)
Holle	1974	784	5 (0.64)
Grossi	1975	787	2 (9.25)
Johnston	1975	107	0
Holst-Christensen	1977	260	0
Andrup	1978	273	2 (0.7)
Dorricot	1978	116	0
Goligher	1978	508	2 (0.4)
Junginger	1979	563	1 (0.18)
Liavag	1979	565	1 (0.18)
Nillsell	1979	137	2 (1.5)
Imperati	1980	849	1 (0.12)
Hollinshead	1982	114	1 (0.9)
De Miguel	1982	158	1 (0.6)
Knight	1983	310	0
Müller	1982	875	4 (0.46)
Moreno-Gonzales	1983	829	2 (0.2)
Clark	1986	272	1 (0.4)
Enskog	1986	326	0
Johnston	1990	750	1 (0.13)
Overall		8583	26 (0.3%)

Table 2. Visick classification of controls and patients 5 years after HSV because of duodenal ulcer (from [10])

Visick classification	Controls ($n = 561$)		HSV patients ($n = 451$)	
	n	%	n	%
I	362	64.5	267	64.3
II	162	28.9	115	27.7
III	36	6.4	18	4.4
IV	1	0.2	15	3.6

review assessing HSV in over 8000 patients, mortality (0.3%) was extremely low (Table 1) complication rate equally low. With regard to unwanted side effects, Müller et al. [10] examined 415 patients with duodenal ulcer 5 years after HSV and compared them with a group of 561 healthy blood donors (Table 2). After a careful case history followed by a listing (according to the Visick classification) he surprisingly found no difference between the two groups except for Visick grade IV. Here the rate HSV patients was 3.6% in comparison to 0.2% of the control group because of symptomatic ulcer recurrences.

The potential for recurrent ulceration is without doubt the major disadvantage of HSV. The rises in some studies is as high as 30% (Table 3). The question is whether such high recurrence rates are inevitable. Are they an intrinsic feature of the operation? Johnston and Blackett compared various preoperative factors in 48 patients in whom recurrent ulcer developed after HSV with the same factors in 400 patients in whom recurrent ulcer did not develop [9]. They found

Table 3. Duodenal ulcer: reported recurrence rates after HSV

3%–10%		10%–20%		20%–30%	
Fraser	1983	Clark	1986	Kronborg	1975
De Vries	1983	Johnston	1990	Koffmann	1983
Moreno-Gonzales	1983			Hoffmann	1987
Müller	1985			Primrose	1988
Dua	1987				
Johnston	1987				
Jordan	1987				

Period of observation 5–20 years.

no difference between the two groups of patients with respect to age, sex, lengths of ulcer history, previous ulcer complications, or basal or peak acid output. The crucial difference between the two groups was at operation; there was a significant correlation between subsequent recurrent ulcer and (a) the individual surgeon who had performed the operation and (b) the postoperative acid response to insulin 1 week postoperatively. In short, recurrence correlated with complete vagotomy and was thus related to operative technique. A second important factor is patient selection in terms of ulcer location, i.e., is HSV in all ulcer locations, pre-, inter- and postspyloric equally effective?

HSV is technically demanding if complete vagotomy of the parietal cell mass is to be achieved consistently. A critical point is the extent of dissection of the esophagus and on the esophagogastric junction. Here a number of anatomical variations of the vagal nerve are seen. Special attention should be paid to vagal fibers, such as Grassi's ramus criminalis, which penetrate high into the esophagus and are carried intramurally and are thus secluded from the eye of the surgeon operating only on the lesser curvature and the esophagogastric junction. Therefore, thorough mobilization of the esophagus is essential so that it may be rotated easily between the thump and fingers, thereby demonstrating all vagal fibers which can then be severed. About 6 cm distal esophagus should be cleared of all fibers as Hallenbeck et al. [7] and others have shown with respect to HSV, but it is equally true for all other types of vagotomy (Table 4). If only 1–2 cm esophagus is dissected, the recurrence rate lies significantly higher, with over 20% in comparison to a dissection of 4–7 cm with a rate well under 10%. Since the dissection of the esophagus can be technically difficult, substantial personal experience of the surgeon is required.

Table 4. Extent of dissection of distal esophagus and reported recurrence rates

Authors	Recurrence rate dissection esophagus		Observation period (years)
	1–2 cm	4–7 cm	
Hallenbeck et al. (1976)	15.4%	6%	1–4.5
Holst-Christensen et al. (1977)	23%	8%	1–4
Kronborg et al. (1977)	23%/24%	–	5–8
Mühe (1982)	–	5·6%	5
Blackett and Johnston (1982)	–	10.7%	5–12

Enskog et al. [5] also regard the performing surgeon as the single most important prognostic factor concerning recurrence rate, with all other factors being of lesser influence. Enskog et al. noticed in their study that while one surgeon had a cumulative recurrence rate of nearly 50%, that of another of comparable operative experience was below 5%.

To help the surgeon in achieving a complete vagotomy, or to compel him to meticulousness, a number of intraoperative tests for completeness have been devised. Of clinical relevance is especially the pH-test of Grassi et al. [6] and the vagomotoric electrotest of Burge and Vane [4]. Whether these tests are helpful to the experienced surgeon is open to discussion, but to the surgeon in training it should be a necessary addition to the operation, even if it prolongs operation time by up to 30 min.

As noted above, the other factor influencing recurrence rate is patient selection. As early as 1978 the study group of Amdrup observed a recurrence rate of 22% in the presence of prepyloric ulcer compared to one of 6% in duodenal ulcer following HSV [2]. While up to then the prepyloric gastric ulcer was classified among duodenal ulcers, following this study doubts arose as to the relevance of this classification. In study of ours in which we analyzed gastric secretion, stomach emptying, gastrin secretion quantitatively, and histological assessment of gastric antrum mucosa in patients with different ulcer locations, definite differences between prepyloric gastric ulcer and duodenal ulcer were seen [3]. Patients with prepyloric ulcer had less acid secretion, slower emptying time, but higher gastrin secretion. The histological analysis of antral mucosa, also showed a high proportion of patients to have changes such as chronic atrophic gastritis and intestinal metaplasia (Table 5). By comparison, duodenal ulcer patients showed the signs only of a superficial gastritis. According to these results the prepyloric ulcus ventriculi seems to be a different entity from duodenal ulcer, with its own pathophysiological constellation. Selection is the key to success: selection of the correct operation for the individual patient by a very experienced surgeon.

It is beyond doubt that conservative therapy is nowadays the method of choice in the treatment of uncomplicated peptic ulcer. However, with recurrences or even complications the physician looking after the patient should not overextend the conservative approach. He should bear in mind that if a ulcer complication occurs which makes an operative intervention unavoidable, mortality rises to 10% following perforation, 15%–30% following bleeding and

Table 5. Characteristics of peptic ulcer in relation to localization (from [3])

	Duodenal ulcer	Prepyloric gastric ulcer
Secretion	↑	↓
Motility	↑	↓
Gastrin	↓	↑
Age of patient	↓	↑
Men:women	↑	↓
recurrence rate after HSV	↓	↑
Histology of antral stomach	Superficial gastritis	Chronic atrophic gastritis, intestinal metaplasia (23%/39%; 59%)

50% in a combination of these. If an assessment of the probability of recurrence or complications in advance is to be achieved, results of the study recently published by Blum and coworkers provide the following risk factors which predispose to a relapsing course [8] smoking, stress, heavy physical labor, previous history of high recurrence rate, scarred duodenal bulb, persistent complaints despite ulcer healing, tea, coffee, and alcohol consumption, and hypercaloric nutrition. If more than eight of these factors are present, the recurrence rate is over 30%; if none is found, the rate lies around 5%. Especially for the first group of patients mentioned above the crucial question of long-term drug therapy or operation must be assessed.

Despite medical progress we must keep in mind that even with omeprazol a definite healing of peptic ulcer disease is still achieved only by surgical means. Finally, the following indications for a HSV can be named: (a) failure of long-term conservative therapy, (b) lack of patient compliance in long-term treatment, (c) drug intolerance or disturbing side effects of medical therapy, (d) severe ulcer complications, and (e) inability to pay the costs. As long as possible a conservative approach should be taken in the following conditions: (a) youth, (b) short ulcer history, (c) atypical pain as the only symptom, (d) absence from work for long periods because of pain, (e) heavy smoking and drinking, and (f) use of medication for nervousness or depression.

In summary, should a optimal result in treatment of peptic ulcer disease be achieved, a careful assessment of therapy by conservative or operative means is necessary. These treatment modalities should not compete with one another but should harmonize and complement one other.

References

1. Alexander-Williams J (1991) A requiem for vagotomy. BMJ 302: 547–548
2. Amdrup E, Andersen D, Hostrup H (1978) The Aarhus County Vagotomy Trial. I. An interim report on primary results and incidences of sequelae following parietal cell vagotomy and selective gastric vagotomy in 748 patients. World J Surg 2: 85–90
3. Bittner R, Meves M, Bittner L, Beger HG (1983) Das peptische Ulcus. Pathophysiologische Aspekte des präpylorischen Ulcus ventriculi. Dtsch Med Wochenshr 4: 137–141
4. Burge H, Vane JR (1958) Method of testing for complete nerve resection during vagotomy. BMJ i. 615–618
5. Enskog L, Rydberg B, Adami HO, Enander L, Ingvar C (1986) Clinical results 1–10 years after highly selective vagotomy in 306 patients with prepyloric and duodenal ulcer disease. Br J Surg 73: 357–360
6. Grassi G, Brecchia C, Cantarelli I, Grassi GB (1975) Development and results of our studies of vagotomy, from selective total vagotomy to ultraselective vagotomy. Chir Gastroenterol 9: 23–28
7. Hallenbeck GA, Gleysteen JJ, Aldrete JS, Slaughter RL (1976) Proximal and gastric vagotomy: effects of two operative techniques on clinical and gastric secretory results. Ann Surg 184: 435–442
8. Holtmann G, Armstrong AL, Blum AL, et al (1991) Effects of 2-year maintenance therapy with ranitidine on the natural course of duodenal ulcer (DU) disease. Gastroenterology 102: A84
9. Johnston D, Blackett R (1988) A new look at selective vagotomies. Am J Surg 156: 416–427
10. Müller C, Engelke B, Fiedler B, Marrie A, Muhe E, Schmitz-Hardauer W, Zumtobel V (1983) How do clinical results after proximal gastric vagotomy compare with the Visick grade pattern of healthy controls? World J Surg 7: 610–615

Effect of Single-Shot Antibiotic Treatment on *Helicobacter pylori* in Patients Undergoing Ulcer Operation*

M. Büchler[1], H. Frieß[1], F. Flock[1], A. Stanescu[2], K. Baczako[3], and P. Malfertheiner[2]

Introduction

The significance of *Helicobacter pylori* in the pathogenesis of duodenal ulcer has broadened the spectrum of drug therapy for ulcers. Preliminary results of treatment with bismuth compounds with or without antibiotics and the recent results of therapy with omeprazole combined with antibiotics indicate that treatment with these drugs is superior to therapy using H_2 receptor blockers [2, 13, 24]. After the eradication of *H. pylori*, fewer recurrences of duodenal ulcer occur in a period of at least 12 months [2, 15, 24]. Although proximal gastric vagotomy (PGV) has a lower rate of ulcer relapse in comparison with conservative drug therapy – based on a follow-up period of up to 20 years – surgical treatment continues to play only a subordinate role in the elective treatment of duodenal ulcer [11, 12, 16, 26, 29]. In two studies, antral *H. pylori* infections were described in 94%–100% of patients 6 months–20 years after PGV [10, 19]. In contrast, Steer et al. observed a reduction in *H. pylori* density 3–12 months after PGV [27].

The objective of the present prospective study was to investigate the influence of PGV with and without simultaneous perioperative single-shot antibiotics on *H. pylori* infection, the degree of infection, and the rate of gastric metaplasia in the duodenum.

Patients and Methods

Twenty-four patients (21 men, 3 women; mean age 43 years, range 21–74 years) with chronic duodenal ulcer were entered in the prospective study. The mean history of ulcer disease was 13 years (range 1–40 years). Based on preoperative randomization the patients received perioperatively a single-shot of 4 g mezlocillin and 500 mg metronidazole (Bayer, Leverkusen, FRG) or no antibiotic.

[1] Department of Surgery, University of Ulm, 89075 Ulm, Germany
[2] Department of Gastroenterology, University of Ulm, 89075 Ulm, Germany
[3] Department of Pathology, University of Ulm, 89075 Ulm, Germany

* Part of this report was published earlier as an abstract in *Gastroenterology* (1991), 100: A67.

Gasbarrini/Pretolani (Eds.)
Basic and Clinical Aspects of H. pylori Infection

Patients were excluded if they had been taking antibiotics, omeprazole, or drugs containing bismuth during the 12 weeks prior to the study. *Group A+* (PGV, single-shot of mezlocillin and metronidazole) included 13 patients (11 men, 2 women; mean age 46 years, range 27–74 years) with a mean history of ulcer disease of 12.6 years (range 1–30 years). Thirty minutes before the operation began, the patients received a single dose of 4 g mezlocillin and 500 mg metronidazole as an intravenous infusion for 30 min. *Group A–* (PGV, no perioperative antibiotics) included 11 patients (10 men, 1 woman; mean age 39 years, range 21–71 years). The mean history of ulcer disease was 13.5 years (4–40 years). The *control group* (5 men, 6 women; mean age 52 years, range 45–78 years) consisted of patients with biopsy-confirmed gastritis associated with *H. pylori*; here the effect of a single intravenous shot of 4 g mezlocillin and 0.5 g metronidazole on the *H. pylori* was analyzed. The antibiotic was administered in the scope of an extragastric abdominal operation.

After approval by the independent ethics committee of the University of Ulm and informed written consent of the patient had been obtained, a gastroduodenoscopy was performed before PGV as well as 2 weeks and 3 months after. The control group underwent postoperative follow-up endoscopy after 4 weeks. Following a standardized examination schedule in all of the patients four biopsies were collected from the antrum, one biopsy from the gastric body, and two biopsies from the duodenum. An antral biopsy was used for the *H. pylori* rapid urease test. Two more antral biopsies were used for the *H. pylori* culture. Both duodenal biopsies, the gastric body biopsy, and one antral biopsy were included in the histopathological evaluation. No duodenal biopsy was performed in the control group.

Histology. The mucosal biopsies were fixed in 4% buffered formalin for 24 h and embedded in paraffin. These samples were cut in 5-μm sections and stained for hematoxylin and eosin to judge the degree of mucosal inflammation and the presence of gastric metaplasia in the duodenum. The degree of inflammation was scored from grade 0 to grade III according to a modified classification proposed by Whitehead [30]:

Grade 0: lymphocytes and plasma cells in the tunica propria; No or only few polymorphonuclear leukocytes (PMNS)
Grade I: increased number of PMNS in the tunica propria with definite infiltration of foveluar epithelium
Grade II: strongly increased number of PMNS in the tunica propria with definite infiltration of foveluar epithelium
Grade III: extremely dense infiltration of PMNS in the tunica propria with infiltration of foveluar epithelium, often with glandular microabscesses

Gastric metaplasia was considered positive if cells were found with aspects of surface mucous cells with secretary granules and stunted microvilli. The degree of *H. pylori* colonization was analyzed following Warthin-Starry silver-staining and was classified from grade 0 to 3:

Grade 0: histopathologically no bacteria detectable
Grade 1: few bacteria, mainly in the superficial mucous layer;

Grade 2: moderate number of *H. pylori*, focally or evenly distributed in the superficial mucous layer and/or colonization of the gastric pits and glands

Grade 3: dense *H. pylori* colonization of the mucous layer and gastric pits along with obvious tendency to intercellular infiltration between the mucous cells

Culture. H. pylori were cultured under microaerobic conditions and at 37°C on Wilkens-Chalgren blood agar with Skirrow's supplement (code SR 69 oxoid) containing polymixin B (1250 IU/l), trimethoprim (2.5 mg/l), vancomycin (5 mg/l), and with 10% human erythrocyte concentration. The growth of *H. pylori* was assessed every 3 days. The earliest point at which a culture was considered negative was 10 days. The bacteria were identified by means of Gram's staining and biochemical tests for urease, oxidase, and catalase.

Helicobacter *Rapid Urease Test.* For rapid urease test we used a commercial test system (CUT, Temmler Pharma, Marburg, FRG), which is based on the cleavage of urea in ammonia by urease produced by *H. pylori.* This test was considered positive if the pH indicator turned from yellow to pink within 24 h.

Statistical Analysis. The results are expressed as mean ± SE. For statistical comparison the paired Student's *t* test with 0.05 as the level of significance was used. For quantitative outcome variables the chi-square test was taken.

Results

A total of 16 patients in whom a PGV was performed (nine patients from group A +, seven from group A −) completed the entire examination protocol. Two patients (A + and A −) refused to undergo the early (2-week) postoperative endoscopy, six patients (A + two; A − four) who were clinically asymptomatic refused the endoscopy after 3 months.

A florid duodenal ulcer was detected in 14 of the 24 (56%) patients who underwent preoperative endoscopic control. In one patient the florid duodenal ulcer persisted in the first (1/22) and second (1/18) postoperative follow-up examinations. The remaining patients showed normal endoscopic and clinical findings after PGV.

All of the patients (24/24) presented with *H. pylori* infection prior to the operation. *H. pylori* colonization in the stomach was found in the group receiving perioperative single-shot double antibiotic therapy 2 weeks after PGV in 5/12 (42%) and 3 months after PGV in 2/11 patients (18%; Table 1). In 4/5 patients who were found postoperatively (2 weeks) to be *H. pylori* positive by at least one of the three *H. pylori* detection methods used, no *H. pylori* infection was detected after 3 months. All of the patients undergoing vagotomy without perioperative single-shot antibiotic treatment (group A −) were positive for *H. pylori* 2 weeks (10/10 patients) and 3 months (11/11) following PGV. All of

Table 1. Rate of infection, degree of colonization and inflammation, and frequency of gastric metaplasia in patients undergoing gastric vagotomy with (A +) and without (A –) a perioperative single shot of 4 g mezlocillin and 0.5 g metronidazole

	A +			A –		
	Pre-operative	2 weeks post-operative	3 months post-operative	Pre-operative	2 weeks post-operative	3 months post-operative
Rate of infection	13/13	5/12	2/11	11/11	10/10	7/7
Degree of colonization	2.2 ± 0.8	0.5 ± 0.9	0.2 ± 0.7	1.8 ± 0.9	1.4 ± 1.0	2.0 ± 0.7
Degree of inflammation	1.7 ± 0.6	0.4 ± 0.5	0.6 ± 0.8	1.4 ± 0.5	1.4 ± 0.7	1.7 ± 0.5
Rate of gastric metaplasia	9/11	4/11	3/10	6/6	3/6	2/7

the patients in the control group (11/11) showed *H. pylori* infection preoperatively. In 8/11 (73%) patients a persisting *H. pylori* infection was found 4 weeks after surgery.

Analysis of the degree of infection (Table 1) produced results similar to the those regarding the frequency of *H. pylori* colonization. Prior to PGV, the two treatment groups had the same degree of infection: A + with 2.2 ± 0.8; A – with 1.8 ± 0.9. The PGV in combination with a perioperative single-shot of 4 g mezlocillin and 0.5 g metronidazole reduced the degree of infection to $0.5 + 0.9$ after 14 days and to 0.2 ± 0.7 after 12 weeks, which indicates a significant reduction ($\alpha < 0.01$). In the patients who received no antibiotics perioperatively the degree of infection 2 weeks and 3 months after proximal gastric vagotomy was $1.4 + 1.0$ and 2.0 ± 0.7, respectively. The degree of infection in the control group decreased slightly from 1.9 ± 0.8 before the operation to 1.0 ± 0.9 after surgery ($\alpha = 0.06$).

The degree of inflammation of the gastric mucosa prior to proximal gastric vagotomy was $1.7 + 0.6$ in group A + and 1.4 ± 0.5 in group A – (Table 1). In these cases as well, the perioperative administration of antibiotics reduced the degree of inflammation to 0.4 ± 0.5 after 14 days and 0.6 ± 0.8 after 3 months. The patients receiving no antibiotics showed no change in the degree of inflammation (1.4 ± 0.7 after 14 days; 1.7 ± 0.5 after 3 months). The control group showed a slight change in degree of inflammation from 1.7 ± 0.5 to 1.3 ± 0.7 after 1 month, respectively.

Gastric metaplasia in the duodenum was analyzed in 19 patients (Table 1). In two patients a stenosed stomach outlet prohibited passage of the endoscope, making preoperative biopsy of the duodenum impossible. Preoperatively, 15/17 patients (88%) presented with gastric metaplasia in the duodenal mucosa. Two weeks after PGV, the prevalance was still 41% (7/17). In 5/17 patients (29%) included in the late follow-up after 3 months evidence of gastric metaplasia was detected, which indicated a significant reduction of the frequency of metaplasia ($\alpha < 0.05$). The lowered rate of metaplasia was independent on the perioperative single shot of antibiotics.

Discussion

Antibiotics, despite their good in vitro effect, are often unsuccessful in vitro in eradicating *H. pylori* [23, 24]. The clinical efficacy of antibiotic treatment on the *H. pylori* infection has been established chiefly for oral preparations. For antibiotic monotherapies (e.g., amoxycillin, ciprofloxacin, metronidazole) *H. pylori* clearance rates of 0–90% have been reported but only 0%–40% eradication rates [6, 9, 17, 23].

As regards mezocillin, which is available only in parenteral form, there are no clinical reports on its use in the treatment of *H. pylori*. With metronidazole *H. pylori* clearance rates of 20%–30% are reached [9, 23, 34]. An important reason for the failure of treatment with nitroimidazole preparations appears to be an acquired antimicrobial resistance [7, 8, 21]. The development of resistance of *H. pylori* to penicillin has not been determined [5, 7, 8, 21].

In the scope of our study the effect of a single intravenous injection of 4 g mezlocillin and 500 mg metronidazole on *H. pylori* infections associated with nonresecting ulcer surgery was determined. In 85% of the patients treated perioperatively with antibiotics (11/13) an eradication of the organisms was accomplished. When antibiotics treatment without PGV was performed, 73% of patients showed the same degree of *H. pylori* infection as before the therapy. The PGV alone had no effect on the *H. pylori* infection. Responsible for the eradication of the organism is probably the change in gastric milieu in the form of an increase in pH in combination with the bactericidal effect of the antibiotics used. This assumption is supported by the results of the study conducted by Steer et al, who observed a reduction in the *H. pylori* colonization density after PGV alone [27]. In addition, in 4/5 patients who underwent vagotomy under perioperative antibiotic treatment and who proved to be *H. pylori* positive by at least one of the three detection methods immediately after surgery, the bacteria were no longer detectable after 3 months. This effect can hardly be attributed to the administration of antibiotics. The reason for the lack of organism eradication in two patients remains unknown. It should be mentioned, however, that both patients were under 30 years of age.

Independent of the perioperative administration of antibiotics, there is a significant decline in the gastric metaplasia rate in the duodenum after PGV. This metaplasia is considered to be an unspecific response to some sort of stimulus, especially acid, and is regarded as a predisposition to *H. pylori* colonization in the duodenum [14, 31]. It is known from animal experiments that increased secretion of gastric acid or exposure to acid leads to gastric metaplasia in the duodenum [25, 28, 32]. In human patients a qualitative correlation between a high output of gastric acid and the occurrence of gastric metaplasias has been demonstrated [22, 32]. The *H. pylori* infection itself does not seem to exert any influence on the occurrence of gastric metaplasia [4, 33]. It is possible, however, that the infection along with the inflammation of the duodenal mucosa has an effect on the extent of gastric metaplasia [33]. This could result in a vicious circle, which could ultimately lead to a spread of the gastric metaplasia on the one hand, and to inflammation caused by the *H. pylori*, on the other, until the integrity of the mucosa is finally lost. This in connection with other ulcerogenic factors might possibly lead to duodenal ulcer. This hypothesis is corroborated by observations that *H. pylori* is found in 43%–100% of patients with ulcer in the duodenal bulbus, whereas under intact duodenal conditions the organism is found in only 0%–15% of patients [3, 4, 15, 20, 23, 33]. The *H. pylori* colonization of gastric metaplasia of the duodenal mucosa is considered an important risk factor in the formation of duodenal ulcer [3]. As many as 98% of patients with a duodenal *H. pylori* infection have an active or a healed duodenal ulcer.

In the present study the effect of PGV on gastric metaplasia was determined. Preoperatively, 87% of the patients presented with a gastric metaplasia in the duodenal bulb, and after surgery this percentage decreased to 43% after 2 weeks and 33% after 3 months. This effect was not dependent on the perioperative administration of antibiotics and can be explained by the reduction in acid secretion. The *H. pylori* colonization in areas of gastric metaplasia found preoperatively was far lower (41%, 7/17 patients) than is reported in the literature. The reason for this could be that we took biopsy specimens at a distance from the duodenal ulcer, while the authors reffered to above determined the *H. pylori* infection rate directly at the border of the ulcer [3, 15, 23]. *H. pylori* was identified in the duodenum in only 2/17 patients early after surgery and in none of the 17 patients at a later time. Thus, it can be concluded that proximal gastric vagotomy reduces the frequency of gastric metaplasia to a level close to that determined in healthy control patients [3, 4, 14, 20, 33].

References

1. Bayerdörfer E, Ottenjann R (1988) The role of antibiotics in *Campylobacter pylori* associated peptic ulcer disease. Scand J Gastroenterol 23 [Suppl 142]: 93–100
2. Borody T, Noonan S, Cole P, Hyland L, Morgan A, Lenne J et al. (1989) Duodenal ulcer recurrence in patients remaining *C. pylori*-negative long term post-eradication. Gastroenterology 96: A52
3. Carrick J, Lee A, Hazell S, Ralston M, Daskalopoulos G (1989) *Campylobacter pylori*, duodenal ulcer, and gastric metaplasia: possible role of functional heterotopic tissue in ulcerogenesis. Gut 30: 790–797
4. Fitzgibbons PL, Dooley CP, Cohen H, Applemen MD (1988) Prevalence of gastric metaplasia, inflammation, and *Campylobacter pylori* in the duodenum of members of a normal population. Am J Clin Pathol 90: 711–714
5. Glupczynski Y, Burette A (1991) Acquired resistance to antibiotics: an underestimated cause of failure in the treatment of *Helicobacter pylori* infection. In: Menge H et al. (eds) *Helicobacter pylori*. Springer, Berlin Heidelberg New York
6. Glupczynski Y, Burette A, Labbe M, Deprez C, De Reuck M, Deltenre M (1988) *Campylobacter pylori*-associated gastritis: a double-blind placebo-controlled trial with amoxycillin. Am J Gastroenetrol 83: 365–372
7. Goodwin CS, Marshall BJ, Blincow ED, Wilson DH, Blackbourn S, Phillips M (1988) Prevention of nitroimidazole resistance in *Campylobacter pylori* by coadministration of colloidal bismuth subcitrate: clinical and in vitro studies. J Clin Pathol 41: 207–210
8. Hirschl AM, Hentschel E, Schütze K, Nemec H, Pötzi R, Gangl A et al. (1988) The efficacy of antimicrobial treatment in *Campylobacter pylori*-associated gastritis and duodenal ulcer. Scand J Gastroenterol 23 [Suppl 142]: 76–81
9. Hirschl A, Stanek G, Pötzi R, Rotter M, Wende L (1986) Die Empfindlichkeit von Campylobacter pyloridis gegenüber antimikrobiellen Chemotherapeutika und Ulcustherapeutika. ZAC 2: 45–49

10. Hölscher AH, Petkaneschkov G, Bollschweiler E (1989) Effekt der proximal-gastrischen Vagotomie auf die Campylobacter Besiedelung des Magens. Z Gastroenterol 27: A563
11. Jordan PH, Thornby J (1987) Should it be parietal cell vagotomy or selective vagotomy-antrectomy for treatment of duodenal ulcer? Ann Surg 205: 572–587
12. Koruth NM, Dua KS, Brunt WP, Matheson NA (1990) Comparison of highly selective vagotomy with truncal vagotomy and pyloroplasty: results at 8–15 years. Br J Surg 77 (1): 70–72
13. Lamouliate H, Bernard PH, Boulard A, Megraud F (1990) Controlled study of omeprazole-amoxycillin-tinidazol vas ranitidine-amoxicillin-tinidazol in *Helicobacter pylori.* Associated duodenal ulcer preliminary results. Rev Esp Enferm Dig 78 [Suppl 1]: 101
14. Malfertheiner P, Stanescu A, Bode G, Baczako K, Kühl P, Ditschuneit H (1990) Gastric metaplasia in duodenal mucosa – key factor for *H. pylori* colonization and duodenal ulcer pathogenesis? In: Malfertheiner P, Ditschuneit H (eds) *Helicobacter pylori*, gastritis and peptic ulcer. Springer, Berlin Heidelberg New York, pp 292–301
15. Marshall BJ, Goodwin CS, Warren JR, Murray R, Blincow ED, Blackbourn SJ et al. (1988) Prospective double-blind trial of duodenal ulcer relapse after eradication of *Campylobacter pylori.* Lancet ii: 1437–1442
16. Meisner S, Jorgensen LN, Jensen HE (1988) The Kaplan and Meier and the Nelson estimate for the probability of ulcer recurrence 10 and 15 years after parietal cell vagotomy. Ann Surg 207: 1–3
17. Morgan D, Kraft WG, Bender M, Pearson A (1988) Nitrofurans in the treatment of gastritis associated with *Campylobacter pylori.* Gastroenterology 95: 1178–1184
18. Natelson B, Dubois A, Sodetz FJ (1977) Effect of multiple-stress procedures on monkey gastroduodenal mucosa, serum gastrin and hydrogen ion kinetics. Dig Dis Sci 22: 888–897
19. O'Connor HJ, Dixon HF, Wyatt JI, Axon ATR, Ward DC, Dewar EP et al. (1986) Effect of duodenal ulcer surgery and enterogastric reflux on *Campylobacter pylori.* Lancet ii: 1178–1181
20. Offerhaus GJ, Molyvas EN, Hoedenmaeker PJ (1990) *Helicobacter pylori* infection of gastric mucin cell metaplasia: the duodenum revisited. J Pathol 162: 239–243
21. O'Riordan T, Mathai E, Tobin E, McKenna D, Keane C, Sweeney E et al. (1990) Adjuvant antibiotic therapy in duodenal ulcers treated with colloidal bismuth subcitrate. Gut 31: 999–1002
22. Parrish JA, Rawlings DC (1965) Intestinal mucosa in the Zollinger-Ellison syndrome. Gut 6: 286–289
23. Rauws EAJ, Tytgat GNJ (1989) Therapeutic trials of eradication of *Campylobacter pylori.* In: Rauws EAJ, Tytgat GNJ (eds) *Campylobacter pylori.* Den Ouden, Amsterdam, pp 89–100
24. Rauws EA, Tytgat GNJ (1990) Cure of duodenal ulcer associated with eradication of *Helicobacter pylori.* Lancet 335: 1233–1235
25. Rhodes J (1964) Experimental production of gastric epithelium in the duodenum. Gut 5: 454–458
26. Soper NJ, Kelly KA, van Heerden JA, Ilstrup DM (1989) Long term clinical results after proximal gastric vagotomy. Surg Gynecol Obstet 169: 488–494
27. Steer HW, Hawtin P, Newell DG (1988) The effect of surgical treatment of chronic duodenal ulceration on *Campylobacter pylori* colonisation of the stomach. Abstract book workshop gastroduodenal pathology and *Campylobacter pylori* Bordeaux, p 153
28. Tatsuta M, Iishi H, Yamamura H, Yamamoto R, Taniguchi H (1989) Enhancement by tetragastrin of experimental induction of gastric epithelium in the duodenum. Gut 30: 311–315
29. Vom Holstein CS, Graffner H, Oscarson J (1987) One hundred patients ten years after parietal cell vagotomy. Br J Surg 74: 101–103
30. Whitehead R, Truelove SC, Gear MWL (1972) The histological diagnosis of chronic gastritis in fibreoptic gastroscopy biopsy specimens. J Clin Pathol 25: 1–11
31. Wyatt JI (1989) The role of *Campylobacter pylori* in the pathogenesis of peptic ulcer disease. Scand J Gastroenterol 24 [Suppl 157]: 7–11
32. Wyatt JI, Rathbone BJ, Dixon MF, Heatley RV (1987) *Campylobacter pyloridis* and acid induced gastric metaplasia in the pathogenesis of duodenitis. J Clin Pathol 40: 841–848
33. Wyatt JI, Rathbone BJ, Sobala GM, Shallcross T, Heatley RV, Axon ATR et al. (1990) Gastric epithelium in the duodenum: its association with *Helicobacter pylori* and inflammation. J Clin Pathol 43: 981–986
34. Xiao SD, Liu WZ, Xia DH, Jiang SJ, Wang RN, Zhang ZH et al. (1990) The efficacy of furazolidone and metronidazole in the treatment of chronic gastritis associated with *Helicobacter* (*Campylobacter*) *pylori* – a randomized double-blind placebo-controlled clinical trial. Hepato-gastroenterology 37 (5): 503–506

The Aging Stomach

J.H. Baron

This survey is in two parts. The first half presents the midcentury model of acid secretion declining with age. The second half explains how I and others were wrong: gastric secretion does not decline with age but with disease, usually the gastritis caused by *Helicobacter pylori.*

The Mid-century Model of the Aging Stomach

This model of acid decreasing with age in the general population has been described in detail elsewhere [1, 2]. In brief, in the normal population a decrease with age has been noted in response to submaximal stimuli such as low-dose histamine [3], food [4], interdigestive basal [5], submaximal histalog [6], and for maximal histamine stimulated acid output [7]. In my control population peak acid output declined slightly and insignificantly in men and markedly and significantly in women, but with no such change in patients with duodenal ulcer [7, 8]. I assumed that the fall off in acid with age was due to the increased incidence of gastritis as controls grew older, and that this was not occurring in patients with duodenal ulcer.

This problem of gastritis has been studied epidemiologically in biopsy studies of controls and patients by Siurala and colleagues in Finland and Estonia. In their 10% random sample of a Finnish village 25% had superficial and 28% atrophic gastritis, with a prevalence rate of each type increasing by 1.4% a year; it took 18–19 years for a change in one degree of severity, such as from superficial to atrophic gastritis [9–12]. Similarly Kimura [13] gastroscoped 570 Japanese and systematically biopsied five points on the lesser and five on the greater curves. The junction between pyloric and fundic mucosa moved cephalad as metaplastic pyloric glands replaced fundic mucosa. The proportion of normal mucosa decreased with age almost to zero as both lesser and greater curves were replaced by superficial and atrophic gastritis mucosa. Thus the proportion of stomachs with normal mucosa in all ten specimens decreased with age on a semi-log scale, suggesting that a normal stomach is found only under the age of 10 years.

Gastroenterology Unit, St Mary's Hospital, London W2 1NY, UK

Gasbarrini/Pretolani (Eds.)
Basic and Clinical Aspects of H. pylori Infection

The 1990s Model: The Healthy Stomach Does Not Age

Our mid-century model was wrong. Our data were correct, but our conclusions were faulty because we confused sequence and consequence and because we were limited to cross-sectional studies and lacked adequate follow-up of healthy individuals and cohorts. What is needed is repeated studies of gastric acidity and acid output in healthy subjects over the longterm, and there are only scanty data available. Published data of repeated tests on a healthy man from 1949 to 1969 showed no age trend [14], and further (unpublished) studies over the following 20 years have still shown no change.

When the subjects in the studies of acid secretion with age were chosen not from a control population but from subjects who were healthy volunteers with no past or present dyspepsia, there was no decrease of acid with age [15–17]. When acid output was expressed as a fraction of fat-free body weight, there was no significant change with age in male subjects with histologically normal body mucosa, and female subjects showed a slight but significant increased acid output with age [17]. In subjects with histological superficial gastritis of the body of the stomach there were significant falls in acid output with age both in men and women [17]. Similar increases in acid secretion with age have been seen recently in a group of 41 healthy volunteers aged 23–71 years in Dallas, Texas, and with increases in basal serum pepsinogen I and II concentrations [18].

Age, Gastritis and Gastric and Duodenal Ulcer

A random population sample in southern Estonia was endoscoped and biopsied and subjected to the same statistical analyses [19] as had been used in Finland [20]. It was then possible to calculate an age-dependent score for both antral and body gastritis to show the increase from age 15 to 69 in antral and body gastritis just as in Finland [9], and comparable with asymptomatic Hungarians and Italians [21] and Germans and Turks [22].

In patients with gastric ulcer [23] the age-related increase in gastritis in the antrum followed that of controls, whereas gastritis in the body progressed extremely rapidly, 11-fold compared with the population at large, during the three examinations between 1974 and 1982, with most ulcers healed, possibly 'burn-out' from hypoacidity. By contrast, in patients with duodenal ulcer disease, whether with actual ulcers, scars or duodenitis, the antral gastritis behaved similarly to the general population, whereas the body mucosa showed no increase in the prevalence and severity of gastritis with age [24].

It was similarly possible for Sipponen and colleagues to establish that the risk of developing active gastric or duodenal ulcer was dependent upon the relative presence of superficial and atrophic gastritis in antral and body mucosa [25] (Table 1). Thus the relative risk in men having a duodenal ulcer rose to 16-fold with superficial gastritis in the antrum and to 18-fold if it was atrophic, compared to the risk with normal antral histology. The risk increased to nearly fourfold

Table 1. Relative risk of duodenal (DU) and gastric ulcer (GU; body, angulus) (from [25])

	DU		GU	
	Men	Women	Men	Women
Body				
Normal	1.0	1.0	1.0	1.0
Superficial gastritis	3.6	2.1	5.4	6.2
Atrophic gastritis	0.3	0.3	3.1	6.1
Antrum				
Normal	1.0	1.0	1.0	1.0
Superficial gastritis	16.2	5.7	6.5	18.4
Atrophic gastritis	18.4	4.8	32.2	24.4

Table 2. Ten-year risk of peptic ulcer in 454 consecutive patients with endoscopy-negative dyspepsia (from [26])

Body	Antrum	*n*	All peptic ulcer	Duodenal ulcer	Pylorus antrum	Angulus body
N	N	133(29%)	1(1%)	0	1	0
N	SG	49(11%)	9(18%)	5	3	1
SG	SG	197(43%)	22(11%)	13	8	1
AG	AG	75(17%)	3(4%)	0	1	2
		454	35(8%)	18	13	4

N, Normal; SG, superficial gastritis; AG, atrophic gastritis.

if there was superficial gastritis in the body but was reduced to only one-third of normal if the body gastritis was atrophic. By contrast with duodenal ulcer the risk of gastric ulcer in men increased to sevenfold with antral superficial gastritis and more than 30-fold if the antral gastritis was atrophic, whereas in the body the gastric ulcer relative risk was three to fivefold with atrophic or superficial gastritis.

This study [25] was cross-sectional, but it has been possible for this group to confirm this model in a 10-year follow-up in 1989 of 454 consecutive outpatients who had been endoscoped and biopsied for dyspepsia in 1979 [26] (Table 2). Those who had normal mucosa in both body and antrum had not developed a duodenal ulcer and showed minimal (1%) risk of developing a gastric ulcer. If the body mucosa was normal, and the antrum had superficial gastritis, there was an 18% risk of developing duodenal or gastric ulcer. If there was superficial gastritis in both body and antrum, there was an 11% risk of peptic ulcer, but it there was atrophic pangastritis ulcers developed only in the stomach.

Helicobacter pylori, Gastritis and Peptic Ulcer

It has been possible for the Finnish/Estonian group to restudy their material in the light of the evidence that the increase with age of gastric *H. pylori* is the principal cause of the development with age of non-autoimmune gastritis of the

Table 3. *H. pylori* in 139 Estonian controls (from [27])

	1979 (*H. pylori* 85%)	1985 (*H. pylori* 89%)
Antrum	N	0 N
	N	+ SG
	SG	0 isq/better
	SG	+ isq/worse
	AG	+ Worse
Body	N	0 N
	N	+ N/SG
	SG	+ SG
	AG	+ Worse

N, Normal; SG, superficial gastritis; AG, atrophic gastritis; *in statu quo*, unchanged.

antrum and body of the stomach. Villako and colleagues [27] found that in their 1979 random sample of 227 subjects in an Estonian town *H. pylori* could be seen in 85%, which increased to 89% at re-examination in 1985 (Table 3). Those with normal antral and body mucosa and who were free of *H. pylori* retained normal mucosa 6 years later whereas, if *H. pylori* had been present, superficial gastritis developed. Antral superficial gastritis without *H. pylori* remained the same or improved, but with *H. pylori* remained the same or worsened. Those with atrophic gastritis either in the antrum or body with *H. pylori* showed worsening of their histology.

The assessment of the causal role of *H. pylori* in atrophic gastritis is complicated by the low presence of these bacteria in this degree of gastritis [28]. However, although serological and histological evidence of *H. pylori* infection correspond in those with normal mucosa or superficial gastritis, in patients with atrophic gastritis *H. pylori* infection by seropositivity (86%) was significantly commoner than positive staining on histology (33%) [29]. These data support the model of *H. pylori* causing atrophic gastritis, but in this milieu with intestinal metaplasia and hypoacidity the bacteria can no longer survive.

Table 4 summarises the current status of the function and structure of the gastric body and antrum in relationship to *H. pylori*.

Table 4. Acid, ulcers, *H. pylori* and gastritis

	N	PA	Nonimmune	GU	DU
Acid	N	0	Low	Low	+
Body	N	AG	AG	SG/AG	N/SG
Body *H. pylori*	0	0	+	+	+
Antrum	N	N/SG	AG	AG	SG
Antrum *H. pylori*	0	0	+	+	++
G cells	N	+++	Few	N	++
Gastrin	N	+++	Low	N	++

N, Normal; PA, Penicious Anaemia; SG, Superficial gastritis; AG, atrophic gastritis; GU, gastric ulcer; DU, duodenal ulcer.

Conclusions

In the general population gastric secretion decreases with age due to superficial and then atrophic gastritis of the body mucosa which is due mostly to infection with *H. pylori*. Subjects with or without *H. pylori* in the body mucosa without gastritis secrete normal acid and may even show an increase in acid output with age. In patients with gastric ulcer of the body (as opposed to the antrum) acid secretion decreases with age in association with increasing atrophic gastritis in the body mucosa. In patients with duodenal ulcer acid secretion remains high throughout life because although almost all have *H. pylori* the body mucosa rarely atrophies.

Unfortunately it is still unclear why in some of the population whose stomachs are infected with *H. pylori* there follows atrophic gastritis and the risk of gastric ulcer and carcinoma, whereas in others there is only superficial gastritis of the body and antrum with increased antral G cell mass, inappropriate hypergastrinaemia, acid hypersecretion and duodenal ulcer [30].

Acknowledgement. I am indebted to the Finnish/Estonian group for helpful discussions and permission to cite their unique data, much of which has been highlighted in a recent monograph [31].

References

1. Baron JH (1977) Gastric secretion and diseases of the mucosal barrier. Rendicont Gastroenterol 9:41–46
2. Baron JH (1978) Clinical tests of gastric secretion. History, methodology and interpretation. Macmillan, London
3. Bloomfield AL, Keefer CS (1928) Gastric acidity: relation to various factors such as age and physical fitness. J Clin Invest 5:285–294
4. Vanzant FR, Alvarez WC, Berkson J, Eusterman GB (1933) Changes in gastric acidity in peptic ulcer, cholecystitis, and other diseases analysed with help of new accurate technic. Arch Intern Med 52:616–631
5. Levin E, Kirsner JB, Palmer WL (1951) A simple measure of gastric secretion in man. Comparison of one hour basal secretion, histamine secretion and twelve hour nocturnal gastric secretion. Gastroenterology 19:88–98
6. Kirsner JB, Ford H (1955) The gastric secretory response to histalog: one hour basal and histalog secretion in normal persons and in patients with duodenal ulcer and gastric ulcer. J Lab Clin Med 46:307–311
7. Baron JH (1963) Studies of basal and peak acid output with an augmented histamine test. Gut 4:136–144
8. Baron JH (1963) An assessment of the augmented histamine test in the diagnosis of peptic ulcer. Gut 4:243–253
9. Siurala M, Isokosi M, Varis K, Kekki M (1968) Prevalence of gastritis in a rural population. Bioptic studies of subjects selected at random. Scand J Gastroent 3:211–223
10. Siurala M, Kekki M, Varis K, Isokoski M, Ihamaki T (1972) Gastritis and gastric cancer. Br Med J 3:530–531
11. Siurala M, Lehtola J, Ihamaki J (1974) Atrophic gastritis and its sequelae. Results of 19–23 years' follow-up examinations. Scand J Gastroenterol 9:441–446
12. Siurala M, Salmi HJ (1971) Long-term follow-up of subjects with superficial gastritis or a normal gastric mucosa. Scand J Gastroenterol 6:459–463
13. Kimura K (1972) Chronological transition of the fundic-pyloric border determined by stepwise biopsy of the lesser and greater curvatures of the stomach. Gastroenterology 63:584–592

14. Baron JH (1970) Gastric secretion in a healthy man, 1949–1969. Lancet 2: 547–549
15. Cleator IGM, Stoller JL, Nunn PN, Holubitsky IB, Johnstone FRC, Harrison RC (1973) Discriminant analysis of data in ulcer and non-ulcer population. Am J Dig Dis 18: 301–310
16. Hobsley M, Whitfield PF, Faber RG, Parkin JV (1975) Hypersecretion and length of history in duodenal ulceration. Lancet 2: 101–104
17. Kekki M, Samloff IM, Ihamaki T, Varis K, Siurala M (1982) Age and sex-related behaviour of gastric acid secretion at the population level. Scand J Gastroenterol 17: 737–743
18. Goldschmiedt M, Barnett CC, Schwarz BE, Karnes WE, Redfern JS, Feldman M (1991) Effect of age on gastric acid secretion and serum gastrin concentrations in healthy men and women. Gastroenterology 101: 977–990
19. Kekki M, Villako K, Tamm A, Siurala M (1977) Dynamics of antral and funsal gastritis in an Estonian rural population sample. Scand J Gastroenterol 12: 321–324
20. Kekki M, Ihamaki T, Sipponen P, Hovinen M (1975) Heterogenerity in susceptibility to chronic gastritis in relatives of gastric cancer patients with different histology of carcinoma. Scand J Gastroenterol 10: 737–745
21. Cheli R, Simon L, Aste H, Figus IA, Nicola G, Bajtai A, Puntoni R (1980) Atrophic gastritis and intestinal metaplasia in asymptomatic Hungarian and Italian populations. Endoscopy 12: 105–108
22. Massarrat S, Paidlick A, Pittner P, Schmitz-Moormann P, Wurbs M (1983) The role of certain habits and various diseases in the occurrence of gastritis. Hepatogastroenterology 30: 249–253
23. Maaroos HI, Salupere V, Uibo R, Kekki M, Sipponen P (1985) Seven-year follow-up study of chronic gastritis in gastric ulcer patients. Scand J Gastroenterol 20: 198–205
24. Kekki M, Sipponen P, Siurala M (1984) Progression of antral and body gastritis in patients with active and healed duodenal ulcer and duodenitis. Scand J Gastroenterol 19: 382–388
25. Sipponen P, Seppala K, Aarynen M, Helske T, Kettonen P (1989) Chronic gastritis and duodenal ulcer: a case control study of risk of coexisting duodenal or gastric ulcer in patients with gastritis. Gut 30: 922–929
26. Sipponen P, Varis K, Fraki O, Korri UM, Seppala K, Siurala M (1990) Cumulative 10-year risk of symptomatic duodenal and gastric ulcer in patients with or without chronic gastritis. A clinkal follow-up study of 454 outpatients. Scand J Gastroenterol 25: 966–973
27. Villako K, Maaros H, Tammur R, Keevallik R, Peetsalu M, Sipponen P. Kekki M, Siurala M (1990) *Helicobacter* (*Campylobacter*) *pylori* infestation and the development and progression of chronic gastritis. Results of long-term follow-up examination of a random sample. Endoscopy 22: 114–117
28. Siurala M, Sipponen P, Kekki M (1988) *Campylobacter pylori* in a sample of Finnish population: relations to morphology and functions of the gastric mucosa. Gut 29: 909–915
29. Karnes WE, Samloff IM, Siurala M, Kekki M, Sipponen P, Kim SWR, Walsh JH (1991) Positive serum antibody and negative tissue staining for *Helicobacter pylori* in subjects with atrophic gastritis. Gastroenterology 101: 167–174
30. Dixon MF (1991) *Helicobacter pylori* and peptic ulceration: histopathological aspects. J Gastroenterol 6: 125–130
31. Kekki M (ed) (1991) Gastritis, peptic ulcer and gastric cancer. Scand J Gastroenterol 26 [Suppl]: 186

Pathogenic Mechanisms of *Helicobacter pylori* Infection: Virulence

Construction of a Molecular Population Genetic Framework for the Characterization of *Helicobacter pylori* Pathogenesis by Multilocus Enzyme Electrophoresis

M.F. Go, D.Y. Graham, and J.M. Musser

Introduction

Helicobacter pylori is now recognized as the most common cause of gastritis. *H. pylori* has also been implicated in the pathogenesis of duodenal ulcer disease and gastric ulcer disease and may play an important role in the development of precursor lesions of gastric cancer. It remains unclear whether the differences in the presentation of *H. pylori* associated diseases are due to infection with different genetic strains of *H. pylori*, variation in the host response, or both. Studies attempting to identify *H. pylori* strains associated with specific *H. pylori* diseases have recently begun (e.g., chromosomal and plasmid DNA restriction endonuclease profiling analyses). DNA–DNA solution hybridization of genomic DNA from *H. pylori* isolates found that *H. pylori* isolates from patients with duodenal ulcer, on average, formed a different hybridization group from isolates from patients with asymptomatic gastritis [3]. Recent studies of many other pathogenic bacterial species have shown that genetic subpopulations of bacteria are nonrandomly associated with certain clinical disorders [2] and that, even for species that are genetically highly variable, the majority of cases of serious disease are caused by a small proportion of the total bacterial cell lineages.

Chromosomal DNA restriction endonuclease profiling is a useful technique when relatively few isolates are to be characterized or classified. However, when large samples of strains must be analyzed to generate statistically robust data, the technique of choice currently is multilocus enzyme electrophoresis. Multilocus enzyme electrophoresis [1] measures genetic relationships or allelic diversity among strains by indexing variation in the primary structure or amino acid sequence of polypeptides affecting net electrostatic charge. The key concept is that electromorphs or mobility variants of enzymes can be equated with alleles at the corresponding structural gene loci; hence, electrophoretic types can be equated with multilocus chromosomal genotypes. Allelic variation is unaffected by environmental conditions, including host, culture medium, and laboratory storage.

Departments of Medicine and Pathology, Baylor College of Medicine and VA Medical Center, Houston, TX 77030, USA

Gasbarrini/Pretolani (Eds.)
Basic and Clinical Aspects of H. pylori Infection

Table 1. Allelic profiles of enzyme loci of seven *Helicobacter pylori* isolates

ET	Isolate	Allele at indicated enzyme locus								
		IPO	IDH	ADK	CAK	GLD	LGG	NSP	ACO	G6P
1	638	5	1	1	13	1	1	8	1	5
2	26	5	5	2	3	5	3	1	9	2
3	40	5	6	7.5	6	4	7	3	13	13
4	54	5	5	7	7	9	7	7	9	3
5	84	5	3	8	8	13	3	1	3	7
6	90	3	5	3	5	4.5	7	8	9	3
7	108	5	5	8	9	7	7	13	9	13

The nine complete enzyme profiles on these isolates indicate that each isolate represents a different mobility variant or electrophoretic type. ET, Electrophoretic type; IPO, indophenol oxidase; IDH, isocitrate dehydrogenase; ADK, adenylate kinase; CAK; carbamylate kinase; GLD, glutamate dehydrogenase; LGG, leucylglycylglycine peptidase; NSP, nucleoside phosphorylase; ACO, aconitase; glucose-6-phosphate dehydrogenase.

Methods and Results

We have begun to use multilocus enzyme electrophoresis to characterize *H. pylori* populations to identify representative genotypes for pathogenesis studies. We are analyzing genetic diversity among strains of *H. pylori* isolates from patients with asymptomatic gastritis, duodenal ulcer, and gastric ulcer disease to determine whether there are specific genotypes associated with each disorder. To date we have studied seven different *H. pylori* isolates from patients with asymptomatic gastritis, duodenal ulcer disease, and gastric ulcer disease.

Isolates were grown in broth under standard conditions, and variation in 12 metabolic enzymes were examined. Distinctive electromorphs of each enzyme, numbered in order of decreasing rate of anodal migration, were equated with alleles at the corresponding structural gene locus. Each isolate was characterized by its combination of alleles at the 12 enzyme loci, and distinctive multilocus enzyme genotypes were designated as electrophoretic types (Table 1). Each isolate has been designated as a distinct electrophoretic type based on the allelic diversity in its enzyme profile. The mean genetic diversity per locus was very high (0.820), indicating that isolates are strongly heterogeneous in overall levels of chromosomal diversity. This value means that two isolates chosen at random from the *Helicobacter* population differ on average at about 80% of their chromosomal loci, demonstrating that isolates are strongly differentiated from one another. Based upon studies from other pathogens the level of genetic diversity identified in our sample suggests that there are perhaps a number of different species of *H. pylori.*

Conclusion

We have demonstrated that (a) *H. pylori* isolates are strongly heterogeneous in overall levels of chromosomal diversity, (b) multilocus enzyme electrophoresis can be used to construct a population genetic framework for this microorganism, and (c) this technique provides a powerful means to examine genomic relationships among isolates and will allow investigation of the strength of association between bacterial genotypes and specific *H. pylori* diseases.

Acknowledgements. This work was supported by the Department of Veterans Affairs, by grant DK 39919 from the National Institute of Diabetes and Digestive and Kidney Diseases, by the generous support of Hilda Schwartz, and by grant R01–AI33119–01, and Biomedical Research Support Grant RR-05425.

References

1. Selander RK, Caugant DA, Ochman H, Musser JM, Gilmour MN, Whittam TS (1986) Methods of multilocus enzyme electrophoresis for bacterial population genetics and systematics. Appl Environ Microbiol 51: 873–884
2. Selander RK, Musser JM, Caugant DA, Gilmour MN, Whittam TS (1987) Population genetics of pathogenic bacteria. Microb Pathog 3: 1–7
3. Yoshimura HH, Evans DG, Graham DY (1990) *H. pylori* strains from duodenal ulcer patients differ at the genomic level from those from patients with simple gastritis. Enferm Dig 78 [Suppl 1]: 22

The Flagella of *Helicobacter pylori*: Molecular Analysis and Potential in Pathogenesis

C.W. Penn and C.J. Luke

Flagellar Structure and Composition

The flagella of *Helicobacter pylori* are unipolar and usually number three to five per organism [1]. They are remarkable in being covered by a sheath layer, which appears relatively fluid and membrane-like judged by its electron microscopic appearance in negatively stained preparations of the organism [2]. Such flagellar sheaths are not common among bacteria; a well-known parallel is the sheathed flagellum of *Vibrio cholerae*, and sheathed flagella are sometimes present, although not always, in *V. parahaemolyticus* which appears to express alternative flagellar structures depending on its flagellar phase (multiple peritrichous–swarmer phase, or single polar–swimmer phase), apparently controlled by a developmental switch [3]. In the latter case the single polar flagellum is sheathed whereas the multiple peritrichous flagella are naked. Little is known of flagellar sheath structure composition in *H. pylori*; however, in *V. cholerae* [4] it is believed that the sheath is continuous with the outer membrane, and there is some evidence for the presence of outer membrane components in the sheath. There is also evidence that in *Beneckea* spp. and *Photobacterium fischeri* [5] and in *Bdellovibrio bacteriovorus* [6] which also possesses sheathed flagella, the sheath is continuous with the outer membrane.

On the other hand, the flagellar shaft, comprised of the flagellin proper, has been well characterised by several groups. Geis et al. [7] first reported the purification of flagella, comprising a fraction of flagellar fragments which had spontaneously lost their sheaths and were purified by density gradient ultracentrifugation; a predominant protein of 51-kDa was obtained. In our hands [2], detergent treatment of flagella sheared by high-speed homogenisation from the surface of the organism, and purified by differential centrifugation, produced a clean preparation of naked flagellar fragments which showed a molecular weight for the flagellin of 54 kDa. Immunoblotting and immunogold labelling with a monospecific antiserum cofiirmed that only the naked flagella showed exposure of the 54-kDa protein, confirming the identity of this protein with the major structural flagellin. More recently Kostrzynska and colleagues [8] reported that two flagellin molecular species could be obtained: a major component of 56 kDa and a minor component of 57 kDa which was shown by immunogold electron microscopy to be confined to the hook-proximal region of the flagellum. The consensus, then, is of a major structural flagellin of about 55 kDa, probably

School of Biological Sciences, University of Birmingham, Birmingham B15 2TT, UK

Gasbarrini/Pretolani (Eds.)
Basic and Clinical Aspects of H. pylori Infection

with some variation in molecular weight between strains – observed, for example, by ourselves (unpublished).

Flagellin Genes

Until this meeting there had been no published report of cloning *H. pylori* flagellin genes (the first such report was presented as a poster at this meeting: [9]). Examination of the properties of flagellin genes from closely related organisms which have already been characterised may, however, give clues to the likely organisation of these genes in *H. pylori*.

The genus *Campylobacter* has recently received detailed attention to the structure, function and genetics of flagella. Trust and colleagues [10, 11] have focussed on the flagellins of *C. coli*, and Nuijten et al. [12, 13] and Fischer and Nachamkin [14] on those of *C. jejuni*. Flagellins of both organisms have been cloned and sequenced. Adjacent tandemly repeated flagellin sequences are present in both cases, and the 5′ copy (*flaA*) encodes normal flagellin and is transcribed from a sigma-28-type promoter. The downstream copy *flaB* appears to be transcribed but at a lower level and normally only in *C. coli*, and while it appears to be necessary for correct flagellar assembly its exact role is unclear [11]. In *C. jejuni*, expression of *flaB* appears enhanced in *flaA*$^-$ mutants, and short flagella are formed which appear unable to confer motility [15]. Interestingly, the latter mutants appear affected in their ability to invade cultured cells [15], one of the indications of the role of flagella in pathogenicity in this group of organisms. The study of motility variants and flagellin antigenicity in *Campylobacter* has indicated that both phase changes involving rapid switching of flagellar expression [16] and variability in flagellar antigenicity [9] may occur. Sequence data and antibody binding experiments indicate that antigenic variability, in both *C. coli* [10] and *C. jejuni* [14], is the consequence of sequence rearrangements in the central part of the *flaA* gene. Whether the flagellin sequence now reported by Haas et al. [9] is homologous in its operon organisation with *flaA* of *Campylobacter* spp., whether there are tandem repeats of flagellin sequences, and whether the influence of flagellin gene sequences of *H. pylori* on the biological role of its flagella parallel those of the *Campylobacter* spp., remains to be determined. In particular, it will be of considerable interest to learn whether the sheathed structure of the *Helicobacter* flagellum is accompanied by significant differences in the flagellin genetic sequence and organisation.

The Flagellar Sheath

Electron microscopy suggests that the flagellar sheath is a pliable structure, presumably membrane-like in its organisation; characteristically, the distal ends or broken termini of sheathed flagella often assume an appearance of a "terminal bulb", which has been referred to by some workers as a "paddle" [17]. It may be that the flagellar sheath is fluid enough to move distally along the rigid flagellar shaft, leading to accumulation of sheath material at the tip which is no longer constrained to be associated tightly with the shaft and is free to assume a more spherical shape.

The composition of the flagellar sheath is as yet uncertain, as is its precise structural relationship with the outer membrane of the organism. Studies of other organisms suggest that the outer membrane and the flagellar sheath are likely to be continuous [3], but our own observations remain equivocal. Evidence from our laboratory [2] suggests that proteins of 26, 30, 58, 62, 66 and 80 kDa may be components of the flagellar sheath, based on the release of proteins by detergent treatment of sheathed flagella removed from the organisms by shearing. The presence of native outer membrane material in such preparations cannot, however, easily be excluded. Furthermore there is still not a definitive identification of outer membrane proteins. We have recently observed, however, that a monoclonal antibody isolated in our laboratory, which is reactive with a moderately abundant protein of 29 kDa, appears to bind specifically to sheathed flagella (C.J. Luke, S. Ward, C.W. Penn, unpublished). The antibody does not bind to unsheathed flagella. Some labelling, of a patchy nature, is sometimes seen on the cell surface; this may be due to the relocation of clearly labile flagellar sheath material from its normal position. An important question raised by this observation is the relationship of such an apparently flagellar component with the prominent urease subunit known to have a molecular weight of about 30 kDa; it has been suggested that urease activity is associated with partially purified flagella [18]. We have tested the monoclonal antibody with semi-purified urease kindly provided by A. Cockayne, and found no cross-reaction; on the other hand antiserum (kindly provided by Dr. C. Clayton) to recombinant urease reacted strongly with the urease preparation. We therefore believe that there is a flagellar sheath protein, which is probably not normally present in the outer membrane, of about 29 kDa. The possibility of confusion of this protein with the smaller subunit of urease is significant.

Additional characterisation of the flagellar sheath awaits the purification of the native structure by physical separation methods.

Flagella and Pathogenesis

The flagella of *H. pylori*, like those of the *Campylobacter* spp., are a significant antigenic component of the organism and feature prominently in the antibody response of humans following infection.

There is evidence that in several pathogenic species of bacteria either possession of flagella or capacity for motility is necessary for full pathogenic potential of these species to be fulfilled. For example, non-motile mutants of *Vibrio cholerae*-O1 have been shown to exhibit diminished virulence [19]. There have also been several reports that the flagella and motility of *Pseudomonas aeruginosa* are necessary for the full virulence of this bacterium. Non-motile, aflagellate mutants of *P. aeruginosa* were found to retain the ability to colonise the wound in the burned mouse model of infection, but characteristic bacteraemia and systemic invasion were absent, suggesting that, unless motile, the bacteria could not invade the blood and therefore could not reach internal organs [20].

It was initially reported by Carsiotis et al. [21] that the flagella, and not motility or chemotaxis, of *Salmonella typhimurium* were necessary for virulence, and also that the flagella conferred upon the organism the ability to survive within murine macrophages [22]. It has since, however, been reported that a mutation in a newly determined virulence factor gene, designated *mviS*, which lies adjacent to the *fla* flagellar genes in *S. typhimurium*, is responsible for the earlier observations [23].

Motility is necessary for strains of *Campylobacter jejuni* to colonise the intestine. In a study undertaken by Morooka et al. [24] non-motile flagellate strains, strains lacking a flagellar filament and aflagellate strains of *C. jejuni* were all rapidly cleared from the intestine following infection, whereas a strain possessing shortened flagellar filaments could only colonise if the challenge inoculum was increased. More recently, there have been reports that the flagella of *C. jejuni* themselves may have a significant role in colonisation and invasion in the host intestinal tract [15, 25].

In many pathogenic bacteria, flagellar antigens have been found to be of immunological significance. Vaccination of mice with flagellar preparations of *P. aeruginosa* and antibody therapy with anti-flagellar antisera have been shown to be protective against lethal challenges with motile, flagellate strains of *P. aeruginosa* [26]. This protective effect of flagellar antigens has also been demonstrated in *Clostridium chauvoei* [27], *Borrelia* [28] and *Campylobacter* spp. [16].

Flagellar antigens have also been exploited in the serodiagnosis of certain infections, although the cross-reactivity of the *H. pylori* flagellin with that of *C. jejuni* means that this may be of limited use in the case of *H. pylori* infection [29]. It may be that flagellar sheath antigens of *H. pylori* are more specific.

There is evidence that motility of *H. pylori* contributes to virulence in infection of gnotobiotic piglets. Aflagellate variants of *H. pylori* obtained by repeated subculture were less effective in colonising the gastric mucosa of these animals than flagellate, motile strains [30]. Flagella themselves may be important in pathogenic processes by acting as adhesins or by enhancing adhesive capacity, for example, by bridging the electrostatic repulsion barrier between bacterial and host cell or mucosal surfaces. Motility and chemotaxis of *H. pylori*, conferred by the presence of flagella, may be significant in pathogenesis by delivering the organisms to the site of adhesion and colonisation of the mucosal surface, for example, by allowing penetration of gastric mucus and/or localisation at intercellular junctions on the gastric epithelium. For these reasons, the flagella, their function and the immune response to them are worthy of investigation so that our understanding of their role in pathogenesis and as potential diagnostically useful antigens can be enhanced.

References

1. Warren JR, Marshall B (1983) Unidentified curved bacilli on gastric epithelium in active chronic gastritis. Lancet ii: 1273–1275
2. Luke CJ, Kubiak E, Cockayne A, Elliott TSJ, Penn CW (1990) Identification of flagellar and associated polypeptides of *Helicobacter* (formerly *Campylobacter*) *pylori*. FEMS Microbiol Lett 71: 225–230

3. McCarter L, Silverman M (1990) Surface-induced swarmer cell differentiation of *Vibrio parahaemolyticus.* Mol Microbiol 4: 1057–1062
4. Fuerst JA, Perry JW (1988) Demonstration of lipopolysaccharide on sheathed flagella of *Vibrio cholerae* O: 1 by protein A-gold immunoelectron microscopy. J Bacteriol 170: 1488–1494
5. Allen R, Baumann P (1971) Structure and arrangement of flagella in species of the genus *Beneckea* and *Photobacterium fischeri.* J Bacteriol 10: 295–302
6. Thomashow LS, Rittenberg SC (1985) Isolation and composition of sheathed flagella from *Bdellovibrio bacteriovorus.* J Bacteriol 163: 1047–1054
7. Geis G, Leying H, Suerbaum S, Mai U, Opferkuch W (1989) Ultrastructure and chemical analysis of *Campylobacter pylori* flagella. J Clin Microbiol 27: 436–441
8. Kostrzynska M, Betts JD, Austin JW, Trust TJ (1991) Identification, characterization and spatial localization of two flagellin species in *Helicobacter pylori* flagella. J Bacteriol 173: 937–946
9. Haas R, Leying H, Meyer TF, Geis G, Suerbaum S, Opferkuch W (1991) Cloning of a *Helicobacter pylori* gene and construction of a non-flagellated mutant by transformation-mediated allelic exchange. Ital J Gastroenterol 23 [Suppl 2]: 31–32
10. Guerry P, Logan SM, Thornton S, Trust TJ (1990) Genomic organisation and expression of *Campylobacter* flagellin genes. J Bacteriol 172: 1853–1860
11. Guerry P, Alm RA, Power ME, Logan SM, Trust TJ (1991) Role of two flagellin genes in *Campylobacter* motility. J Bacteriol 173: 4757–4764
12. Nuijten PJM, van Asten FJAM, Gaastra W, van der Zeijst BAM (1990) Structural and functional analysis of two *Campylobacter jejuni* flagellin genes. J Biol Chem 265: 17798–17804
13. Nuijten PJM, van der Zeijst BAM, Newell DG (1991) Localization of immunogenic regions on the flagellin proteins of *Campylobacter jejuni* 81116. Infect Immun 59: 1100–1105
14. Fischer SH, Nachamkin I (1991) Common and variable domains of the flagellin gene, *flaA*, in *Campylobacter jejuni.* Mol Microbiol 5: 1151–1158
15. Wasenaar TM, Bleumink-Pluym NMC, van der Zeijst BAM (1991) Inactivation of the *Campylobacter jejuni* flagellin gene by homologous recombination demonstrates that *flaA* but not *flaB* is required for invasion. EMBO J 10: 2055–2061
16. Caldwell MB, Guerry P, Lee EC, Burans JP, Walker RI (1985) Reversible expression of flagella in *Campylobacter jejuni.* Infect Immun 50: 941–943
17. Goodwin CS, McCulloch RK, Armstrong JA, Wee SH (1985) Unusual cellular fatty acids and distinctive ultrastructure in a new spiral bacterium (*Campylobacter pyloridis*) from the human gastric mucosa. J Med Microbiol 19: 257–267
18. Dunn BE, Perez-Perez GI, Blaser MJ (1989) Two-dimensional gel electrophoresis and immunoblotting of *Campylobacter pylori* proteins. Infect Immun 57: 1825–1833
19. Guentzel MN, Berry LN (1975) Motility as a virulence factor for *Vibrio cholerae.* Infect Immun 11: 890–897
20. Drake D, Montie TC (1988) Flagella, motility and invasive virulence of *Pseudomonas aeruginosa.* J Gen Microbiol 134: 43–52
21. Carsiotis M, Weinstein DL, Karch H, Holder IA, O'Brien AD (1984) Flagella of *Salmonella typhimurium* are a virulence factor in infected C57BL/6J mice. Infect Immun 46: 814–818
22. Weinstein DL, Carsiotis M, Lissner CR, O'Brien AD (1984) Flagella help *Salmonella typhimurium* survive within murine macrophages. Infect Immun 46: 819–825
23. Carsiotis M, Stocker BAD, Weinstein DL, O'Brien AD (1989) A *Salmonella typhimurium* virulence gene linked to *flg*. Infect Immun 57: 3276–3280
24. Morooka T, Umeda A, Amako K (1985) Motility as an intestinal colonisation factor for *Campylobacter jejuni.* J Gen Microbiol 131: 1973–1980
25. McSweegan E, Walker RI (1986) Identification and characterisation of two *Campylobacter jejuni* adhesins for cellular and mucous substrates. Infect Immun 53: 141–148
26. Montie TC, Drake D, Sellin H, Slater O, Edmonds S (1987) Motility, virulence and protection with a flagellar vaccine against *Pseudomonas aeruginosa* infection. Antibiot Chemother 39: 233–248
27. Tamura Y, Minamoto N, Tanaka S (1984) Demonstration of protection antigen carried by flagella of *Clostridium chauvoei.* Infect Immun 28: 1325–1332
28. Barbour AG, Hayes SF, Heiland RA, Schrumpf ME, Tessier SL (1986) A *Borrelia*-specific monoclonal antibody binds to a flagellar epitope. Infect Immun 52: 549–554
29. Newell DG (1987) Identification of outer membrane proteins of *Campylobacter pyloridis* and antigenic cross-reactivity between *C. pyloridis* and *C. jejuni.* J Gen Microbiol 133: 163–170
30. Eaton KA, Morgan DR, Krakowka S (1989) *Campylobacter pylori* virulence factors in gnotobiotic piglets. Infect Immun 57: 1119–1125

Identification of Potential S Layer Proteins of *Helicobacter pylori*

B. Eschweiler[1], B. Gerstenecker[1], T. Moriki[2], B. Bohrmann[3], and M. Kist[1]

Introduction

Reports on surface layers (S layers) of gram-negative and gram-positive eubacteria and archaebacteria have increased in recent years [2, 3, 16, 17, 22, 23]. These structures are regarded as important virulence factors mediating serum resistance [3] and protection against proteolytic attack and phagocytosis [4, 16, 18]. Furthermore, bacterial adhesion, autoaggregation, and recognition of the host cells are promoted by S layers [23]. This report describes the preparation and structural analysis of surface-associated proteins of *Helicobacter pylori* (*H. pylori*).

Material and Methods

Growth of the Bacteria. H. pylori was grown under microaerophilic conditions in *Brucella* broth (Difco) supplemented with 3% fetal calf serum for 24 h at 37°C. Cells were harvested by centrifugation (3000 *g*, 10 min) and washed twice with phosphate-buffered saline (PBS), pH 7.4.

Electromicroscopical Studies. Freshly harvested *H. pylori* cells were cryofixed according to the method of Hobot [12]. After transfer into 2% (w/v) OsO_4 dehydration was performed in pure acetone in the presence of a molecular sieve. After an incubation for 80 h at − 87°C, the temperature was increased to 0°–4°C ($\Delta t = 6.7$°C/h). The specimen was further processed as previously described. Serial sections (50–60 nm thickness) were prepared using a LKB Ultratome IV ultramicrotome equipped with a diamond knife, collected on Formvar carbon-coated grids, and poststained with uranylacetate. For examination a Zeiss EM 10 electron microscope was used.

H. pylori cells were fixed with 3% glutardialdehyde/0.2 *M* cacodylate, pH 7.2 at 4°C for 2 h and postfixed in 1% OsO_4 and 1.5% KFeCN at 4°C for 1 h. Dehydration was performed in ascending ethanol concentrations and the specimens embedded in Spurr's mixture.

[1] Department for Microbiology and Hygiene, Institute for Medical Microbiology and Hygiene, University of Freiburg, Germany
[2] Institute for Pathology, University of Freiburg, Germany
[3] Institute for Microbiology, Biozentrum Basel, Switzerland

Gasbarrini/Pretolani (Eds.)
Basic and Clinical Aspects of H. pylori Infection

Extraction, Characterization, and Purification of Superficial Proteins. For the isolation of potential S layer proteins, intact *H. pylori* cells were treated with 10% 2-butanol in water for 15 min. After sedimentation at 5000 *g* the cells were reextracted with 10% 2-butanol. The supernatant and the remaining pellet were analyzed by SDS-PAGE according to the method of Laemmli [14]. The extractable proteins were characterized by (a) surface labelling with ^{125}I according to Newell [19, 20] (b) trypsine treatment of intact cells, (c) preparation of *N*-lauolsarcosinate insoluble outer membranes according to Filip et al. [8], and (d) after solubilization with Triton X-114 [5]. To investigate the importance of hydrogen bondings, cells were treated with 2 *M* urea according to Beveridge [2]. The extracted proteins were purified by anion exchange chromatography (Mono Q HR 5/5, Pharmacia/LKB, Uppsala, Sweden; buffer A, 20 m*M* Tris/HCl pH 7; buffer B, A + 3 *M* NaCl, flow: 1 ml/min, linear gradient 0%–33% B, 1 h) and tested for urease activity with 100 m*M* urea and phenol red as indicator [11].

Nearest-Neighbor Analysis. Structural association of surface proteins was investigated by cross-linking studies with the homobifunctional cleavable agent dimethyl 3,3′-dithiobispropionimidate (DTBP) according the method of Newhall [21]. Briefly, log-phase grown *H. pylori* cells were incubated with the cross-linker (0.5–5 m*M* in 50 m*M* triethanolamine (pH 8.5), 5 m*M* $MgCl_2$, 100 m*M* KCl) for 1 h. The reaction was stopped with 100 m*M* NH_4Cl. Cross-linked samples were solubilized (3% SDS, 7% sucrose) and separated by SDS-PAGE under nonreducing conditions (8% T, first dimension). For two-dimensional analysis the lane was excised and reduced by incubation with 100 m*M* β-mercaptoethanol for 1 h and layered on the second dimension polyacrylamide gel (8% T).

Analysis of Lipopolysaccharides. We isolated lipopolysaccharides (LPS) by the phenol-water method, according to Westphal [24] and analyzed by DOC-PAGE [13].

Results

Electron microscopic examination of thin-sectioned *H. pylori* cells detected an electrondense layer on the outer membrane (Fig. 1). By cryofixation this surface structure was seen to be approximately 10 nm thick and seemed to be unstructured (Fig. 1a). After fixation of the bacteria with glutardialdehyde and conventional dehydration, the S layer-like structure offered a regularly spiked structure (Fig. 1b). This S-layer-like structure was completely removed by treatment with 2-butanol while the integrity of the *H. pylori* cells was not affected (Fig. 1c). DOC-PAGE of the LPS of this particular *H. pylori* strain 151 showed a semirough LPS type, consisting mainly of homogeneous long-chain polysaccharides (data not shown).

To analyze the protein constituents of the extracted S layer, corresponding supernatants were collected and analyzed by SDS-PAGE (Fig. 2). Three proteins with 70, 60, and 30-kDa were selectively removed from the cells by treatment with alcohol (Fig. 2, lane c). In contrast, the 55-kDa protein, most probably

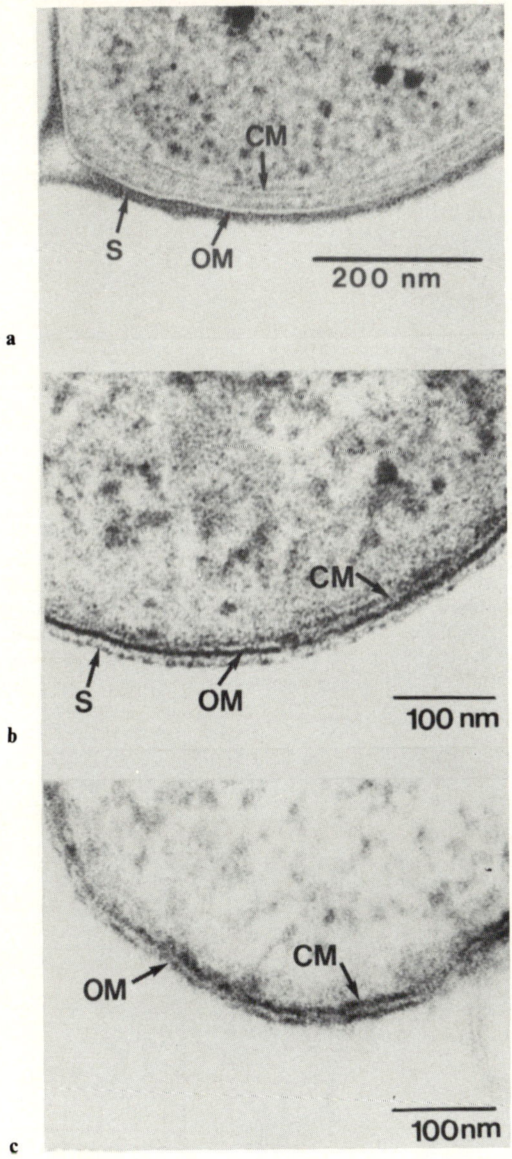

Fig. 1a–c. Electronmicroscopic features of the surface of *H. pylori*. **a** Living bacteria were cryofixed and embedded in epon after freeze substitution in 3% glutardialdehyde in aceton. **b** Bacteria were fixed by the conventional method with glutardialdehyde in cacodylate buffer and embedded in epon. **c** Same as **b** after treatment with 10% 2-butanol. *CM*, Cytoplasmatic membrane; *OM*, outer membrane; *S*, surface layer

the flagellin [10], was still present in the remaining cell-pellet and not affected by this treatment (Fig. 2, lane b). For further characterization the proteins were purified by anion exchange chromatography and tested for urease activity (Fig. 3) Whereas the 70-kDa and the copurifying 30-kDa proteins showed a strong urease activity, the 60-kDa was completely negative in the urease test.

Localization of the extracted proteins was examined applying various methods. After radioactive surface labeling of intact *H. pylori* cells all three major extractable proteins were detected by autoradiography (Fig. 4). Whereas

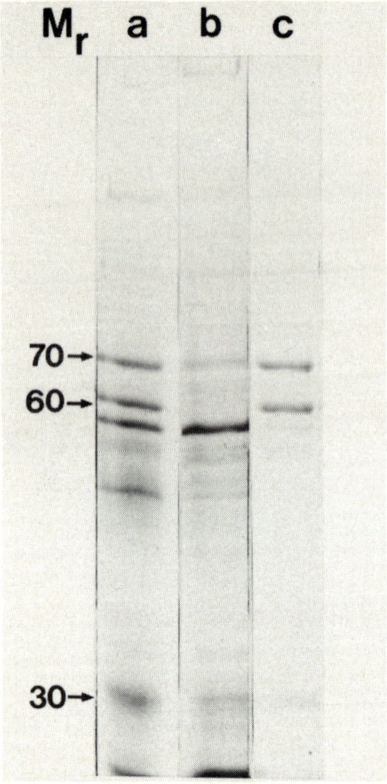

Fig. 2. The 8% SDS-PAGE of *H. pylori* proteins after treatment of intact cells with 10% 2-butanol. *Lane a*, untreated whole cell lysate; *lane b*, cell pellet after 2-butanol treatment; *lane c*, protein pattern of the supernatant

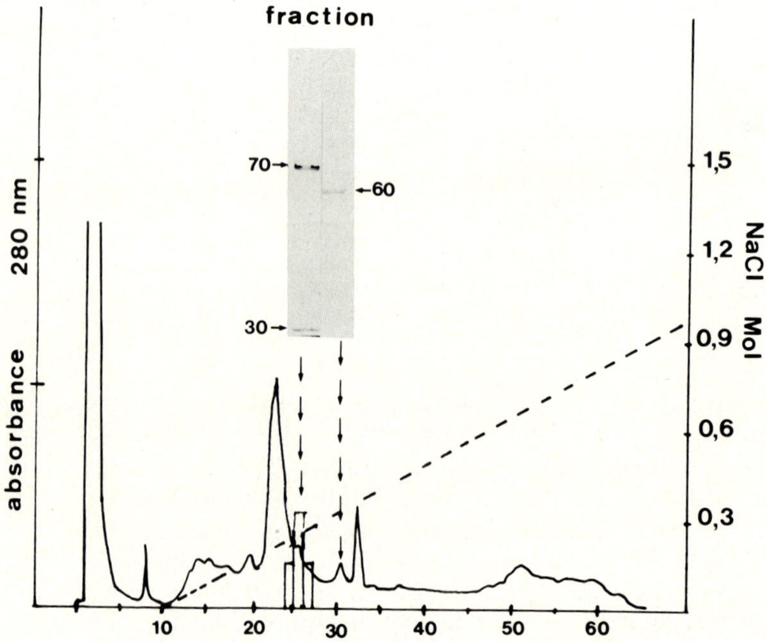

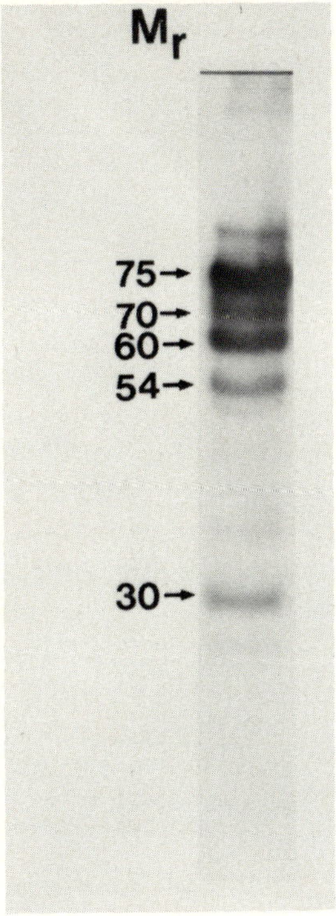

Fig. 4. Surface labeling of *H. pylori* with ^{125}I. Intact *H. pylori* were labeled with ^{125}I (50 μCi/800 μg protein). Autoradiography of the SDS-PAGE was performed by exposition for 4 h by double-screening technique

Table 1. Extractable major proteins by 10% 2-butanol

	70 kDa	60 kDa	30 kDa
Surface exposure ^{125}I	+	+	+
Trypsine sensitivity	−	+	−
Outer membrane preparation	+	−	+
2 *M* urea pellet	+	−	+
Urease activity	+	−	+

the 70- and 30-kDa proteins seemed to be outer membrane constituents, the 60-kDa protein was absent in the sarcosyl-insoluble outer membrane fraction (Table 1). Furthermore, the 60-kDa protein was totally removed from the insoluble membrane material after treatment of *H. pylori* with 2 *M* urea (data not shown).

After cross-linking of log-phase grown *H. pylori* cells high molecular weight complexes above 170 kDa were detectable in the stacking gel after SDS-PAGE under nonreducing conditions (Fig. 5, lane b). The high molecular weight complexes were cleaved in situ and further analyzed by a two-dimensional gel system

Fig. 3. Anion exchange chromatography (Mono Q HR 5/5) of the second supernatant after 2- butanol treatment of *H. pylori*. Fraction 25–27 showed urease activity (□) and contained the 70- and 30-kDa proteins. Fraction 31 represents the 60 kDa protein as indicated

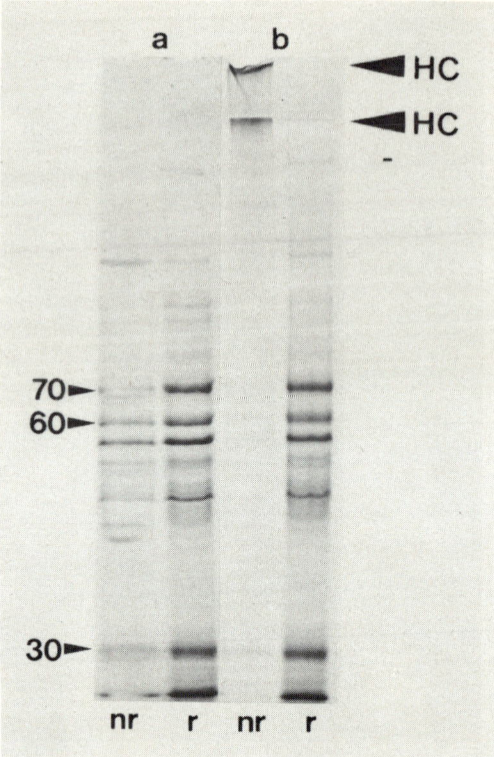

Fig. 5. First-dimension SDS-PAGE (8%) of intact *H. pylori* cells cross-linked with the homobifunctional, cleavable agent dimethyl-3,3′-dithio-bis-propionimidate (DTBP), range 1.2 nm. *Lane a*, control without cross-linker; *Lane b*, cross-linked proteins with 5 m*M* DTBP in 50 m*M*, triethanolaminbuffer (5 m*M* $MgCl_2$, 100 m*M* KCl), pH 8.5. *nr*, Nonreducing conditions; *r*, reducing conditions (100 m*M* β-mercaptoethanol); *HC*, high molecular weight complexes

(Fig. 6). The 70-, 60-, and 30-kDa proteins turned out to be main constituents of the cross-linked complexes (Fig. 6b). However, a few minor proteins were present, including the immunodominant 120- and a 50-kDa protein.

For control, untreated *H. pylori* cells were lysed and separated by two-dimensional SDS-PAGE. No high molecular weight complexes were detected when nonreducing conditions were applied (Fig. 6a). However, two polypeptides with apparent molecular weights of 26- and 50-kDa were sensitive for mercaptane treatment, indicating their dimerization by disulfide bridges. The 26-kDa protein was used as internal standard to control the effectiveness of the reduction.

Discussion

The presented investigations yield evidence that *H. pylori* carries an external surface layer, visible after thin sectioning. Depending on the fixation and dehydration conditions the S layer shows a different morphology. After cryofixation

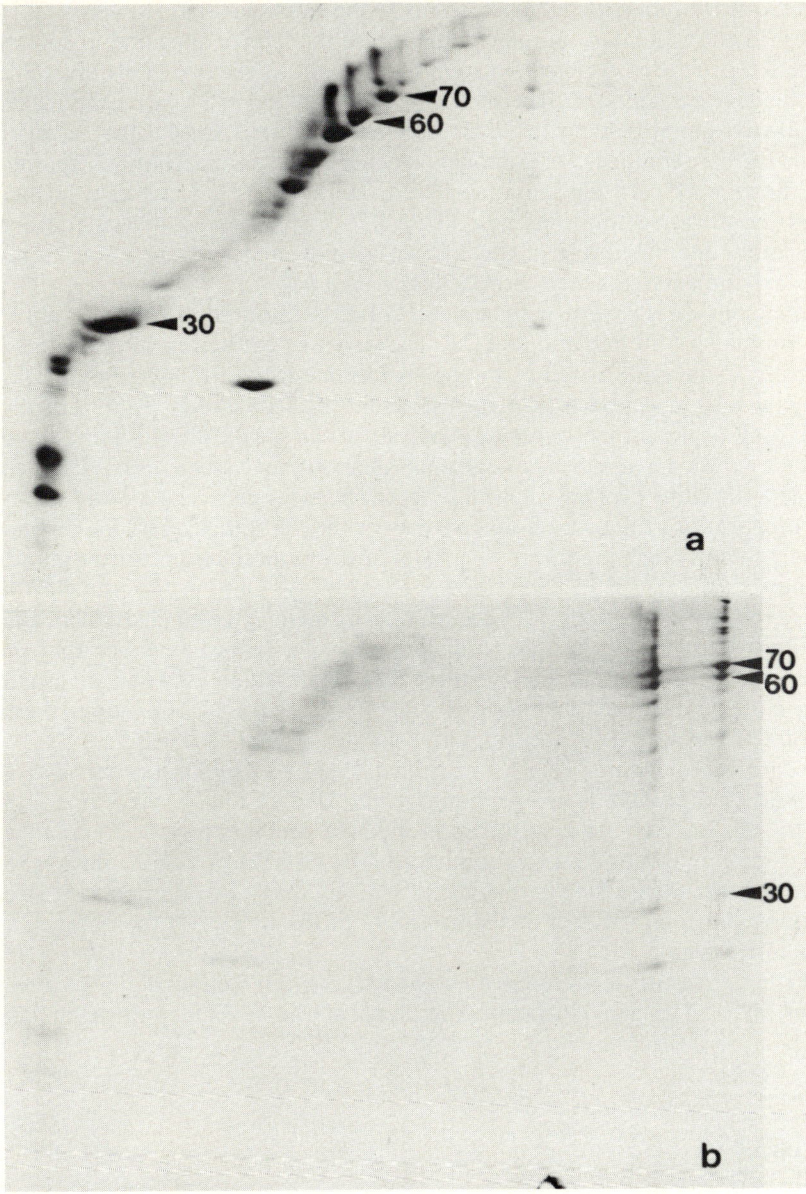

Fig. 6a, b. Second-dimension SDS-PAGE (10%) of the cross-linked *H. pylori* proteins separated in the first dimension (Fig. 5) after reducing with 100 m*M* β-mercaptoethanol. **a** Control without cross-linker. **b** cross-linked with DTBP (as indicated in Fig. 5)

and freeze-substitution the S layer seems to be homogenous. However, after chemical fixation and conventional dehydration the S layer appeared to consist of spikelike structures. A possible explanation might be the loss of watersoluble components (e.g., sugars). Furthermore, the cross-linking of S layer components by the fixative glutardialdehyde could result in a structured shape of the S layer.

The LPS are composed of homogenous long-chain polysaccharides, characteristic for S layer carrying gram-negative bacteria [6, 15]. These data further support the ultrastructural findings. These LPS types seem to be essential for the assembly and anchoring of the S layer, as indicated by transposon mutagenesis experiments with Aeromonas *salmonicida* [1].

Treatment of *H. pylori* with organic solvents (2-butanol) extracted three major proteins of 70, 60, and 30 kDa. The selective extraction of these three proteins by 2-butanol as well as the persisting integrity of the remaining cells missing the S layer, supports the hypothesis that the S layer of *H. pylori* possibly is composed of these three proteins. Analysis of the localization of these three proteins by radioactive labeling confirmed their surface association. As shown in Table 1 the three proteins showed different features concerning outer membrane preparations by sarcosyl. In contrast to the 60-kDa protein, the 70 and 30-kDa proteins were present in the outer membrane fraction. Furthermore, they showed differences in their trypsin accessibility. Only in the presence of high trypsin concentrations was the 60 kDa protein affected, hypothetically indicating a "hidden" localization of this protein. After nearest-neighbor analysis by cross-linking surface proteins the three major extractable proteins are found to be in close contact. All these findings suggest a close association among these three proteins as well as to the outermost surface of *H. pylori* cells.

According to Dunn [7], who identified a 62- to 66-kDa protein and a 29.5- to 30-kDa protein as urease subunits, the 70- and 30-kDa proteins could represent this enzyme. After purification of these proteins by anion exchange chromatography this finding was confirmed. The 60-kDa protein seems not to be necessary for urease activity but hypothetically may play in important role concerning the conformation or the assembly of the urease on the outermost surface of *H. pylori.*

Further investigations concerning mainly the interaction of these three proteins, as well as the biochemical analysis of the 60-kDa protein, are in progress.

References

1. Belland RJ, Trust TJ (1984) Analysis of the synthesis, export, and assembly of the A-layer of *Aeromonas salmonicida* analyzed by transposon mutagenesis. J Bacteriol 163: 871–881
2. Beveridge TJ (1979) Surface arrays on the wall of *Sporosarcina urease*. J Bacteriol 139: 1039–1048
3. Blaser MJ, Smith PF, Hopkins JA, Heinzer I, Bryner JH, Wang W-LL (1987) Pathogenesis of *Campylobacter fetus* infections: serum resistance associated with high-molecular-weight proteins. J Infect Dis 155: 696–706
4. Blaser MJ, Smith PF, Repine JE, Joiner KA (1988) Pathogenesis of *Campylobacter fetus* infections. Failure of encapsulated *C. fetus* to bind C3b explains serum and phagocytosis resistance. J Clin Invest 81: 1434–1444

5. Bordier C (1981) Phase separation of integral membrane proteins in Triton X-114. J Biol Chem 256: 1604–1607
6. Chart H, Shaw DH, Ishiguro EE, Trust TJ (1984) Structural and immunochemical analysis of *Aeromonas salmonicida* lipopolysaccharides. J Bacteriol 158: 16–22
7. Dunn E, Campell GP, Perez-Perez G, Blaser MJ (1990) Purification and characterization of urease from *Helicobacter pylori*. J Biol Chem 265: 9464–9469
8. Filip C, Fletcher G, Wulff JL, Erhart CF (1973) Solubilization of the cytoplasmic membrane of *Escherichia coli* by ionic detergent sarcosyl. J Bacteriol 115: 717–722
9. Fogg GC, Yang L, Wang E, Blaser MJ (1990) Surface array proteins of *Campylobacter fetus* block lectin-mediated binding to type A lipopolysaccharides. Infect Immun 58: 2738–2744
10. Geis G, Leying H, Suerbaum S, Mai U, Opferkuch W (1989) Ultrastructure and chemical analysis of *Campylobacter pylori* flagella. J Clin Microbiol 27: 436–441
11. Hallman L, Burkhardt F (1974) Klinische Mikrobiologie. Thieme, Stuttgart
12. Hobot JA, Villiger W, Escaig J, Maeder M, Ryter A, Kellenberger E (1985) The shape and fine structure of the nucleoid observed on sections of ultrarapid frozen and cryosubstituted bacteria. J Bacteriol 162: 960–971
13. Komoro T, Galanos C (1988) Analysis of lipopolysaccharides by sodium deoxychelate-polyacrylamide gel. electrophoresis. J Chromatogr 450: 381–387
14. Laemmli UK (1970) Cleavage of structural proteins during assembly of the head of bacteriophage T4. Nature 227: 680–685
15. Logan SM, Trust TJ (1984) Structural and antigenic heterogeneity of the lipopolysaccharides of *Campylobacter jejuni* and *Campylobacter coli*. Infect Immun 45: 210–216
16. McCoy E C, Doyle D, Burda K, Corbeil B, Winter AJ (1975) Superficial antigens of *Campylobacter* (*Vibrio*) *fetus*: characterization of an antiphagocytotic component. Infect Immun 11: 517–525
17. Messner P, Sleytr UB (1988) Separation and purification of S-layers from gram-positive and gram-negative bacteria. In: Hancock IC, Poxton IR (eds) Bacterial cell surface techniques. Wiley, New York
18. Munn CB, Ishiguro EE, Kay WW, Trust TJ (1982) Role of surface components in serum resistance of virulent *Aeromonas salmonicida*. Infect Immun 36: 1069–1075
19. Newell DG (1984) The identification of outer membrane proteins and flagella of *Campylobacter jejuni*. J Gen Microbiol 130: 1201–1208
20. Newell DG (1987) Identification of the outer membrane proteins of *Campylobacter pyloridis* and antigenic cross-reactivity between *Campylobacter pyloridis* and *Campylobacter jejuni*. J Gen Microbiol 133: 163–170
21. Newhall WJ, Sawyer WD, Haak R (1980) Cross-linking analysis of the outer membrane proteins of *Neisseria gonorrhoe*. Infect Immun 28: 785–791
22. Pei Z, Ellisont RT, Lewis RV, Blaser MJ (1988) Purification and characterization of a family of high molecular weight surface-array proteins of *Campylobacter fetus*. J Biol Chem 263: 6416–6420
23. Sleytr UB, Messner P (1983) Crystalline surface layers on bacteria. Am Rev Microbiol 37: 311–339
24. Westphal O, Jann K (1965) Bacterial lipopolysaccharides. Methods Carbohydr Chem 5: 83–91

Urease as a Colonisation Factor in *Helicobacter*

A.A. McColm, J. Bagshaw, C. O'Malley, and A. McLaren

Urease secretion by *Helicobacter* species may be a mechanism for survival against acid in the stomach. However, since the bacteria reside predominantly underneath the overlying mucus layer on the mucosa, the major exposure to acid is likely to be during transit across the gastric lumen upon initial colonisation. It is probable, therefore, that urease inhibition during this period may interfere with gastric mucosal colonisation. We have studied the role of urease in the colonisation of naive, infant ferrets with *H. mustelae* (Hm) using four different approaches: (a) challenge with a urease negative mutant, (b) challenge with Hm grown in the presence of a urease inhibitor, (c) dosing of animals with a urease inhibitor prior to challenge and (d) dosing of animals with inhibitor after suppression of Hm with a bismuth salt.

Methods

In Vitro. In order to distinguish the challenge strain from any subsequent, naturally acquired colonisation, a spontaneous rifampicin-resistant (to 50 μg/ml) strain was used throughout (URP/Rif R). A urease negative variant (URN) of this strain was selected by urea pressure [1]. Urea was measured non-enzymatically using a diacetyl monoxime assay. The presence or absence of the urease protein was determined by western blot (see Table 1).

In Vivo. Infant ferrets (3–5 days old) were challenged with either URP or URN Hm cultured in brain heart infusion broth (BHIB) supplemented with 5% foetal calf serum. Colonisation was assessed by rapid urease testing and semi-quantitative culture of antral punch biopsies (4 mm diameter) removed from three to five animals at various times post-challenge. Biopsies were homogenised in 1 ml BHIB and serial dilutions plated onto chocolate Columbia agar and cultured microaerophilically for 5–6 days. In some experiments, [^{14}C]-urea breath test analysis was also performed [2]. Adult ferrets (6–9 months old) naturally infected with Hm were sampled by gastroscopy and antral biopsies cultured as above.

Glaxo Group Research Ltd., Greenford, UK

Gasbarrini/Pretolani (Eds.)
Basic and Clinical Aspects of H. pylori Infection

Results

Challenge with Urease Negative Mutant. Our findings (Tables 1, 2; Fig. 1) can be summarised as follows. (a) Challenge with URN gave considerably lower frequency of colonisation than URP. (b) Pretreatment with an H_2 antagonist did not improve URN colonisation rate. (c) In the few animals successfully colonised with URN, the initial numbers of Hm isolated from the antrum were

Table 1. Strain comparison

	Rif-R URP	Rif-R URN
Urease activity (μmol min^{-1} ml^{-1}/10^8 CFU)	0.73	0
Urea MIC (m*M*)	15	> 50
Rif MIC (μg/ml)	> 100	> 100
Presence of urease protein	+	+

Table 2. Challenge of baby ferrets with urease-positive or-negative rifampicin resistant (URN Rif R) variant *H. mustelae*

Challenge[a]	No. infected no. challenged	Percentage colonisation	No. (%) reverted urease positive
URP Rif/R[b] (parent strain)	26/26	100%	–
URN Rif R[c] (+ ranitidine)	2/46	4%	0
URN Rif R	10/33	30%	3/33 (9%)
URN (total)[d]	12/79	15%	3/79 (4%)

[a] All challenges 5×10^7–10^8 CFU.
[b] 12, single challenge; 14, triple challenge on days 0, 1 and 2.
[c] Ranitidine HCl, 50 mg/kg, 1 h pre-challenge.
[d] 3/13 (23%) single challenge; 6/66 (9%) triple challenge.

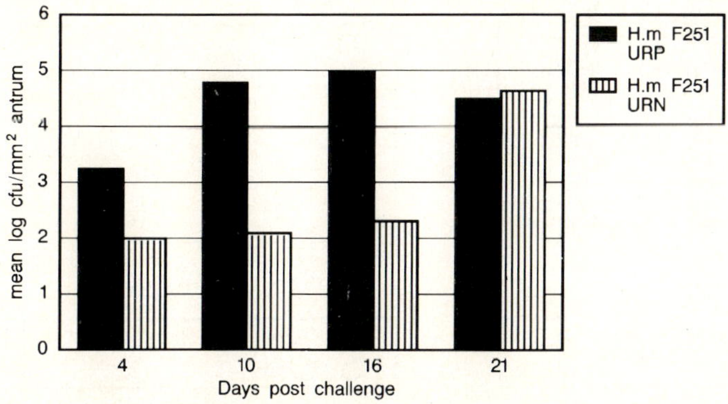

Fig. 1. Degree of antral colonisation in ferrets successfully infected with URP or URN Hm

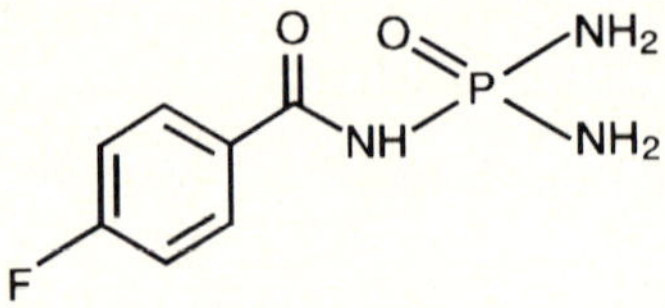

Fig. 2. Structure of flurofamide

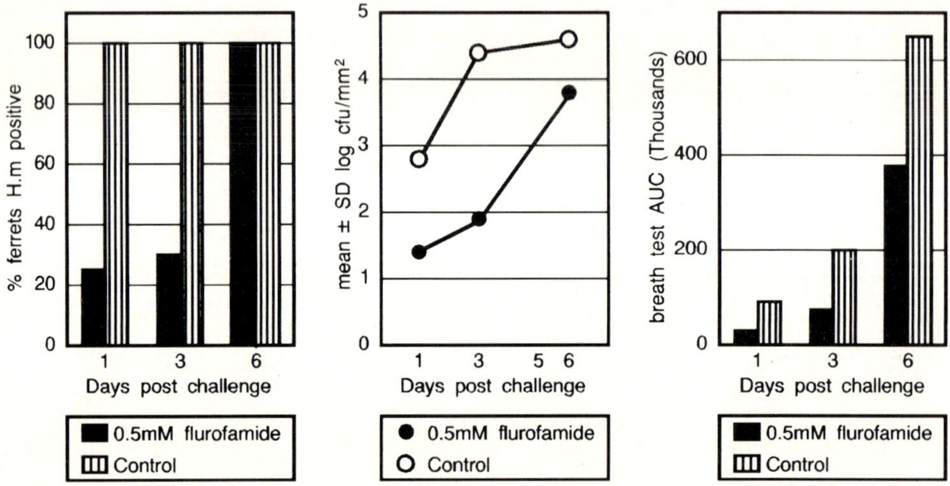

Fig. 3. *Left*, Number of animals Hm positive. *Middle*, Extent of antral colonisation, *Right*, Urea breath test response

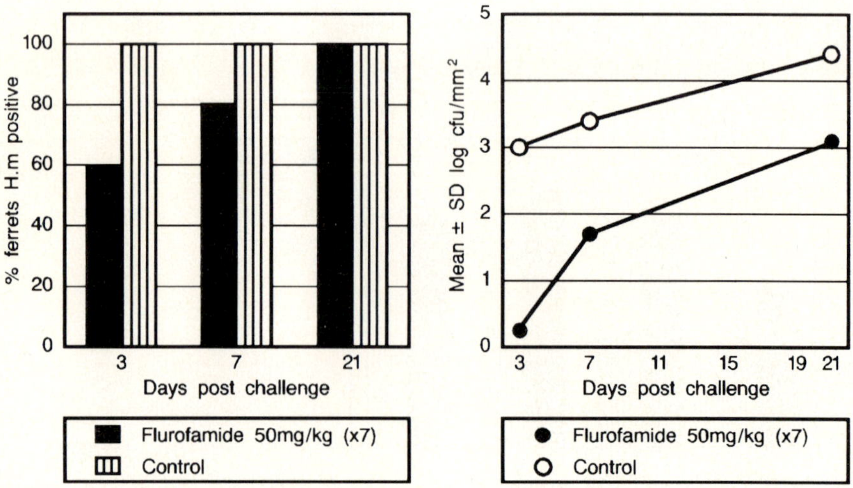

Fig. 4. *Left*, Number of animals Hm positive. *Right*, Extent of antral colonisation

Table 3. Treatment of ferrets with ranitidine bismuth citrate (24 mg/kg b.d., days 0–27) followed by continued treatment with either flurofamide or placebo

		Dosed with ranitidine bismuth citrate[a]		Pre-follow up therapy: day 28[b]		Follow-up phase: day 33	
	Pre-treatment	day 14	Day 28	Flurofamide	Placebo	Flurofamide	Placebo
Number of ferrets *H. mustelae* positive	24/24 (100%)	17/23 (74%)	8/24 (33%)	3/12 (25%)	5/12 (42%)	11/12 (92%)	11/12 (92%)
Log CFU/biopsy (mean ± SD)	4.4 ± 0.6	2.9 ± 1.0	2.2 ± 1.1	2.0 ± 1.0	2.4 ± 1.2	3.8 ± 1.3	4.4 ± 1.1

[a] Endoscopy performed 24 hr after previous ranitidine bismuth citrate dose.

[b] On day 28 all ferrets are randomised into two follow-up groups of 12 animals dosed with either flurofamide (50 mg/kg, b.d.) or placebo (0.5% sodium carboxymethyl cellulose, 1 ml/kg).

markedly lower than for the URP-challenged ferrets; however, by day 21 the degree of colonisation was similar in the two groups.

Challenge with Hm Cultured in Flurofamide. Flurofamide (Fig. 2) is one of the most potent urease inhibitors yet described (IC_{50} 0.4 nM, approximately 100 times the activity of acetohydroxamic acid). It has no direct anti-*Helicobacter* activity (MIC = > 1000 μg/ml). The concentration used (0.5 m*M*) completely inhibited detectable whole cell urease activity in vitro, and the organism became susceptible to acid in the presence of urea. Hm 251 Rif-R was grown in 0.5 m*M* flurofamide for 24 h prior to challenge of infant ferrets (Fig. 3). (a) Flurofamide initially decreased the numbers of colonising Hm to below detectable levels (< 10 cfu/biopsy). (b) This was seen over the first 3 days as an apparent reduction in the numbers of colonised animals, the degree of antral colonisation and [^{14}C] urea breath test activity. (c) By day 6 the colonisation rate in the urease inhibited group had attained that of the control animals.

Pretreatment of Infant Ferrets with Flurofamide Prior to Hm Challenge. Infant ferrets were dosed with 50 mg/kg flurofamide orally b.d. on days −3, −2, −1 and 0; the last dose was given 1 h before challenge. Breath test results showed that this concentration completely inhibits the enzyme for a least 24 h [2] (Fig. 4). Flurofamide predosing resulted in a similar outcome to inclusion of the inhibitor in the cultures, i.e. a reduction in the rate and degree of Hm colonisation.

Effect of Flurofamide on Relapse. Treatment of ferrets with flurofamide after Hm clearance by ranitidine bismuth citrate did not reduce the relapse rate compared to placebo (Table 3).

Conclusion

Our results can be summarised as follows. (a) A functional urease appears to be necessary for effective colonisation of the gastric mucosa by *Helicobacter*. (b) The fact that in some cases URN organisms could colonise is probably a function of the large challenge inocula used in these studies. (c) Urease does not appear to be important in relapse of a suppressed *Helicobacter infection*. In previous in vitro acid tolerance and in vivo therapy studies we have shown that under physiological urea concentrations, urease inhibition would kill *Helicobacter* only at low pH [3]. The present experiments support this belief by demonstrating a role for urease in initial colonisation – where acid is present – but not in relapse where acid is presumably deficient as the bacteria are already beneath the gastric mucus.

References

1. Cox DM, McLaren A, Snowden M (1990) Rev Esp Enferm Dig 47
2. McColm AA, Bagshaw J, O'Malley C (1990) Rev Esp Enferm Dig 78: [Suppl 1]: 97
3. McColm AA, Bagshaw J, O'Malley C, McLaren A (1991) Microb Ecol Health Dis 4: S145

Affinity and Ion Exchange Chromatography in the Purification and Characterization of *Helicobacter pylori* Cytotoxin-Associated Proteins

I. Luzzi[1], M. Bugnoli[2], C. Pezzella[1], N. Figura[3], I. Benedetti[1], D. Armellini[2], and A. Rossolini[3]

Introduction

The study of the virulence characteristics of *Helicobacter pylori* (HP) seeks to contribute to explaining why only few persons infected with HP develop peptic ulcers. Cytotoxicity plays a crucial role in the pathogenetic mechanisms of most infections of the digestive system. Some HP isolates produce one or more substances which induce intracytoplasmic vacuolization in mammalian cells in culture. Several studies have shown that vacuolating activity or cytotoxicity of these isolates is associated with proteins of apparent molecular weights of 130, 95, and 82 kDa in SDS-PAGE [3, 4]. This association is based mainly on the presence of these proteins in concentrated broth culture filtrates of cytotoxic strains and their absence in those of noncytotoxic ones. In addition, by immunoblotting with human sera a serological recognition of these proteins is more prevalent among subjects infected with cytotoxic strain than in persons colonized by non-cytotoxic HP [1]. Sera from patients infected with HP are also able to neutralize the vacuolization suggesting that cytotoxin is produced in vivo [5].

The aim of this study was to verify the suitability of two chromatographic techniques, affinity and ion exchange chromatography, in the purification of cytotoxin-associated proteins.

Material and Methods

Cytotoxic HP CCUG 17874 and noncytotoxic HP clinical isolate G21 were tested for affinity chromatography. Bacteria were cultured microaerobically at 37°C in *Brucella* broth containing 5% of fetal calf serum on a gyratory shaker at 100 rpm for 48 h. Broth culture filtrates were concentrated with Ficoll 400 and absorbed on Affigel blue. After washing proteins were eluted from the resin with 0.75 *M* MgCl in 50 m*M* Tris-HCl, pH 7.4. Fractions were tested for vacuolating activity on HeLa cells and run in 4%–16% SDG-PAGE. Proteins were

[1] Laboratorio di Batteriologia e Micologia Medica Istituto Superiore di Santià, Viale R. Elena, 299 00161 Rome, Italy
[2] Immunobiologic Research Institute–Siena, 53100 Siena, Italy
[3] Istituto di Malattie Infettive, Università di Siena, 53100 Siena, Italy

Gasbarrini/Pretolani (Eds.)
Basic and Clinical Aspects of H. pylori Infection

transferred onto nitrocellulose paper and blotted with two serum samples diluted 1:800; one neutralized the in vitro vacuolization of cytotoxic HP, the other did not. Alkaline phosphatase conjugate of anti-human IgG was used to show the reactions. For ion exchange chromatography, broth culture filtrate of cytotoxic HP CCUG 17874 was concentrated 20-fold using a 50-kDa ultrafiltration membrane.

To verify whether cytotoxicity is maintained at different pH and to assess which pH value allows the cytotoxin-associated proteins to be bound to an anion exchange resin (Trisacryl M) the starting material was dialized against 50 m*M* Tris-HCl, pH 7.5 and 8.5. A test tube method was used. Briefly, 1 ml of the two dialized samples was incubated with 1 ml resin equilibrated at the same pH values. After 10 min of incubation at room temperature and with shaking, the resin was allowed to settle, and the supernatant together with starting material and the two dialized samples were tested for vacuolization in HEp-2 cells, run in 7.5% SDS-PAGE, and immunoblotted with both neutralizing and nonneutralizing human serum samples as described above.

Results

Neutralizing sera reacted with proteins of about 130, 95, and 82 kDa molecular weight of the eluted fractions and in small amount in nonabsorbed material on Affigel blue; these proteins were lacking in the fractions of noncytotoxic HP. Only fractions containing these three major proteins possessed vacuolating activity. Neutralizing sera reacted also with starting material and the two dialized samples used for ion exchange chromatography. A weak reaction with only the 82-kDa protein was visible in the supernatant obtained after incubation with the resin at pH 7.5 whereas no reaction was found with supernatant at pH 8.5, the only sample negative for vacuolating activity.

Discussion

The results of this study confirm the association of vacuolating activity with proteins of 130, 95, and 82 kDa and show that ion exchange chromatography can represent a useful technique for separation and purification of HP cytotoxin. Unfortunately, purification of the cytotoxin-associated proteins is affected by their low concentration in broth filtrates; efforts must be made to enhance the production in liquid media. Recently an antigenic protein of 120-kDa detectable in whole cell and ultrasonicated cultures of some HP isolates has been proposed as a marker of pathogenicity of these strains as its mucosal IgA and systemic IgG recognition is associated with peptic ulceration [2]. Whether this protein is the same as the 130-kDa protein present in the supernatant of cytotoxic HP strains is not known.

The application of ion exchange chromatography to ultrasonicated cultures of cytotoxic HP strains other than to broth culture can represent an important step for the study of the localization of the cytotoxin-associated proteins in the bacterial cell and their role in the pathogenesis of gastroduodenal disease.

References

1. Cover TL, Dooley CP, Blaser MJ (1990) Characterization of and human serological response to proteins in *Helicobacter pylori* broth culture supernatants with vacuolizing cytotoxin activity. Infect Immun 58: 603–610
2. Crabtree JE, Taylor JD, Wyatt JI, Heatley RV, Shallcroos TM, Tompkins DS, Rathbone BJ (1991) Mucosal IgA recognition of *Helicobacter pylori* 120 kDa protei, peptic ulceration, and gastric pathology. Lancet 338: 332–335
3. Figura N, Guglielmetti P, Rossolini A, Barberi A, Cusi G, Musmanno RA, Russi M, Quaranta S (1989) Cytotoxin production by *Campylobacter pylori* strains isolated from patients with peptic ulcers and from patients with chronin gastritis only. J Clin Microbiol 27: 225–226
4. Leunk RD, Johnson PT, David BC, Kraft WG, Morgan DR (1988) Cytotoxic activity in broth culture filtrates of *Campylobacter pylori*. J Med Microbiol 26: 93–99
5. Leunk TL, Ferguson MA, Morgan DR, Low DE, Simor AE (1990) Antibody to cytotoxin in infection by *Helicobacter pylori*. J Clin Microbiol 28: 1181–1184

Neutralization of the Vacuolating Toxin from *Helicobacter pylori* by Antisera from Patients with Duodenal or Gastric Ulcer

H. Goossens, Y. Glupczynski, J.P. Lambert, A. Burette, L. Vlaes, and J.P. Butzler

Introduction

Helicobacter pylori has been considered to cause type B gastritis and perhaps peptic ulcer disease, but the mechanisms which infection may lead to tissue inflammation and damage are poorly understood. Broth culture supernatants may induce vacuolation of cells in vitro, and it has been shown that the toxic substance(s) are statistically significantly more frequently produced by *H. pylori* isolated from patients with peptic ulcer [2]. Human serum samples from patients infected with *H. pylori* are able to neutralize the vacuolating activity [4]. Recently, the vacuolating activity of *H. pylori* culture supernatants has been attributed to urease activity rather than to a specific cytotoxin. The ammonia liberated following the degradation of urea by urease is known to induce vacuolation. However, it has also been shown that the vacuolating activity of *H. pylori* broth culture supernatants is not mediated solely by urease activity [1]. We studied the production of the cytotoxic factor in *H. pylori* strains isolated from clinically well defined groups of patients and looked for the presence of neutralizing antibodies in the patients' serum specimens.

Materials and Methods

Clinical Data and Strains. We assayed 286 *H. pylori* strains isolated from the gastric mucosa of 130 different patients; 89 showed gastritis, and 41 were found to have duodenal and/or gastric ulcer.

Cytotoxin Assay Procedure. Isolates of *H. pylori* were grown in *Brucella* broth, supplemented with 1% vitox, 5% fetal calf serum, and Skirrow's antibiotic supplement, in a microaerophilic atmosphere at 150 oscillations per minute for 48 h. After centrifugation (10 000 rpm, 10 min at $\pm 4°C$), the broth culture supernatants were tested on cell lines. Vero cells (ATCC no. CCL81) and intestine 407 cells (ATCC no. CCL6) were used for cytotoxin assays. The method of Figura et al. [2] was used for screening of cytotoxin production by *H. pylori*. *H. pylori* broth culture supernatants showing discordant results on both cell lines were repeatedly tested after ammonium sulfate precipitation (70% w/v).

University Hospital Antwerp; Sint-Pieters and Brugmann University Hospital, Nouvelle Clinique de la Basilique, Brussels, Belgium

Gasbarrini/Pretolani (Eds.)
Basic and Clinical Aspects of H. pylori Infection

Neutralization Assay. Uptake of neutral red dye by cell vacuoles was used to quantitate the amount of toxin present in the broth culture supernatant [1]. For neutralization, sera, diluted twofold in cell culture medium in 100-μl amounts, were incubated with 100 μl of a preparation of cytotoxin previously determined to be the highest dilution showing a maximal OD (100% vacuolization) by the neutral red dye cytotoxin assay. The mixtures were incubated for 2 h at 37°C and added to the cells. After 24 h of incubation, the uptake of neutral red was determined as previously described. Neutralization was defined as the highest dilution of a serum completely neutralizing vacuolation, which corresponds to the lowest OD. Sera from blood donors without *H. pylori* antibodies were used as controls. *H. pylori* antibodies were determined by means of a second-generation Roche EIA [3].

Statistical Analysis. Results were considered significantly different for *p* values of less than 0.05.

Results and Discussion

We found that 22 out of 89 (24.7%) strains of *H. pylori* isolated from patients with chronic gastritis only were producing a cytotoxin, and that 20 out of 41 (48.7%) strains isolated from patients with peptic ulcer were cytotoxic. Table 1 reports on the correlation between diagnosis and cytotoxin results. Statistical analysis are showing that cytotoxin production is statistically significantly associated with the presence of duodenal and gastric ulcer ($\chi^2 = 6.16$, $p = 0.01$, df = 1). These results confirm findings by Figura et al. [2] that cytotoxigenicity is involved in the development of peptic ulcerations.

We compared the sensitivity of the intestine 407 and Vero cells for the detection of the cytotoxic factor in broth culture supernatants. It appears that intestine 407 cells are more sensitive than Vero cells (97.7% versus 86.4%). All *H. pylori* strains showing discordant results on both cell lines were tested again after ammonium sulfate precipitation; identical results were obtained as with the nonconcentrated supernatants.

We evaluated the reproducibility of the toxin assay by blindly testing *H. pylori* strains isolated simultaneously from the antrum and body of the stomach of 55 patients. We found that all *H. pylori* strains isolated simultaneously from the different sites of the stomach in the same patient showed identical results for the cytotoxin production: 14 patients were found to harbor cytotoxin positive

Table 1. Cytotoxin production by *H. pylori* isolated from patients with gastritis or peptic ulcer disease

	Cytotoxin		Total
	+	−	
Ulcer	20	21	41
Gastritis	22	67	89
Total	42	88	130

strains whereas in 41 patients cytotoxin negative strains were isolated. Moreover, a follow-up study was performed in 28 patients with subsequent endoscopy and culture of gastric biopsy specimens. Discordant cytotoxin results were obtained with strains isolated during the first and second endoscopy in only one patient (results not shown). This may be due to lack of sensitivity, a technical error, the loss of the potential to produce cytotoxin, or to the fact that the strains isolated during the first and second endoscopy were different. Therefore, the cytotoxin test is highly reproducible and reliable.

Finally, antibody to *H. pylori* and to the cytotoxin in serum was investigated. The presence of IgG antibodies was detected by means of the Cobas Core EIA from Roche [3]. The presence of antibody to the cytotoxin was measured by neutralization. Table 1 illustrates the neutralization of a cell culture supernatant by the homologous and a heterologous serum specimen, but not with the serum specimen from a healthy blood donor. Neutralization of the cytotoxin activity was obtained with all eight serum specimens from peptic ulcer patients infected with cytotoxin-producing *H. pylori* strains, and with six out of eight serum specimens from peptic ulcer patients, infected with *H. pylori* strains not producing a cytotoxin. Neutralization was not obtained with serum specimens from nine healthy blood donors (absence of *H. pylori* infection in these blood donors was shown by absence of specific *H. pylori* antibodies by means of the second generation EIA from Roche). These data suggest that the cytotoxin in produced in vivo. It may therefore be involved in the production of the disease associated with *H. pylori*.

Presence of neutralizing antibodies in patients infected with *H. pylori* strains not producing the cytotoxin in vitro was also observed by Leunk et al. [4]. This might be explained by a loss of the ability to produce cytotoxin upon cultivation in vitro, an insensitive assay for the cytotoxin, infection by toxigenic and nontoxigenic isolates, or by switching the gene(s) involved in cytotoxin production of and off. These data suggest that more isolates of *H. pylori* produce the cytotoxin than is suggested by the direct in vitro assay alone.

In conclusion, *H. pylori* produces a cytotoxin which was found to be statistically significantly associated with peptic ulcer disease. Neutralizing antibodies were found in peptic ulcer patients infected with *H. pylori*, suggesting that the cytotoxin is produced in vivo. Thus, these data support further efforts to purify and characterize the cytotoxin.

References

1. Cover TL, Puryear W, Perez-Perez GI, Blaser MJ (1991) Effect of urease of HeLa cell vacuolation induced by *Helicobacter pylori* cytotoxin. Infect Immun 59: 1264–1270
2. Figura N, Guglielmetti P, Rossolini A, Barberi A, Cusi G, Musmanno RA, Russi M, Quaranta S (1989) Cytotoxin production by *Campylobacter pylori* strains isolated from patients with peptic ulcers and from patients with chronic gastritis only. J Clin Microbiol 27: 225–226
3. Goossens H, Glupczynski Y, Burette A, Van den Borre C, Butzler JP (1992) Evaluation of a commercially available second-generation immunoglobulin G enzyme immunoassay for detection of *Helicobacter pylori* infection. J Clin Microbiol 30: 176–180
4. Leunk RD, Ferguson MA, Morgan DR, Low DE, Simor AE (1990) Antibody to cytotoxin in infections by *Helicobacter pylori*. J Clin Microbiol 28: 1181–1184

Helicobacter pylori: Phospholipase C and Haemolysis

M.A. Daw, H.X. Xia, and C. O'Morain

Introduction

Helicobacter pylori is a unique organism and produces many virulence factors such as enzymes, adhesins and cytotoxins that have been linked with its pathogenicity. The organism exerts a damage to the gastric mucus in the patients with *H. pylori* associated diseases [1].

Haemolysis, lysis of the erthrocytes, is an ubiquitous capacity of gram-negative and gram-positive bacterial species [2]. The in vivo action of haemolysis causes physical damage to a variety of eukaryotic cells. Extracellular enzymes are responsible for haemolysis of some bacteria [3].

Phospholipase C (lecithin or phosphorylcholine phosphorylase) catalyses the hydrolysis of lecithin into phosphorylcholine and 1, 2 digylceride [4]. Bacterial phospholipase C was first described in *Clostridium Perfringes* and is well known as the lethal, haemolytic and dermonecrotic factor responsible for tissue destruction associated with this organism [5]. Phospholipid, the substrate, is a component of most biological membranes. Phospholipase-hydrolysing enzymes occur naturally in mammalians and bacterial cells.

Phospholipase C as a bacterial virulence factor capable of mediating cell, tissue and organism toxic effects has been a subject of much interest recently [6]. Phospholipase C also directly disrupts the cells and leads to the release of biologically active contents into the local tissue. Therefore phospholipase C is a bacterial virulence factor that may cause direct and indirect tissue damage. Various haemolytic organisms produce phospholipase C including gram-positive bacteria such as *Clostridium perfringes, C. novyi, Staphylococcous aureus, Bacillus cereus, B. listeria* and *B. monocytogenes* and gram-negative bacteria such as *Acinetobacter, Pseudomonas, Proteus, Escherichia coli*, and *Serrtia marcescens* [1].

We have shown that *H. pylori* can produce different phospholipases including phospholipase C which may contribute to its ulcerogenic activity [7]. In this study we report on the ability of *H. pylori* to produce haemolysin, which mediates its haemolytic activity in relation to phospholipase C production.

Departments of Medical Microbiology, Faculty of Medicine, Tripoli, Libya and Gastroenterology, Meath/Adelaide Hospitals, Dublin

Gasbarrini/Pretolani (Eds.)
Basic and Clinical Aspects of H. pylori Infection

Materials and Methods

Clinical Isolates. Fifteen clinical isolates of *H. pylori* were cultured from antral biopsies of different patients (nine male, six female) aged 22–65 years, all these patients had duodenal ulcer at the endoscopy. The isolates were stored at −70°C in suspension of 10% serum, 40% glycerol and 50% trypton soya broth.

Preparation of Culture Filtrates. Cell free culture supernates were prepared by the method described by Daw et al. [8]. Each supernate was then suspended in Tris hydrochloride buffered saline (pH 7.2), the protein concentration was standardised and each isolate was sonicated for 5 min (45 s brust) in an ice bath. Each supernate was dialysed using a hypertonic saline overnight at 4°C. The culture supernates were stored at −20°C and tested for haemolysis and phospholipase C activities within a week of preparation.

Haemolysis. Four different species of (2% v/v) erythrocytes (RBCs) collected from human, horse, sheep and guinea pig were used. The erythrocyte suspension was washed twice with isotonic saline and then suspended in Tris hydrochloride buffered saline. The haemolytic activity of each isolate was tested by adding 50 μl of (2% v/v) of each erythrocyte suspension to the 50 μl dialysed supernates which is usually serially diluted in tubes containing 50 μl Tris hydrochloride buffered saline. The mixture was then incubated for 3 h at 37°C water bath (Grant Instruments) shaking constantly at 90 RPM and at 4°C for 30 min. The mixture was centrifuged at 1 500 g and, the amount of haemolysin released in the supernates was measured with spectrophotometer (Titretek Multiskan MCC) at 540 nm against controls (100% haemolysis, where 0.5 distilled water mixed with 0.5 ml erythrocyte to give the maximum haemolytic dose (MHD). The isolate was considered to be haemolytic if it showed at least 25% of MHD. Guinea pig erythrocytes was used for the effect of dilution, EDTA 10^{-3} *M* and heating (boiling for 10–15 min) on the haemolytic activity.

Enzyme Assay. Phosolipase C was measured by hydrolysis of synthetic substrate of *p*-nitrophenylphosphorylcholine as previously described [9] at an optical density (OD) of 410 nm. The amount of phospholipase C was expressed in picomoles/second. Phospholipase C levels were correlated with the haemolytic activity in each isolate, and the effect of heat (boiling the lysates for 10–15 min) and EDTA 10^{-3} *M* on phospholipase C was also determined.

Results

Phospholipase C production and the haemolytic activity of *H. pylori* collected from different patients were studied. The haemolysis was tested using four different erythrocytes collected from guinea pig, horse, sheep and human. The haemolytic activity measured in the dialysed supernates was expressed as the percentage of total haemolysis of the same amount of erythrocytes. All the isolates showed different levels of haemolysis, and the erythrocytes were also

Table 1. Phospholipase C (PLC) and haemolytic activities of *H. pylori*

No. of isolates	PLC (OD)[a]	Haemolysis (%)
1	0.150	35
2	0.203	63
3	0.263	70
4	0.270	76

[a] PLC, 55–91 p mol/s.

Table 2. Effect of heat and EDTA 10^{-3} *M* on the haemolytic activity (percentage) of *H. pylori*

No. of isolates	Unheated	Heated	With EDTA
1	35	0	30
2	63	30	0
3	70	53	0
4	76	62	66

different in their sensitivity to the supernates tested. The proportion of haemolysis for guinea pig RBCs was 60% ± 17%, horse RBCs 40% ± 9%, human RBCs 35% ± 3% and sheep RBC 5% ± 8%. *H. pylori* exerted a less degree of haemolysis on sheep erythrocytes in comparison to the other erythrocytes while guinea pig erythrocytes were the most susceptible of all. Eight (51%) isolates showed more than 75% of haemolysis, 2 (25%) isolates were weakly haemolytic, and 5 (30%) isolates showed 25%–75% haemolysis.

Ten isolates (75%) that were variable in their haemolytic activities were found to have different levels of phospholipase C (Table 1). The OD ranged from 0.150 for one (10%) isolate (haemolysis 35%) to 0.270 (haemolysis 76%) for 4 (40%) isolates and phospholipase C as expressed in picmols ranged from 55–91 p/s. The isolates with a higher phospholipase C (OD = 0.275) were found to be more haemolytic (76%).

Table 2 shows the effect of heat and EDTA on the haemolytic activity of *H. pylori*. Heating reduced the haemolytic activity of 2 (20%) isolates to 33%, 3 (30%) isolates to 17%, 4 (40%) isolates to 14%, and totally inhibited it in one (10%) isolate. EDTA, however, reduced the haemolytic activity of all the isolates. Phospholipase C activity was also inhibited by EDTA and was reduced by heating to 20%–40% in the isolates tested.

Discussion

H. pylori has been implicated as a cause of duodenal ulcer. A variety of virulent factors may contribute to its pathogenecity [10]. *H. pylori* was found to be an adherent organism [11] which can attach to the mucosal surface of the antram and elaborates urease which protects it from acidic environment; hence other enzymes such as phospholipases could be produced and cause damage to the antral mucosa [12].

In this study *H. pylori* isolates were found to be haemolytic. The haemolytic effect varied according to the erythrocytes used. Of the four different erythrocytes (human, horse, sheep and guinea pig) tested and found to be susceptible to the haemolysin(s) produced by *H. pylori.* Guinea pig erythrocytes were the most responsive. The degree of haemolysis was also variable among the isolates tested, and the titer of the haemolysis of the isolates was low.

Production of the haemolysins has been reported throughout a broad spectrum of organisms including anaerobic and aerobic bacteria. The in vivo action of the haemolysins ultimately causes physical damage to the surrounding tissue [13]. Another study [14] on the haemolysis of *H. pylori* also indicated that the haemolytic activity was most pronounced against guinea pig erythrocytes.

Bacterial production of phospholipase C may hydrolyse cell membrane and cause complete lysis to the affected cells. We have previously reported that strains isolated from duodenal ulcer patients produced a higher level of phospholipase C compared to those isolated from patients with gastritis [15]. In this study the level of phospholipase C was associated with the degree of haemolysis. The initial characterisation of the haemolytic activity of *H. pylori* showed the haemolytic activity was reduced by heating and inhibited by EDTA. The phospholipase level was also inhibited by EDTA and reduced by heating, which may suggest the association of phospholipase with the haemolytic activity of *H. pylori.*

Phospholipids form a major content of the erythrocytes membrane. They are not symmetrically distributed between the outer and inner halves of the lipid bilayer. Most of the choline-containing phospholipids are located in the extertior half [16] in the case of sheep erythrocytes, which were less susceptible to the haemolysis by *H. pylori* and contain little or no phosphotidylcholine.

While phospholipase C activity may be involved in the haemolytic activity of *H. pylori*, it does not necessarily indicate that the haemolysis was eventually caused by phospholipase C. EDTA, however, is a chelating agent capable of inactivating other enzymes and proteins which may have a role to play in this complex phenomenon.

The nomenclature of the haemolysins is usually derived from the producing organism [13], for instance, *Areomonas hydrophila* produces aerolysin and *Listeria monocytogens* produces listerrolysin; the haemolysin produced by *H. pylori* may be called "helicolysin". Whether this helicolysin attributes to the cytotoxic activity of *H. pylori* [17] has not been determined. Further studies on the purification and characterisation of this helicolysin(s) are required [18].

Acknowledgment. The authors would like to thank Mrs. B. Turner for typing the manuscript.

References

1. Peterson WL (1991) *Helicobacter pylori* and peptic ulcer disease. N Engl J Med 423: 1043–1048
2. Koronakis V, Cross M, Senior B, Koronakis E, Hughes C (1987) The secreted haemolysins of *Proteus mirablis, Proteus vulgaris* and *Morganella marganii* are genetically related to each other and to alpha-haemolysin of *Escherichia coli.* J Bacteriol 169: 1509–1515

3. Berka MR, Gray GL, Vasil ML (1981) Studies of phospholipase C (heat-labile haemolysin) in *Pseudomonas aeruginosa.* Infect Immun 34: 1071–1074
4. Mollby R (1978) Bacterial phospholipases. In: Jelgaszewicz J, Wodstrom T (eds) Bacterial phospholipases, bacterial toxins and cell membranes. Academic, New York, 367
5. McDonal JL (1986) Toxins of *Clostridium perfringens* type A, B, C, D, and E. In: Dorner F, Drews J (eds) Pharmacology of bacterial toxins. Pergamon, Oxford, 477
6. Levine L, Xiao DM (1988) Increased arachidonic acid metabolites from cells in culture after treatment with the phosphotidylcholine-hydrolyzing phospholipase C from *Bacillus cereus.* Prostaglandins 34: 633–643
7. Daw MA, Cotter L, Healy M, O'Moore R, Keane C, O'Morain C (1990) Phospholipases and cytotoxic activity of *Helicobacter pylori.* Rev Esp Dig [Suppl] 1: 25–26
8. Daw MA, O'Moore R, O'Morain C (1992) Detection of phospholipases and cytotoxic activity of *Helicobacter pylori.* In: Pajars *et al*; (ed) *Helicobacter pylori* and Gastroduodenal Pathology. Berlin Heidelberg New York, 101
9. Daw MA, Keane C, O'Moore R, O'Morain C (1991) Phospholipase C activity; new pathogenicity marker for *Helicobacter pylori.* Ital J Gastroenterol 23 (S2): 37–38
10. Goodwin CS, Armstrong JA, Marshall BJ (1986) *Campylobacter pylori,* gastritis and peptic ulceration. J Clin Pathol 39: 353–365
11. Hemalath SG, Drumm B, Sherman P (1991) Adherence of *Helicobacter pylori* to human gastric epithelial cells *in vitro.* J Med Microbiol 35: 197–202
12. Daw MA, Deegan P, Leen E, O'Morain C (1991) The effect omeprazole on *Helicobacter pylori* and associated gastritis. Aliment Pharmacol Ther 5: 435–439
13. Chakraborty T, Kathariou S, Hacker J et al. (1987) Molecular analysis of bacterial cytolysins. Rev Infec Dis 9 [Suppl 5]: 456–466
14. Wetherall BL, Johnson AM (1989) Haemolytic activity of *Campylobacter pylori.* Eur J Clin Microbiol Infect Dis 8: 706–710
15. Daw MA, Cotter L, Healy M, O'Moore R, Keane CT, O'Morain C (1991) Are *Helicobacter pylori* strains isolated from duodenal ulcer patients more virulent than those isolated from gastritis? Gastroenterology 100: 572A
16. Bernheimer AW (1974) Interactions between membranes and cytolytic bacterial toxins. Bio Phys Acta 344: 27–50
17. Leunk RD, Johnston PT, David BC, Kraft WG, Morgan DR (1988) Cytotoxic activity in broth culture filtrates of *Campylobacter pylori.* J Med Microbiol 26: 93–99
18. Daw MA, Xia HX, O'Morain C (1992) Characterisation of the haemolytic activity of *Helicobacter pylori.* Irish J Med Sci 161 (S10): 48

Haemagglutinins of *Helicobacter pylori* and Adherence to HEp-2 Cells

C.S. Goodwin

Introduction

Adherence to surface receptors is an essential step in pathogenesis for many bacteria. Attachment is mediated by adhesions or ligands which may be soluble or cell-associated, and which can be demonstrated by haemagglutination of various species of erythrocyte. Mannose-resistant haemagglutination by *H. pylori* has been described by Evans et al. [3] and others [2, 4]. However, these reports disagree on the properties of the haemagglutinins. Furthermore, different workers have used different methods of testing for HA; Evans et al. used slide haemagglutination [3], but Huang et al. used a micro-titre method [4]. It is probable that some of these differences are explained by the presence of different adhesins so that more than one type of receptor is involved.

Soluble Haemagglutinins

Some plate-grown strains of *H. pylori* that were harvested into phosphate-buffered saline and left for 1 h released soluble haemagglutinins [7]. These caused high-titre agglutination of human and guinea-pig erythrocytes, whereas chicken, sheep and bovine erythrocytes were agglutinated at various titres. Six of ten strains which had been subcultured repeatedly did not possess soluble haemagglutinins. Slide agglutination of bacterial suspensions demarcated the strains into two groups. By micro-titre assay, all group 1 strains and only two group 2 strains produced a soluble haemagglutinin. The soluble haemagglutinin was inhibited by sialoproteins containing predominantly the *N*-acetylneuraminyl (2–3) galactopyranosyl [NeuAc(2–3)Gal] structure. Bovine submaxillary mucin was strongly inhibitory; it contains several structures with sialic acid linked 2–6 to oligosaccharides. These results suggest that the soluble haemagglutinin recognises a NeuAc(2–3)Gal structure but has high affinity for another, as yet undetermined, sialic acid containing structure.

Department of Medical Microbiology, Faculty of Medicine and Health Science, United Arab Emirates University, P.O. Box 17666, Al Ain, United Arab Emirates

Gasbarrini/Pretolani (Eds.)
Basic and Clinical Aspects of H. pylori Infection

Importance of Soluble Haemagglutinins for Adherence of *H. Poylori*

Among six strains of *H. pylori*, two different modes of bacterial adherence to HEp-2 cells were found [1]. Strains that possessed soluble haemagglutinin such as NCTC 11637 adhered intimately to the cell surface, producing adherence pedestals similar to those found in vivo. Strains of *H. pylori* without soluble haemagglutinin such as NCTC 11638 also attach, but when viewed by electron microscopy their appearance resembled tennis balls on a surface and there was no membrane cupping or glycocalyx fusion. Thus, possession of the soluble haemagglutinin could be a marker of adherent strains of *H. pylori*. It is tempting to speculate that all strains possess soluble haemagglutinin and adherence ability when first isolated, but that some strains lose these two features. Certainly we have seen one strain which underwent loss of soluble haemagglutinin during subculture in the laboratory.

Latest Reports of Adherence by *H. pylori*

Lingwood et al. [6] have demonstrated that *H. pylori* specifically binds to a glycerolipid receptor present in human stomach antrum, which has been identified as a form of phosphatidylethanolamine [5]. Clinical isolates of *H. pylori* have been found to bind specifically and with high affinity not only to phosphatidylethanolamine but also to asialo-GM1. Similar binding has been shown for exoenzyme S (EXO S) [6]. Western blots have revealed cross-reactive proteins between this product of *Pseudomonas aeruginosa* and *H. pylori*. It is therefore proposed that an EXO S related adhesin mediates the lipid binding specificity of *H. pylori*. *H. pylori* may itself produce EXO S.

The same workers have shown that 25 bacterial pathogens show a similar receptor binding activity concomitant with an expression of an EXO S phenotype.

References

1. Armstrong JA, Cooper M, Goodwin CS et al. (1991) Influence of soluble haemagglutinins on adherence of *Helicobacter pylori* to HEp-2 cells. J Med Microbiol 34: 181–187
2. Emödy L, Carlsson Â, Ljungh Â et al. (1988) Mannose-resistant haemagglutination by *Campylobacter pylori*. Scand J Infect Dis 20: 353–354
3. Evans DG, Evans DJ, Moulds JJ et al. (1988) *N*-Acetylneuraminyllactose-binding fibrillar haemagglutinin of *Campylobacter pylori*: a putative colonization factor antigen. Infect Immun 56: 2896–2906
4. Huang J, Smyth CH, Kennedy NP et al. (1988) Haemagglutinating activity of *Campylobacter pylori*. FEMS Microbiol Lett 56: 109–112
5. Krivan HC, Nilsson B, Lingwood CA et al. (1991) *Chlamydia trachomatis* and *Chlamydia pneumoniae* bind specifically to phosphatidyelethanolamine in HeLa cells and to GalNAc beta 1-4Gal beta 1-4GLC sequences found in asialo-GM1 and asial-GM2. Biochem Biophys Res Commun 175: 108–109
6. Lingwood CA, Woods DE, Krivan HC (1991) *Helicobacter pylori*: its lipid receptors and adhesin. Microb Ecol Health Dis 4 (Special Issue): S123
7. Robinson J, Goodwin CS, Cooper M et al. (1990) Soluble and cell-associated haemagglutinis of *Helicobacter (campylobacter) pylori*. J Med Microbiol 33: 277–284

Partial Purification and Characterization of Sialic Acid Specific Soluble Haemagglutinin(s) of *Helicobacter pylori* Strain NCTC 11637

J. Lelwala-Guruge, A.S. Kreger, W. Shen, and T. Wadström

Introduction

Bacterial surface haemaglutinins and lectins play a significant role in pathogenesis of many mucus-associated infections. A number of reports describe cell surface haemagglutinins of *Helicobacter pylori* [2, 3, 8, 10, 11] that may mediate adhesion to stomach tissues. Robinson et al. [10] recently reported that some strains of *H. pylori* incubated in phosphate-buffered saline (PBS) released soluble haemagglutinins (SHAs) active against human and guniea pig erythrocytes that specifically bind to a NeuAc(2–3)Gal structure and also have high affinity for another sialic acid containing structure. Evans et al. [3] has described a fibrillar haemagglutinin of *H. pylori* which binds to NeuAc(2–3)Gal isomer of NeuAc-lactose. In this study we describe the partial purification and characterization of soluble haemagglutinin(s) of *H. pylori* strain NCTC 11637.

Materials and Methods

Bacteria. H. pylori strain NCTC 11637 was stored in tryptic soy broth at − 80°C and cultivated on brain heart infusion agar (Difco Laboratories, Detroit, MI) supplemented with 7% (w/v) saponinlysed horse blood, under microaerophilic atmosphere containing CO_2 8%, O_2 5%, H_2 and N_2 80% [10] for 3 days.

Soluble Haemagglutinin(s). The growth from each agar plate was collected with deionized water (5 ml/plate) by rubbing the surface of the medium with an L-shaped glass spreader. The bacterial cells were immediately sedimented by centrifugation (23,500 *g* for 20 min at 4°C). The supernatant fluids were filtered (0.45 μm) and lyophilized (stage 1 preparation). The stage 1 preparation was centrifuged at 4°C for 1 h at 100,000 *g* in a VTi 65.2 Beckman rotor.

Erythrocytes. Bovine, chicken, dove, guinea pig, horse, human (group A), African green monkey, mouse, pig, rabbit, and sheep erythrocyte suspensions were standardized according to Bernheimer [1]. Briefly, citrated blood was washed twice in PBS, pH 7.2, and the concentration of erythrocytes in the PBS suspen-

Department of Medical Microbiology, University of Lund, Sölvegatan 23, S-223 62, Lund, Sweden

Gasbarrini/Pretolani (Eds.)
Basic and Clinical Aspects of H. pylori Infection

sion was adjusted so that saponin-induced lysis of 1 ml suspension diluted with 1 ml water yielded a solution with an absorbance at 545 nm of 0.8 in a 1-cm light-path cuvette (ca. 0.7% erythrocytes, v/v).

Haemagglutination. Equal volumes of two-fold dilutions of stage 1 SHA preparations in PBS and erythrocyte suspensions (250 μl) were mixed in polystyrene tubes (12 × 55 mm) and allowed to settle at room temperature for 60–90 min. PBS was used as a negative control. One haemagglutinating unit (HAU) is the amount of SHA which causes complete agglutination.

Haemagglutination Inhibition. Four HAU of the stage 1 preparation in 250 μl PBS was mixed with 30 μl orosomucoid from human plasma (Scottish National Blood Transfusion Association, Protein Fractionation Centre, Edinburgh UK), fetuin and asialofetuin (type II) from fetal calf serum (Sigma, St. Louis, MO), NANLac from bovine colostrum (Sigma) solutions (10 mg/ml) and guinea pig erythrocytes were added and allowed to settle at room temperature.

Enzyme Treatment of Erythrocytes. Incubated with 1 ml guinea pig erythrocyte suspension at 37°C for 20 min were 100 ml PBS containing various concentrations of neuraminidase from *Clostridium perfringens* (Sigma) and *Vibrio cholerae* (Sigma) and the following enzymes at 1 mg/ml in PBS (all enzymes from Sigma): pepsin from porcine stomach mucosa, protease type XIV and protease type XXV (pronase E) from *Streptomyces griseus*, protease type X from *Bacillus thermoproteolyticus*, trypsin and α-chymotrypsin type VII from bovine pancreas, and protease XI-S (proteinase K) from *Tritirachium album*. Untreated cells (control) and treated cells were washed three times, suspended to the original volume and used to determine their residual sensitivity to Haemagglutination (HA) with 4 HAU stage 1 SHA preparation.

Enzyme Treatment of SHA. The stage I SHA preparation was treated with the following enzymes coated on latex beads (Sigma); chymotrypsin (0.15 U), protease (4 U), and neuraminidase (0.05 U) for 20 min at 37°C. The beads were sedimented at 12,000 *g* for 10 min, and the supernatant fluids were assayed for HA activity. Untreated RBCs and SHA were used as the negative control.

Heat Treatment. Stage 1 SHA was heated at 37°C for 30 min, 40°C for 30 min, 56°C for 15 min, and 100°C for 15 min, and residual activity was assayed with guinea pig erythrocytes.

Protease Activity. Protease activity of the stage 1 SHA preparation was determined against azocasein according to Kothary and Krager [5].

Phospholipase Activity. Phospholipase activity of the stage 1 SHA preparation against egg yolk agar and against *p*-nitrophenylphosphorylcholine [6] was tested.

Haemolytic Activity. Haemolytic activity of the stage 1 SHA was tested according to Bernheimer [1].

Protein Determination. Protein was estimated using Coomassie brilliant blue G-250 dye reagent (Bio-Rad, Richmond, UK) with bovine serum albumin (Sigma) as the standard.

Ammonium Sulphate Precipitation. All steps were performed at 4°C. Ammonium sulphate (KEBO Lab, Stockholm, Sweden) was dissolved in 10 ml stage 1 preparation to a final concentration of 60% saturation (420 g/l). After storage overnight the precipitate was collected by centrifugation (23,500 *g* for 20 min) and dissolved in 2 ml PBS. A small amount of insoluble matter was removed by centrifugation, and the solution was assayed for HA activity against guniea pig erythrocytes.

Purification of SHA. The lyophilized material (stage 1 preparation) was dissolved in PBS and subjected to gel filtration at 4°C on a Sephacryl S-200 in a column (96 × 1 cm) (Pharmacia, Uppsala, Sweden) using PBS containing 0.02% Na azide and 0.1 m*M* phenylmethylsulphonyl fluoride for elution. The fractions with peak HA activity were pooled (stage 2 preparation). Blue dextran (Pharmacia) was used to determine the column void volume. The stage 2 preparation was subjected to anionic-exchange chromatography on a *Q*-Sepharose fast flow column (7 × 0.01 cm; Pharmacia) using a salt gradient (0.15–1 *M* NaCl) for elution. Peak HA activity fractions (stage 3 preparation) were pooled, dialysed against PBS, and stored at −80°C.

SDS-PAGE. SDS/PAGE was performed by the method of Laemmli [7]. The stage 1 and 2 preparations were examined with a 12.5% polyacrylamide separating gel (7 × 8 cm) and a 3% stacking gel at a constant voltage of 200 V for 45 min. Proteins were denatured and reduced at 100°C for 3 min with Tris-HCl buffer (pH 6.8) containing SDS and 2-mercaptoethanol. Loaded onto the gel were 4 μg protein/well stage 3 preparation and 8 μg protein/well stage 1 preparation. Protein standards were obtained from Bio-Rad Laboratories.

Isoelectric Focusing. Lyophilized crude SHA preparation (50 mg) was fractionated by high-speed isoelectric focusing [13] at 4°C in at pH 3.5–10 sucrose density gradient containing 1% ampholine buffer (Pharmacia). The pH gradient was formed at a constant power of 15 W and 1600 V for ca. 18 h in a model 8100-1 electrofocusing column (Pharmacia). The pH of each fraction (4 ml) was determined at 4°C and the fractions were assayed for HA activity against guinea pig erythrocytes.

Results and Discussion

HA and HA Inhibition. The erythrocyte spectrum of whole cells and stage 1 preparations is shown in Table 1. The SHA has broad-spectrum activity against chicken, guinea pig, human, mouse, pig, sheep, rabbit and dove erythrocytes in that order, but is inactive against horse, bovine and monkey erythrocytes. HA of stage 1 SHA preparation with guinea pig erythrocytes was totally inhibited by orosomucoid, fetuin, and NANLac, but not by asialofetuin (300 μg/ml). Both

Table 1. Erythrocyte spectrum and specific activity of whole cells and stage 1 soluble haemagglutinin(s)

Erythrocyte species	Specific activity (total HAU/mg protein	
	Whole cells	Stage 1 SHA preparation
Bovine	12	–
Chicken	23	23
Dove	6	0.2
Guinea pig	23	12
Horse	0.7	–
Human	12	3
Monkey	3	–
Mouse	12	3
Pig	0.7	0.7
Rabbit	0.7	0.2
Sheep	6	0.4

orosomucoid and fetuin contain largely the NeuAcα-(2–3)-Gal isomer [4, 9] and 85% of NANLac from bovine colostrum is NeuAcα-(2–3)-Gal isomer. Thus, the SHA recognizes the (2–3) structure on sialylated glycoconjugates on the erythrocyte membrane.

Heat and Enzyme Treatment. HA of the stage 1 SHA preparation was heat labile (56°C, 15 min), and the only immobilized enzyme tested that deleteriously affected HA activity was α-chymotrypsin.

Treatment of guinea pig erythrocytes with 0.03 U of neuraminidase from *C. perfringens* abolished HA, while the HA titer decreased with treatment by pepsin and α-chymotrypsin. All other enzyme treatment were without effect. Neuraminidase from *C. perfringens* specfiically cleaves NeuAc(2–3)Gal(1–4)Glu, again indicating that the (2–3) structure of the sialylated glycoconjugate is recognized by the SHA preparation. Both the soluble haemagglutinins [10] and the fibrillar haemagglutinin [3] of *H. pylori* recognise the (2–3) structure sialylated glycoconjugate on the erythrocyte membrane.

Purification of SHA. SHA activity is not associated with a particulate fraction sedimented by centrifugation at 100,000 *g* for 1 h at 4°C. The SHA activity is stable to lyophilization and ammonium sulphate precipitable (60% w/v). Density gradient electrofocusing of SHA revealed a single peak of HA activity (pI ca. 3.7;

Table 2. Purification of soluble haemagglutinin(s) of *H. pylori* strain NCTC 11637

Preparation stage	Volume (ml)	Total HAU	Total protein (mg)	Specific activity (HAU/mg protein)	Percentage recovery
1. Crude SHA preparation	2	8192	56	146	–
2. Gel filtration pool	30	1920	6.9	278	23
3. Q-Sepharose fast flow pool	35	563	1.2	469	7

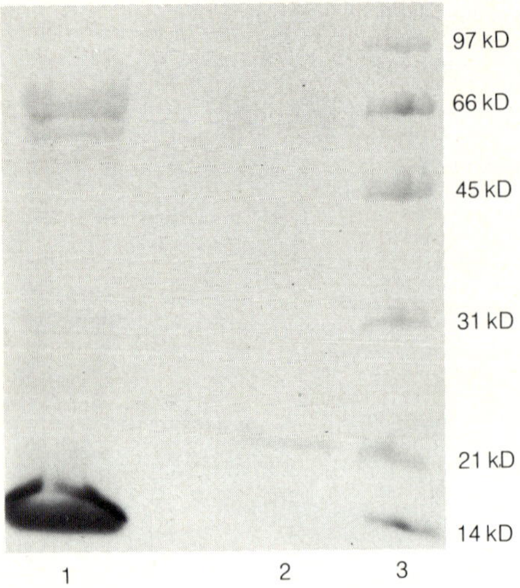

Fig. 1. SDS-PAGE analysis of stage 1 (*lane 1*) and stage 3 SHA preparations (*lane 2*). The bands are stained with Coomassie blue R-250. Marker proteins (*lane 3*)

data not shown). The stage 1 SHA preparation contained urease activity but not protease, phospholipase or haemolytic activity.

Gel filtration of the stage 1 preparation on a Sephacryl S-200 column resulted in several fractions with HA activity at a position corresponding to a molecular weight of approximately 200,000 (data not shown). A nondenaturing silver-stained PAGE of stage 2 preparation showed a protein band at ca. 200,000 (data not shown). About 23% of HA activity was recovered in the pool obtained by gel filtration (stage 2), and the preparation did not contain urease activity (Table 2). Fractionating the stage 2 preparation by anionic-exchange chromatography (stage 3) yielded 7% recovery of the starting HA activity. SDS-PAGE analysis of the stage 3 preparation showed protein bands with molecular weights of ca. 60,000 and 20,000 (Fig. 1). Based on its elution behaviour during gelfiltration, the SHA has an apparent molecular weight (assuming it has a globular shape) of more than 200,000. Unlike the bacterial surface haemagglutinins associated with fimbriae or other surface appendages, SHA of *H. pylori* is easy to disassociate [13].

References

1. Bernheimer AW (1988) Assay of hemolytic toxins. Methods Enzymol 165: 213–225
2. Emödy L, Carlsson Å, Ljungh Å, Wadström T (1988) Mannose-resistant haemagglutination by *Campylobacter pylori*. Scand J Infect Dis 20: 353–354
3. Evans DG, Evans DJ, Moulds JJ, Graham DY (1988) *N*-Acetylneuraminlactose-binding fibrillar hemagglutinin of *Campylobacter pylori*: a putative colonization factor antigen. Infect Immun 56: 2896–2906
4. Isemura M, Schmid K (1971) Studies on the carbohydrate moiety of α_1-acid glycoprotein (orosomucoid) by using alkaline hydrolysis and deamination by nitrous acid. Biochem J 124: 591–604

5. Kothary MH, Kreger AS (1985) Production and partial characterization of an elastolytic protease of *Vibrio vulnificus*. Infect Immun 49: 25–31
6. Kurioka S, Matsuda M (1976) Phospholipase C assay using *p*-nitrophenylphosphorylcholine together with sorbitol and its application to studying the metal and detergent requirement of the enzyme. Anal Biochem 75: 281–289
7. Laemmli UK (1970) Cleavage of structural proteins during the assembly of the head of bacteriophage T4. Nature 227: 680–685
8. Nakazawa T, Ishibashi M, Konishi H, Takemoto T, Shigeeda M, Kochiyama T (1989) Hemagglutination activity of *Campylobacter pylori*. Infect Immun 57: 989–991
9. Nilsson B, Norden NE, Svensson S (1979) Structural studies on the carbohydrate portion of fetuin. J Biol Chem 254: 4545–4553
10. Robinson J, Goodwin CS, Cooper M, Burke V, Mee BJ (1990) Soluble and cell-associated haemagglutinins of *Helicobacter* (*Campylobacter*) *pylori*. J Med Microbiol 33: 277–284
11. Wadström T, Guruge JL, Wei S, Aleljung P, Ljungh Å (1990) *Helicobacter pylori* Hemagglutinin – possible gut mucosa adhesion. In: Malferthiener P, Ditschuneit H (eds) *Helicobacter pylori*, gastritis and peptic ulcer. Springer, Berlin Heidelberg New York, pp 96–103
12. Wadström T, Trust TJ (1984) Bacterial surface lectins. Med Microbiol 4: 287–334
13. Winter A, Karlsson C (1976) Preparative electrofocusing in density gradients. LKB application note 219. LKB-Produkter AB Bromma, Sweden

Pathogenic Mechanisms of *Helicobacter pylori* Infection: Host Response

The Role of *Helicobacter pylori* Gastritis in Ulcerogenesis and Carcinogenesis

E. Solcia[1,2], R. Fiocca[1], L. Villani[2], O. Luinetti[2], A. Gianatti[2], E. Trespi[3], G. Stella[4], M. Cornaggia[5], A. Chiaravalli[5], and C. Capella[5,6]

Recent studies suggest that *Helicobacter pylori* (HP) gastritis is a major risk factor for both peptic ulcer disease [36] and cancer [16,31,32]. However, the histologic factors and mechanisms leading from gastritis to ulcer or cancer are poorly known. Gastritis activity and HP-linked surface epithelium lesions have been suggested to play some role in ulcerogenesis [7,9,12,13,15,34] while intestinal metaplasia (IM) has long been indicated as a factor in cancerogenesis [6,21,22].

In the present paper the morphology of HP-associated gastritis is reinvestigated with special attention to mechanisms involved in gastritis progression, epithelial damage, mucosal ulceration and cancer development.

Material and Methods

The following material has been investigated: (a) surgical specimens from 40 patients free of gastric symptoms undergoing gastric resection for severe obesity; (b) endoscopic biopsies of pyloric and corpus mucosa from 333 patients with dyspepsia (NUD; $n = 146$) duodenal ulcer (DU; $n = 91$) or gastric ulcer (GU; $n = 96$), 50 of which were rebiopsied at the end of and 2 months after an antibiotic therapy (amoxycillin + metronidazole coupled with bismuth or omeprazole) resulting in HP eradication, and (c) gastrectomy specimens of 137 patients with early cancer.

Paraffin sections of formaldehyde-fixed tissues were stained with hematoxylin-eosin, Giemsa, or immunoperoxidase using monoclonal or polyclonal antibodies directed against human IgG, IgA, and IgE (Dakopatts, Denmark), B lymphocytes (L26 antibody recognizing CD20 antigen; Dakopatts), T lymphocytes, and myelomonocytes (MT1 antibody for CD43 antigen, Biotest, FRG; UCHL1 antibody for CD45RO antigen, Dakopatts), and HLA-DR antigen (LN3 antibody, Biotest). Gastritis classification and scoring were performed according to the Sidney system [29]. A similar 4-score (0–3) system has been

[1] Department of Pathology, University of Pavia, Italy
[2] Pathology Service and [3]Digestive Physiopathology Center, IRCCS Policlinico San Matteo, 27100 Pavia, Italy
[4] Pathology Service, General Hospital, Voghera, Italy
[5] Pathology Service, General Hospital, Varese, Italy
[6] Department of Pathology, University of Pavia at Varese, Italy

Gasbarrini/Pretolani (Eds.)
Basic and Clinical Aspects of H. pylori Infection

developed for scoring HP-linked surface epithelium lesions (SEL), where *score 1* corresponds to cellular bulging with irregular but well-preserved luminal surface, *score 2* to focal or multifocal micropapillary change, and *score 3* to extensive micropapillary change or to erosion of the epithelium, either restricted to its luminal part or involving its whole depth with cell desquamation, denudation of the basal membrane, and underlying reactive inflammation (fibrin deposition, hyperemia, edema, granulation tissue).

Results and Discussion

HP Gastritis: Morphology and Pathogenesis

HP was found to adhere to the luminal membrane of epithelial cells lining middle and upper foveolae as well as gastric surface. In 66% of HP-positive antral biopsies cellular edema with luminal bulging, cytoplasmic vacuolization, micropapillary change (Fig. 1a), and erosion of the juxtaluminal cytoplasm, with resultant loss of mucin granules, occurred in HP-colonized epithelium [12, 15], likely as a result of *direct bacterial cytotoxicity* [10, 25]. In the HP-free epithelium covering the deepest foveolae and upper glandular necks signs of activation were usually seen, with mucin loss and increased cytoplasmic basophilia and mitotic rate. HLA-DR antigen was regularly expressed, more or less intensely, in this *activated foveolar-neck epithelium* and also in underlying antral or fundic glands when surrounded by inflammatory cells. Enhanced expression of HLA-DR is known to occur in activated intestinal epithelia involved in antigen transport and presentation at mucosal level, leading to T4 stimulation and massive B cell response [4]. In fact, a massive increase of B lymphocytes in the deep half and plasma cells in the superficial half of the gastric mucosa was the most impressive response of lamina propria cells to HP colonization. *B lymphocytes* accumulated especially in the deep lamina propria of pyloric and transitional pyloric/corpus mucosa, concentrated mainly in and around *activated follicles*. Most *plasma cells* stored IgA antibodies and filled the lamina propria in between superficial epithelium, foveolae, necks, and uppermost gland bodies. IgG plasma cells were as a rule fewer and more variable in number, with a tendency to concentrate around activated deep foveolae and upper necks (Fig. 1b) and, unlike IgA plasma cells, to disappear in granulocytes-free "nonactive" gastritis. HLA-DR positive dendritic cells in association with T lymphocytes also increased focally in perifoveolar and deep lamina propria. In the latter site they formed, together with B lymphocytes, deep aggregates, from which activated follicles are believed to take origin [24].

Several kinds of *effector cells* with a potential to damage the mucosa were easily recognized in conventional hematoxylin-eosin or Giemsa stained sections. *Neutrophilic granulocytes* appeared in 71% of 1032 antral biopsies with gastritis and in 84.3% of 870 biopsies with HP-positive gastritis [13], concentrated mainly in and around activated, HP-free foveolar-neck epithelia and associated with IgG plasma cells (Fig. 1). Direct complement activation by HP [3] may explain the (relatively inconspicuous) granulocyte infiltration of HP-colonized

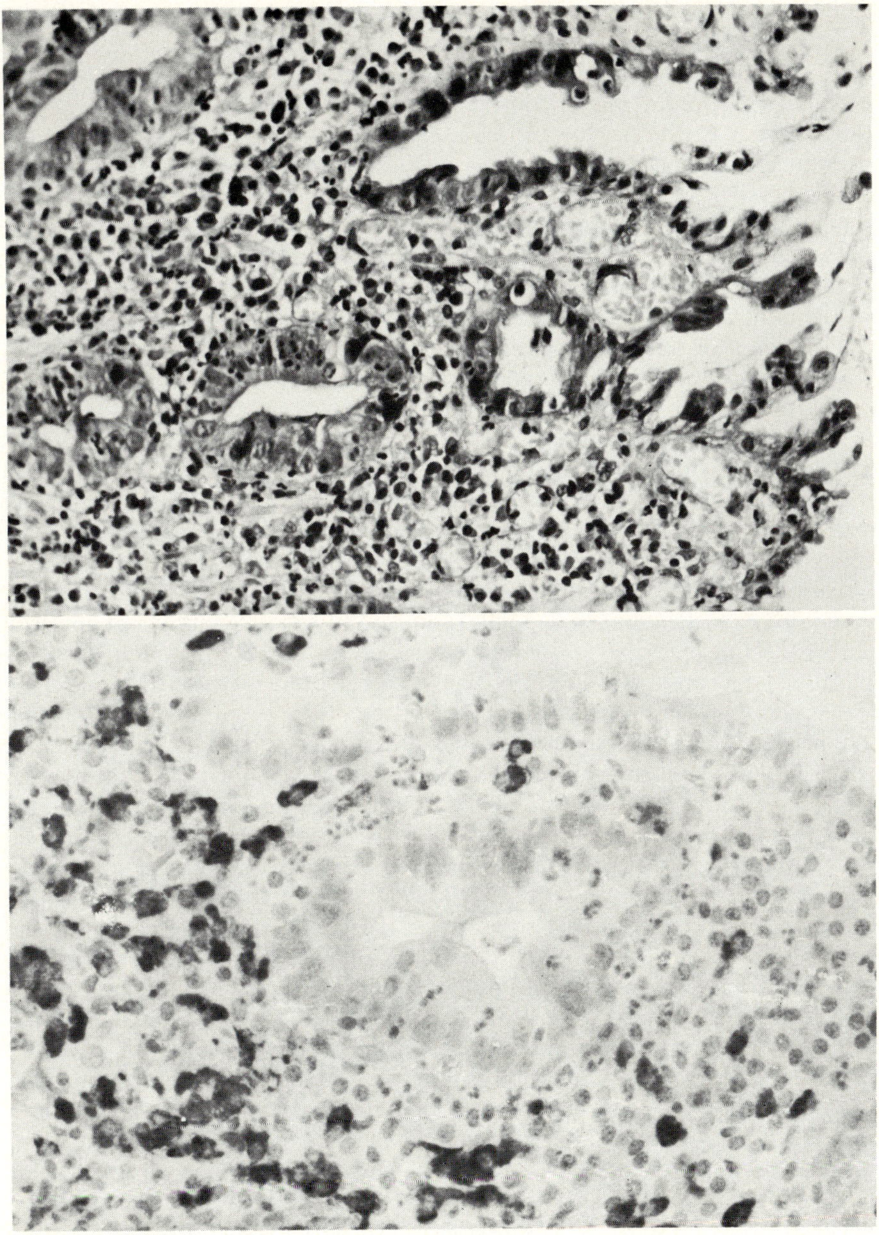

Fig. 1a, b. HP-positive active gastritis. **a** Micropapillary lesions of surface epithelium (*right*), neutrophilic granulocytes infiltration of underlying renewal zone epithelium (*left*), and abundant round cells (mainly plasma cells) infiltration of the lamina propria. Hematoxylin-eosin, × 260. **b** Abundant IgG plasma cells (*left*) in the lamina propria surrounding deep foveolar-neck tubules (found to be HLA-DR positive in a consecutive section, not shown) with peri- and intraepithelial granulocytes (*center*). Note unreactive plasma cells (mostly IgA in a consecutive section) in more superficial lamina propria (*right*). IgG immunoperoxidase, × 420

epithelium, while "necrotaxis" [19] may account for granulocyte infiltrates of heavily damaged surface epithelium. In addition, soluble HP products such as the formyl-methionyl-leucyl-phenylalanine peptide [30] known to attract and activate neutrophils, might contribute to neutrophil infiltration of HP-free foveolar-neck epithelia. However, it seems more likely that the latter is caused mainly by complement activation by IgG (especially of the IgG_1 subclass [38] antibodies linking HP antigens transported through activated epithelia. A similar IgG_1-mediated granulocyte chemotaxis seems to be prominent in the pathogenesis of ulcerative proctocolitis [4], a disease showing many histologic similarities with HP-induced active chronic gastritis, including cytolitic damage to the infiltrated epithelium contributing to mucosal erosion and ulceration. The presence or absence of granulocytes (as well as activated foveolac/necks and IgG plasma cells) allows separation of so-called "*active*" from "*nonactive*" *gastritis*.

In addition, increased amounts of *eosinophilic granulocytes, macrophages* and *mast cells* with membrane-bound IgE antibodies were disseminated in both deep and superficial lamina propria. Edema was frequently found at sites of excessive eosinophil accumulation and degranulation, a finding akin to some edematous states of the skin reputed to be caused by eosinophil activation [18]. Occasionally, epithelial infiltration and damage by eosinophils was also observed. It should be recalled that eosinophils produce and release a number of powerful toxins affecting epithelia, nerves, blood vessels, etc. [17]. A role for both eosinophils [27] and mast cells [1] in HP gastritis has been suggested.

It seems likely that direct, HP-related cytotoxicity of surface epithelium and immune-mediated granulocyte chemotaxis at foveolar-neck level represent the two main damaging processes of HP-gastritis which can lead to mucosal erosion and ulceration. Neutrophil or eosinophil leukocytes, as well as activated macrophages, natural killer cells and sentisized T cells, either acting at renewal zone level to destroy epithelial stem cells or, directly, on mature epithelia of deep glands, may all have a role in producing gland atrophy. Interestingly, the inflammatory process affecting the superficial part of the mucosa (*superficial* gastritis) differs from that located in the deep mucosa (*interstitial* gastritis, with or without *follicular or atrophic* patterns) in many respects, including presence or absence, respectively, of colonizing HP bacteria and neutrophilic granulocytes, prevalent type of immunocompetent cells (plasma cells versus lymphocytes) as well as nature of resulting mucosal lesions (erosion/ulceration rather than gland dysfunction or atrophy). Concerning gland dysfunction, it seems worth recalling that a powerful inhibitory effect of some lymphokines on gastric secretion has been documented [8]. On the other hand, cytoprotective and trophic factors like prostaglandin E_2 [20] and tumor growth factor-α [2] produced by parietal cells might selectively prevent oxyntic glands atrophy and partly explain the overall prevalence of superficial gastritis (61% of our 1177 patients) in corpus mucosa as against interstitial-atrophic gastritis (77%) in antral mucosa [13].

Gastritis Resolution in HP-Eradicated Mucosa

Surface epithelium damage, neutrophil infiltration, and activated foveolar/neck epithelia with HLA-DR expression disappeared 1 week after the end of an

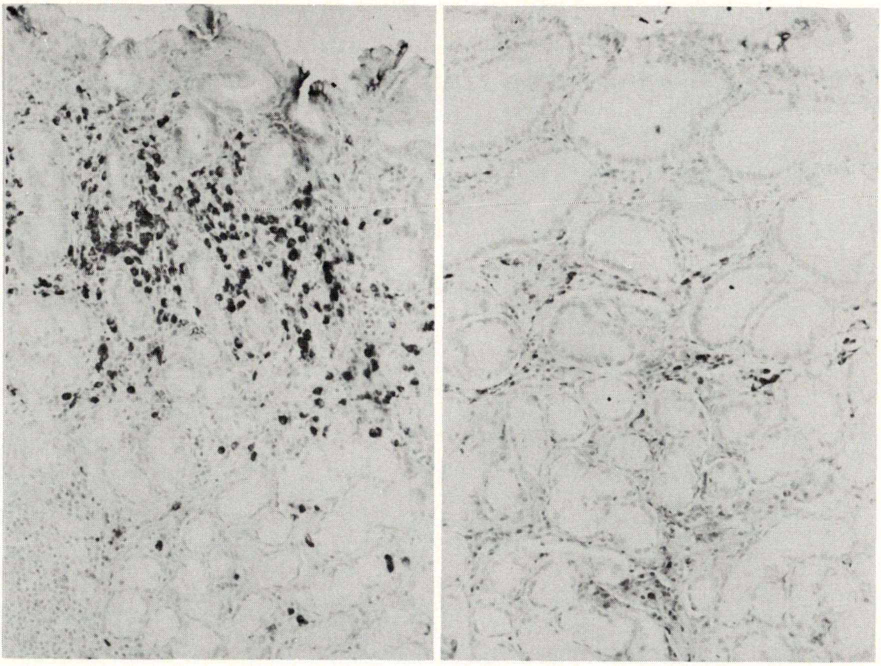

Fig. 2a, b. HP-positive active antritis in a duodenal ulcer patient. Abundant IgG plasma cells concentrated at foveolar-neck level (**a**), which were sharply reduced (**b**) after combined antibiotic (amoxycillin × metronidazole, 2 weeks) and antisecretory (omeprazole, 4 weeks) therapy resulting in HP eradication (assessed 2 months after end of therapy) as well as ulcer healing. IgG immunoperoxidase, × 125

antibiotic treatment causing HP clearance. Most of the remaining components of the inflammatory process (eosinophils, IgG and IgA plasma cells, B lymphocytes, and activated follicles) were markedly reduced when HP eradication was confirmed 2 months after the end of therapy (Fig. 2). Coupled with the reduced rate of ulcer recurrence in successfully eradicated patients [11, 26, 35], these findings suggest a pathogenetic role of bacterial cytotoxicity and granulocytes infiltration in the mucosal process leading to ulceration.

Inflammation and Epithelial Changes of Various Clinical Conditions Scored by the Sidney System

Results obtained by the application of the Sidney system for gastritis scoring [29] to antral and corpus mucosa of HP-negative or HP-positive NUD and HP-positive DU or GU are outlined in Figs. 3 and 4. Statistical analysis by the contingency table test covering the four scores (0–3) showed a highly significant ($p < 0.001$) increase in epithelial lesions and inflammation in both antral and corpus mucosa, as well as of activity in antral mucosa only, when 96 HP-positive

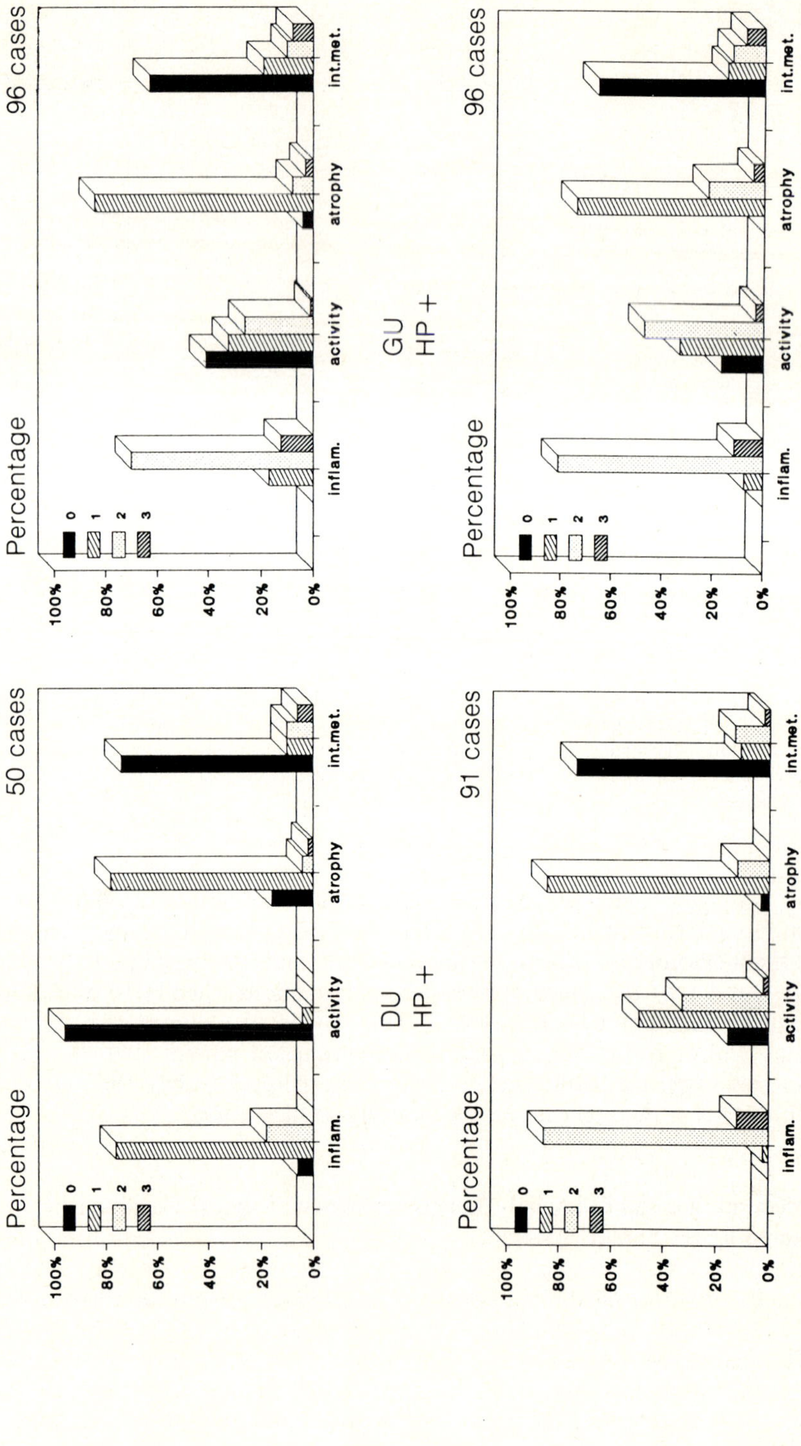

Fig. 3. Sydney system scores of antral mucosa in patients with nonulcer dyspepsia (*NUD*), duodenal ulcer (*DU*), and gastric ulcer (*GU*) From Fiocca et al. [13].

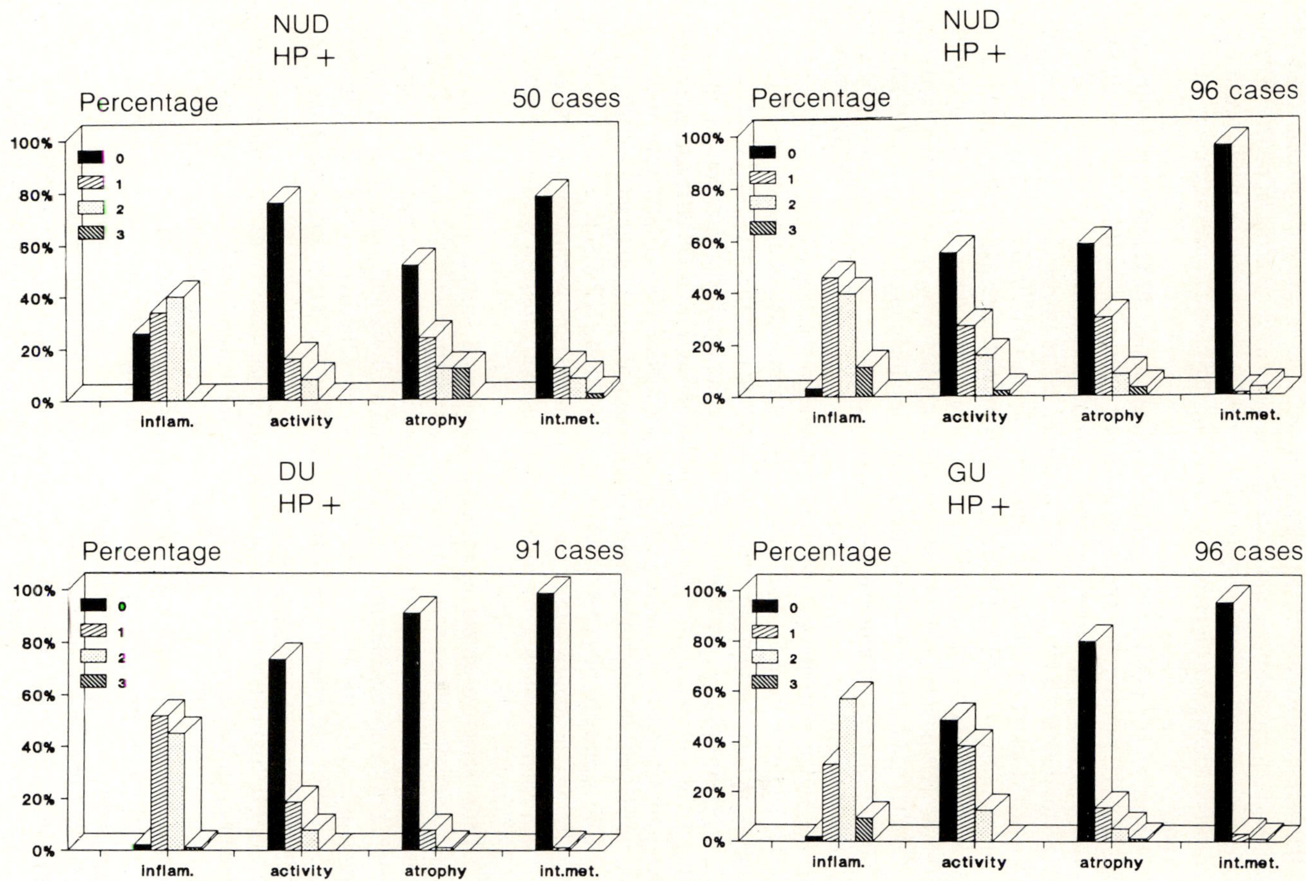

Fig. 4. Sydney system scores of corpus mucosa in patients with nonulcer dyspepsia (*NUD*), duodenal ulcer (*DU*), and gastric ulcer (*GU*)

NUD were compared with 50 HP-negative NUD of the same patient median age (58 years). In addition, gland atrophy showed an increasing trend ($p = 0.078$) in the antrum and a decreasing trend ($p = 0.148$) in the corpus, while intestinal metaplasia showed an increase ($p < 0.01$) in the corpus and no change in the antrum.

When 91 HP-positive DU patients (median age 49 years) were compared with the HP-positive NUDs, increased HP colonization ($p < 0.01$), epithelial lesions ($p < 0.001$), activity ($p < 0.002$), and inflammation ($p < 0.002$) as well as a trend for decreased IM ($p = 0.097$) were seen in the antrum, whereas unchanged HP and IM as well as decreased epithelial lesions ($p < 0.01$), activity ($p < 0.05$), inflammation ($p < 0.05$) and atrophy ($p < 0.001$) were seen in the corpus mucosa.

When 96 HP-positive GU patients (median age 60 years) were compared with the HP-positive NUDs, increased epithelial lesions ($p < 0.001$), activity ($p < 0.001$), and atrophy ($p < 0.02$) as well as unchanged IM ($p = 0.82$) and a trend for increased inflammation ($p = 0.17$) were observed in the antrum, whereas decreased atrophy ($p < 0.02$) and no significant change in HP, epithelial lesions, activity, inflammation, and IM were detected in the corpus.

GU differed from DU only in showing an increase of atrophy ($p < 0.02$) in the antrum and of activity ($p < 0.01$) and inflammation ($p < 0.01$) in the corpus.

When antral and corpus mucosa from the same patients were compared each other, lower antral activity ($p < 0.05$) and inflammation ($p < 0.001$) and increased low-grade coupled with decreased high-grade atrophy ($p < 0.001$) were observed among HP-negative NUD, whereas higher antral inflammation ($p < 0.001$), IM ($p < 0.001$), and atrophy ($p < 0.001$) were seen among HP-positive NUD. In both DU and GU a highly significant increase in antrum versus corpus scores for HP, epithelial lesions, activity, inflammation, atrophy, and IM was found ($p < 0.01$ for HP among GU, $p < 0.001$ in all other cases).

Thus, selective antral increase of HP-linked surface epithelium lesions, gastritis activity and, to some extent, HP colonization were the mucosal changes more specifically associated with ulcer disease. These findings, which are in keeping with those obtained in HP-eradicated patients (see above) and of previous investigations [7, 9, 12, 13, 35] support the hypothesis that epithelial cytotoxicity and gastritis activity are among the main mucosal factors of HP-linked human ulcerogenesis.

In GU patients our findings of an increased activity of juxtaulcer versus distant antral mucosa ($p < 0.001$) and a similar trend for HP-linked epithelial lesions, suggest that these factors may also be important for gastric ulcer localization. However in DU patients, HP colonization, epithelial lesions, and activity were all less severe in juxtaulcer duodenal mucosa, with or without gastric metaplasia, than in ulcer-free antral mucosa of the same patients, suggesting that additional factors (increased acidopeptic secretion, impaired cytoprotection, bile-induced damage of metaplastic gastric-type epithelium, soluble HP toxins and antigens floading from adjacent pyloric mucosa with resultant damage to villous epithelium and immune-inflammatory response) may be involved in duodenal ulcerogenesis.

Cancer-Associated HP Gastritis

Available data concerning HP colonization of cancer-bearing stomachs are rather conflicting, with rates ranging from 20% to 80% due likely to interfering technical problems [6]. Recent investigations showed up to 89% incidence of HP in non cancer mucosa of 37 patients with "intestinal-type" cancer, as opposed to only 32% of 23 patients with diffuse-type cancer [33]. The latter finding apparently contrasts with the results of serologic studies suggesting an highly increased risk for both types of cancer among HP-infected patients [31, 32].

In an attempt to resolve this discrepancy and gain more informative histopathologic data on a possible role of HP in gastric cancerogenesis, we investigated nontumor mucosa of 137 resected stomachs bearing early gastric cancers. In the mucosa adjacent to cancer (2–20 mm from tumor border) HP colonization was detected in all 26 cases of diffuse cancer investigated, in 33 out of 60 (55%) "intestinal" cancers, and in 10 out of 13 (77%) mixed cancers. When specimens of gastric mucosa distant from cancer were also investigated the bacterium was detected in 44 of 60 (73%) cases with intestinal cancer and 11 of 13 (85%) cases with mixed cancers. In 38 early cancers where only the mucosa distant from tumor was investigated, HP was detected in 15 out of 15 diffuse cancers, 3 of 3 mixed, and 15 of 20 (75%) intestinal cancers. On the whole, HP has been detected in 100% of 41 diffuse cancers (median age 57 years), 13 of 16 (81%) mixed cancers (65 years), 59 of 80 (74%) intestinal cancers (66 years), and 113 of all 137 (82.5%) noncardial early cancers (64 years).

Interestingly, HP incidence in the juxtatumor mucosa of the three cancer types was inversely related to the extension of intestinal metaplasia. The median of mucosal area occupied by IM was 35% in intestinal cancers, 17% in mixed, and 14% in diffuse cancers. As HP fails to colonize intestinalized mucosa, the lower mucosal HP colonization of the intestinal type might be due to its extensive IM. Achlorhydria secondary to oxyntic mucosa atrophy, also increased in our intestinal-type cancers, may be another cause of HP eradication [23].

Our finding of an extensive IM just around early intestinal-type cancers confirms previous observations [22] and supports previous suggestions concerning a role of IM in the histogenesis of such cancers [5, 21, 22], especially because dysplasia was frequently seen in juxtatumor intestinalized mucosa. Foci of immature IM expressing the CAR-5 anigen, a possible precursor lesion of frank dysplasia [37], were also prominent in such mucosa. An important histogenetic role of IM in respect to diffuse-type cancers seems unlikely, despite the fact that tumor cells with intestinal phenotypes were equally represented in intestinal and diffuse cancers of advanced stage [14]. Thus, alternate histogenetic pathways remain to be identified in the case of diffuse cancers.

Very high scores of gastritis activity were observed in peritumor (especially around diffuse cancers), nonintestinalized mucosa affected by HP gastritis. Neutrophilic granulocytes were especially abundant at renewal zone level, where increased mitotic rates and DNA precursor (bromodeoxyuridine) incorporation (Luinetti and Fiocca, unpublished findings) were seen in immature epithelial cells. These often showed signs of nuclear activation (enlarged, vesicular, occasionally hyperchromatic, or polymorphic nuclei with prominent nucleoli) promptly disappearing after HP eradication by antibiotic therapy (Fig. 5). As neutrophils

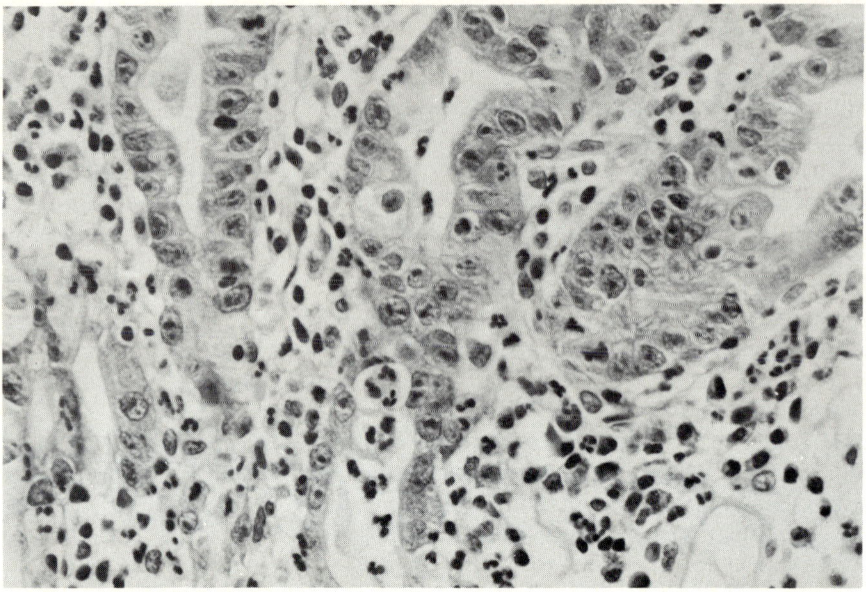

Fig. 5. Corpus mucosa 2 cm proximal to an early cancer of diffuse type: active HP gastritis (note a crypt microabscess) with activated foveolar-neck epithelia showing apparent mild atrophy which disappeared after bacterial eradication and gastritis remission (so-called severe hyperplasia or pseudodysplasia). Hematoxylin-eosin, × 420

are site of intensive oxidative processes producing high amounts of free radicals [39], whose contribution to experimental cancerogenesis is well documented, it seems possible that a long-standing oxidative stress sustained by chronic HP gastritis might contribute to gastric human cancerogenesis. This would explain the protective effect of antioxidants against gastric cancerogenesis [28]. However, as neutrophilic granulocytes were highly represented also inside tumor tissue, especially of diffuse cancers, and decreased in the mucosa distant from tumor, more work is needed to see whether granulocyte infiltration of peritumor mucosa precedes cancer rather than being part of mucosal response to cancer.

Conclusion

In conclusion, available histopathologic evidence suggests that HP gastritis plays a major role in both ulcerogenesis and cancerogenesis. Among various gastritis components, granulocyte infiltration and epithelial lesions, due to direct bacterial cytotoxicity or secondary to HP-activated immune-inflammatory response, may have an important role in the pathogenesis of the ulcerative process. Gastritis activity, epithelial stem cell activation with increased mitotic rate and pseudodysplastic changes, and extensive or immature intestinal metaplasia may all be HP-linked factors promoting cancerogenesis.

Acknowledgements. This work was supported in part by grants from the Italian Health Ministry to the IRCCS Policlinico San Matteo.

References

1. Aceti A, Celestino D, Caferro M, Casale V, Citarda F, Conti EM, Grassi A, Grilli A, Pennica A, Sciarretta F, Leri O, Ameglio F, Sebastiani A (1991) Basophil-bound and serum immunoglobulin E directed against *Helicobacter pylori* in patients with chronic gastritis. Gastroenterology 101:131–137
2. Beauchamp RD, Barnard JA, McCutchen CM, Cherner JA, Coffey RJ (1989) Localization of transforming growth factor alpha and its receptor in gastric mucosal cells. Implications for a regulatory role in acid secretion and mucosal renewal. J Clin Invest 84:1017–1023
3. Bernatowska E, Jose P, Davies H, Stephenson M, Webster D (1989) Interaction of *Campylobacter* species with antibody, complement and phagocytes. Gut 30:906–911
4. Brandtzaeg P, Halstensen TS, Kett K, Krajci, P, Kvale D, Rognum TO, Scott H, Sollid LM (1989) Immunobiology and immunopathology of human gut mucosa: humoral immunity, and intraepithelial lymphocytes. Gastroenterology 97:1562–1584
5. Correa P, Cuello C, Duque E (1970) Carcinoma and intestinal metaplasia of the stomach in Columbian migrants. J Natl Cancer Inst 44:297–306
6. Correa P, Ruiz B (1989) *Campylobacter pylori* and gastric cancer. In: Rathbone BJ, Heatley RV (eds) *Campylobacter pylori* and gastroduodenal disease. Blackwell, Oxford, pp 139–145
7. Crabtree JE, Taylor JD, Wratt JI, Heatley RV, Shallcross TM, Tompkins DS, Rathbone BJ (1991) Mucosal IgA recognition of *Helicobacter pylori* 120 kDa protein, peptic ulceration, and gastric pathology. Lancet 338:332–335
8. Cucala M, Le T, Mugridge K, Parente L, Wallance JL (1991) Inhibitory effects of interleukin-1 on gastric acid secretion are secretagogue-specific. Gastroenterology 100: A49
9. Eidt S, Stolte M (1990) Differences between *Helicobacter pylori* associated gastritis in patients, with duodenal ulcer, pyloric ulcer, other gastric ulcer, and gastritis without ulcer In: Malfertheiner P, Ditschuneit H (eds) *Helicobacter pylori*, Gastritis and Peptic Ulcer. Springer, Berlin Heidelberg New York, pp 228–336
10. Figura N, Guglielmetti P, Rossolini A, Barbieri A, Cusi G, Musmanno RA, Russi M, Quaranta S (1989) Cytotoxin production by *Campylobacter pylori* strains isolated from patients with peptic ulcers and from patients with chronic gastritis only. J Clin Microbiol. 27:225–226
11. Fiocca R, Solcia E, Santoro B (1991) Duodenal ulcer relapse after eradication of *Helicobacter pylori.* Lancet 337:1614
12. Fiocca R, Villani L, De Giacomo C, Perego, M, Trespi E, Solcia E (1989) Morphological evidence of *Campylobacter pylori* pathogenicity in chronic gastritis and peptic ulcer. Acta Gastroenterol Belg 52:324–335
13. Fiocca R, Villani L, Luinetti O, Gianatti A, Perego M, Alvisi C, Turpini F, Solcia E (1992) Helicobacter colonization and histopathologic profile of chronic gastritis in patients with or without dyspepsia, mucosal erosion and peptic ulcer. A morphologic approach to the study of ulcerogenesis in man. Virchows Arch [A] 420:489–498
14. Fiocca R, Villani L, Tenti P, Cornaggia M, Finzi G, Capella C, Prat M, Bussolati G, Solcia E (1988) Widespread expression of intestinal markers in gastric carcinoma: of light and electron-microscopic study using BD-5 monoclonal antibody. J Clin Pathol 41:178–187
15. Fiocca R, Villani L, Turpini F, Turpini R, Solcia E (1987) High incidence of campylobacter-like organisms in endoscopic biopsies from patients with gastritis, with or without peptic ulcer Digestion 38:234–244
16. Forman D, Sitas F, Newell DG, Stacey AR, Boreham J, Peto R, Campbell TC, Li J, Chen J (1990) Geographic association of *Helicobacter pylori* antibody prevalence and gastric cancer mortality in rural China. Int J Cancer 46:608–611
17. Gleich GJ, Adolphson CR (1986) The eosinophilic leukocyte: structure and function. Adv Immunol 39:177–253
18. Gleich GJ, Schroeter AL, Marcoux JP, Sachs, MI, O'Connell EJ, Kohler PF (1984) Episodic angioedema associated with eosinophilia. N Engl J Med 310:1621–1626

19. Gruler H (1988) Necrotaxis and galvanotaxis. Methods Enzymol 162: 115–127
20. Higuchi K, Matsumoto T, Arakawa T, Kitano A, Nagura H, Kobayashi K (1988) Immunohistochemical localization of prostaglandin E_2 (PGE_2), in human gastric mucosa. Gastroenterology 94: AI86
21. Ihamaki T, Sipponen P, Varis K, Kekki M, Siurala M (1991) Characteristics of gastric mucosa which procede occurrence of gastric malignancy: Results of long-term follow-up of three family samples. Scand J Gastroenterol 26 [Suppl 186]: 16–23
22. Johansen A (1981) Gastric carcinoma: a contribution to the pathology and to gastric cancer histogenesis. Bisperbjerg Hospital, Copenhagen
23. Karnes WE Jr, Samloff IM Siurala M, Kekki M, Sipponen P, Kim SWR, Walsh JH (1991) Positive serum antibodies and negative tissue staining for *Helicobacter pylori* in subjects with atrophic body gastritis. Gastroenterology 101: 167–174
24. Kirchner T, Melber A, Fischbach W, Heilmann KL, Muller-Hermelink HK (1990) Immunohistological patterns of the local immune response in *Helicobacter pylori* gastritis. In: Malfertheiner P, Ditschuneit H (eds) *Helicobacter pylori*, gastritis and peptic ulcer. Springer, Berlin Heidelberg New York, pp 213–222
25. Leunk RD, Johnson PT, David BC, Kraft WG, Morgan DR (1988) Cytotoxic activity in broth-culture filtrates of *Campylobacter pylori*. J Med Microbiol 26: 93–99
26. Marshall BJ, Goodwin CS, Warren JR, Murray R, Glincow ED, Blackbourn SJ, Phillips M, Waters TE, Sanderson CR (1988) Prospective double-blind trial of duodenal relapse after eradication of *Campylobacter pylori*. Lancet 11: 1437–1442
27. McGovern TW, Kephart GM, Gleich GJ, Talley NJ (1989) Eosinophil infiltration and degranulation in *Campylobacter pylori* gastritis. Klin Wochenschr 67 [Suppl 18]: 46
28. Mirvish S (1986) Effect of Vitamin C and E on *N*-nitroso compound formation and other theories. J Natl Cancer Inst 58: 1842–1850
29. Misiewicz JJ, Tytgat GNJ, Goodwin CS, Price AB, Sipponen P, Strickland RG, Cheli R (1990) The Sydney system: a new classification of gastritis. Working Party reports, world congresses of gastroenterology, Sydney, pp 1–10
39. Mooney C, Keenan J, Munster D, Wilson I, Allardyce R, Bagshaw P, Chapman B, Chadwick V (1991) Neutrophil activation by *Helicobacter pylori*. Gut 32: 853–857
31. Nomura A, Stemmermann GN, Chyou PH, Kato I, Perez-Perez GI, Blaser MJ (1991) *Helicobacter pylori* infection and gastric carcinoma among Japanese Americans in Hawaii. N Engl J Med 325: 1132–1136
32. Parsonnet J, Friedman GF, Vandersteen DP, Chang Y, Vogelman JH, Orentreich N, Sibley RK (1991) *Helicobacter pylori* infection and the risk of gastric carcinoma. N Engl J Med 325: 1127–1131
33. Parsonnet J, Vandersteen D, Goates J, Sibley RK, Prikikin J, Chang Y (1991) *Helicobacter pylori* infection in intestinal – and diffuse – type gastric adenocarcinomas. J Natl Cancer Inst 83: 640–643
34. Rauws EAJ, Langenberg W, Houthoff HJ, Zanen HC, Tytgat GNJ (1988) *Campylobacter pyloridis*-associated chronic antral gastritis. Gastroenterology 94: 33–40
35. Rauws EAJ, Tytgat GNJ (1990) Cure of duodenal ulcer associated with eradication of *Helicobacter pylori*. Lancet 335: 1233–1235
36. Sipponen P, Varis K, Fraki O, Korri UM, Seppälä K, Siurala M (1990) Cumulative 10-years risk of symptomatic duodenal and gastric ulcer in patients with or without chronic gastritis. A clinical follow-up of 454 patients. Scand J Gastroenterol 25: 966–973
37. Solcia E, Capella C, Fiocca R, Cornaggia M, Rindi G, Villani L, Bosi F, Ambrosiani L (1990) Exocrine and endocrine epithelial changes in types A and B chronic gastritis. In: Malfertheiner P, Ditschuneit H (eds) *Helicobacter pylori*, gastritis and peptic ulcer. Springer, Berlin Heidelberg New York, pp 245–258
38. Stacey AR, Hawtin PR, Newell DG (1990) Local immune responses to *Helicobacter pylori* infections. In: Malfertheiner P, Ditschuneit H (eds) *Helicobacter pylori*, gastritis and peptic ulcer. Springer, Berlin Heidelberg New York, pp 162–166
39. Van der Valk P, Herman CJ (1987) Leukocyte functions. Lab Invest 57: 127–137

Isolation and Phenotypical Characterization of T-Lymphocytes Isolated from the Gastric Mucosa of Patients With and Without *Helicobacter pylori*

W.P. Brooks[1,2], G. Meimarakis[2], R.A. Hatz[2], E. Bayerdörffer[3], G. Enders[1], and H.J. Krämling[2]

Introduction

Infection with the gram-negative bacterium *Helicobacter pylori* is now accepted as a causative agent in antral type B gastritis and in gastric ulcer disease [1–3]. *H. pylori* may also be associated with an increased risk of developing gastric cancer [4–6]. However the pathogenic mechanisms by which *H. pylori* may cause or be involved in these conditions is as yet unknown.

Infection with *H. pylori* elicites a marked activation of the local humoral immune system that is characterized by a primary influx of neutrophils followed by an increase in the numbers of infiltrating lymphocytes [7]. The phenotypical identification of these invading lymphocytes in normal and inflamed mucosa has already been determined by immunohistology [8, 9]. The characterization of the cells that are active and responsive to mitogenic or antigenic stimulation has yet to be investigated. We have isolated T-lymphocytes that outgrow from antral biopsies taken from subjects that are either antibody positive or negative for *H. pylori* outer membrane proteins and characterized these cells with regard to their T-cell subclass profile.

Materials and Methods

Biopsies. Three of four punch biopsies were taken at endoscopy from the antral region of the stomachs of consenting patients that were either positive or negative for antibodies to *H. pylori* acid extracted outer membrane proteins.

Biopsy Culture. Biopsies were washed 10× in Ca^{2+}-, Mg^{2+}-free Hank's buffered salts solution containing streptomycin, penicillin and kanamycin (all 200 μg/ml, Gibco, UK). Biopsies were then divided into approximately 60 smaller pieces and placed with 100 μl culture medium (HEPES buffered RPMI 1640 with 10% foetal calf serum, 10% inactivated human AB serum) plus antibiotics

[1] Institute for Surgical Research, Ludwig-Maximilians Universität, Klinikum Grosshadern, 81377 Munich 70, Germany
[2] Department of Surgery II, Ludwig-Maximilians Universität, Klinikum Grosshadern, 81377 Munich 70, Germany
[3] Medical Clinic II, Ludwig-Maximilians Universität, Klinikum Grosshadern, 81377 Munich 70, Germany

Gasbarrini/Pretolani (Eds.)
Basic and Clinical Aspects of H. pylori Infection

and 10 μg/ml of the T-cell mitogen phytohaemagluttinin (PHA; Seramed, FRG) and cultured at 37°C in a 5% CO_2 incubator. On day 4 and day 10, 2 U/ml recombinant interleukin-2 (IL-2; Boehringer-Mannheim, FRG) was added. Biopsy pieces were then cultured up to 14 days before harvesting.

Cell Harvesting. Cells were harvested by repeated passing up and down through a 23-G syringe. Of the cell culture supernatant 100 μl was collected and stored at − 70°C for cytokine assay. Cells were resuspended in 1 ml phosphate-buffered saline (PBS) and passed over a Ficoll gradient (1.077, Seromed, FRG) for 20 min at 800*g*. The lymphocyte layer was removed, the cells resuspended in PBS, counted and viability tested using trypan blue then prepared for FACS analysis.

Flow Cytometric Analysis. Harvested cells were incubated with either phycoerythrin (PE) or fluorescein isothiocyanate (FITC) labelled antibodies to CD3 (T-pan-cell), CD4 (T-helper-cell), CD8 (T-cytotoxic-cell) and anti-bodies against the T-cell receptors, α/β and γ/δ (all from Becton-Dickson, FRG). Cells were also labelled for the human mucosal lymphocyte marker HML-1 (Dianova, FRG), a marker for intraepithelial lymphocytes [10]. The cells were incubated 30 min at 4°C, lysed and then subjected to two-colour analysis on a Becton-Dickinson FACStar cytometer.

H. pylori *and Cytokine Enzyme-Linked Immunosorbent Assays.* Each patient serum was measured for antibodies to acid extracted *H. pylori* outer membrane proteins in an in-house enzyme-linked immunosorbent assay (ELISA). All titres over 3 × background at a dilution of 1:800 were regarded as positive and over 5 × background as double positive. Culture supernatant (100 μl) from biopsies was assayed for interleukin-6 (IL-6), tumor necrosis factor-alpha (TNF-α) and interferon-gamma (INF-γ) by commercial ELISA kits (Megenex, Belgium); 2 pg/ml was taken to be 1 U/ml.

Results

After 4 days a clear outgrowth of cells could be seen from the biopsy culture. After labelling these cells with a PE-labelled antibody to CD3 most of them were found to be T-cells (Fig. 1). These cells were also to a lesser extent HML-1 positive and also marked for CD-4 or CD-8. The cells were then cultured for another 10 days with IL-2 and PHA before being harvested and labelled for FACS. When the cells from *H. pylori* positive and negative subjects were examined after 14 days, clear differences in the expression of T-cell markers on the cell surface could be observed. There was no change in the overall level of CD3 expression; however, there was an increase in the level of cells expressing the CD4 molecule that was relative to the level of antibody expressed in the ELISA. This increase was matched by a corresponding decrease in the numbers of cells expressing the CD8 molecule (Fig. 2).

This gave a change in the CD4:CD8 ratio from 1:5 to 3:1. This change from $CD8^+$ to $CD4^+$ cells is also reflected in the alterations in the T-cells

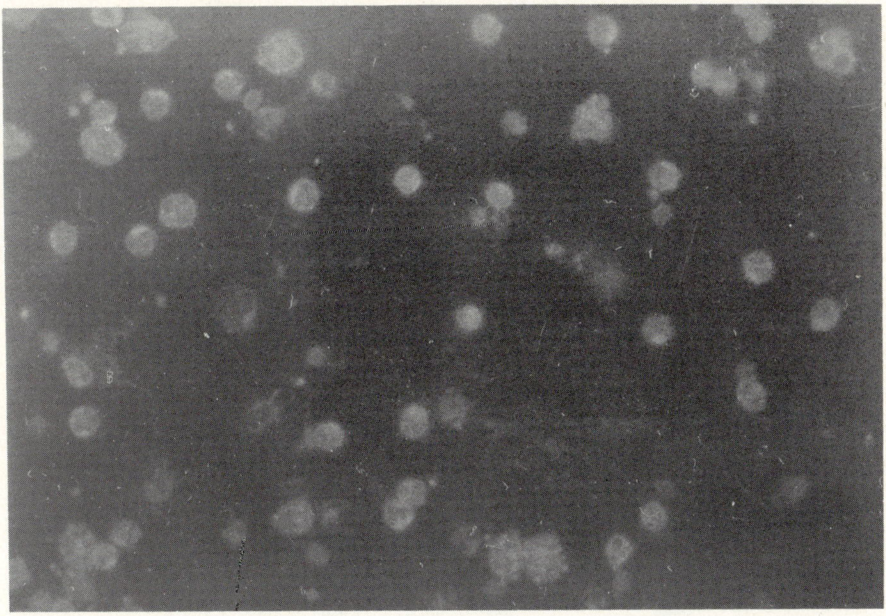

Fig. 1. Cells out-growing from a biopsy culture after 4 days, labelled with the T-pan marker anti-CD3-PE. × 400

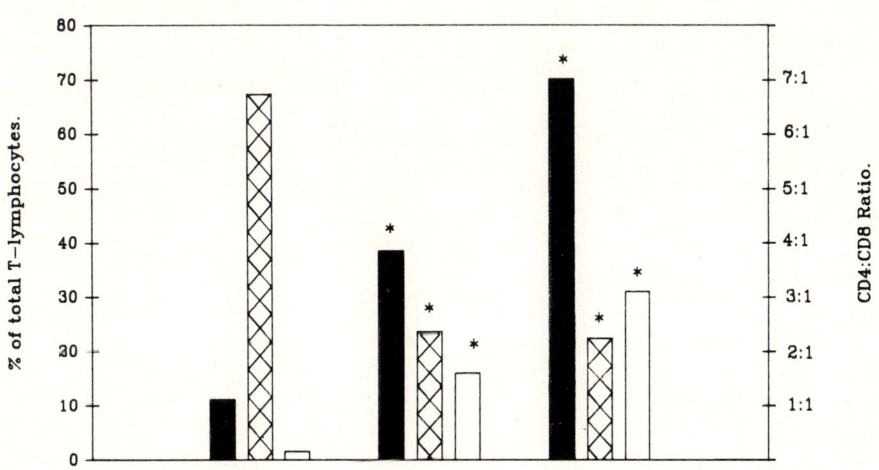

Fig. 2. Changes in the level of $CD4^+$ (■), $CD8^+$ (□) cells after 14 days in culture and the reactive change in the CD4:CD8 ratio (□) of *H. pylori* antibody negative(−), positive(+), and double positive(+ +) patients ($n = 14$). *, Significant difference from control ($p < 0.005$)

receptor classes in the three patient groups. Negative patients have a low expression of the γ/δ TcR (5%) that, after infection, steadily increases (5%–9%) along with the α/β cells (24%–78%) while at the same time there appears to be a decline (75%–50%) in the numbers of intraepithelial lymphocytes (HML-1$^+$), although the level of total lymphocytes is not altered (Fig. 3).

Supernatants taken from the biopsy cultures at day 4 were assayed for different cytokines. There was no difference between positive and negative

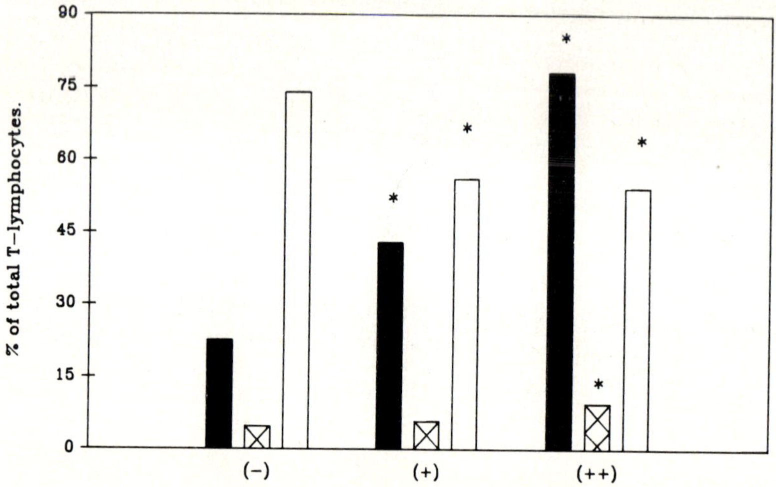

Fig. 3. Differences in the expression of α/β (■) γ/δ (☒) TcR and HML-1 (□), in *H. pylori* antibody negative(–), positive(+), and double positive(+ +) patients after 14 days in culture ($n = 14$). *, Significant difference from control ($p < 0.005$)

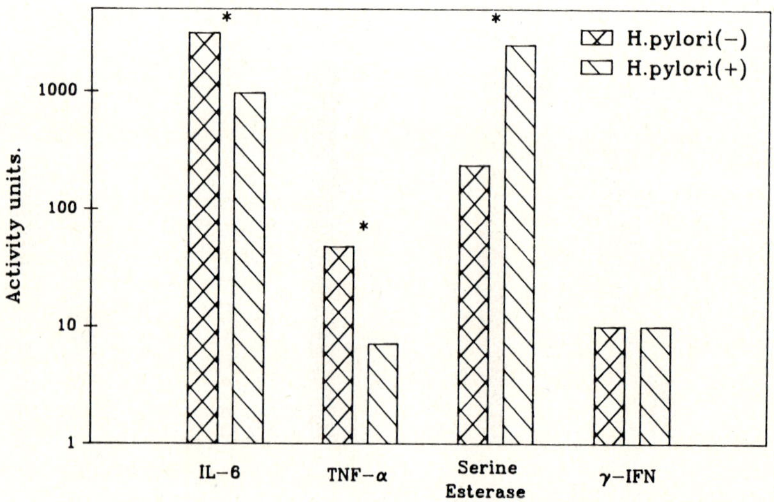

Fig. 4. Levels of cytokines detected in the supernatants of biopsies from *H. pylori* antibody negative(–) and positive(+) patients ($n = 14$). *, Significant difference from normal values ($p < 0.005$)

subjects in their expression of INF-γ, which did not rise above normal levels (< 10 pg/ml). Although both groups showed higher than normal levels of IL-6 (< 10 pg/ml) and TNF-α (< 25 pg/ml), in the supernatants there was a significant difference between the antibody-positive samples (965 U/ml) and the antibody-negative samples (3127 U/ml) in IL-6 and, to a lesser extent, in the TNF-α antibody-positive samples (7.1 U/ml) and antibody-negative samples (47.6 U/ml). When the levels of serine esterase, an indicator of cytotoxiclike activity were measured, the *H. pylori* supernatants showed a ten times greater level of enzyme activity (Fig. 4).

Discussion

It is clear that infection with *H. pylori* causes a major change in the local cellular immune response; however, it can also be seen from the results presented here that the changes that are seen are also indicitive of the functional abilities of these cells.

During an active on-going infective state one expects a recruitment of $CD4^+$ T-cells. It appears from these results that in *H. pylori* positive patients there is a definite proliferation of the $CD4^+$ cell population from biopsy samples, whereas in *H. pylori* negative patients the $CD4^+$ cells present do not proliferate to the same degree. Since the level of $CD8^+$ T-cells is lower in *H. pylori* positive patients, this seems to indicate a development away from the normal population of intraepithelial lymphocytes which are high in $CD8^+$ and low in $CD4^+$. This is similar to the situation in the antibody-negative patients. The argument for recruitment of peripheral or lamina-propria lymphocytes is further enhanced by the fact that there is an antibody dependent increase in the level of α/β T-cell receptor bearing cells and a related decrease in the level of both γ/δ T-cell receptor and HML-1 bearing cells, both of which are strong markers for the normal intraepithelial lymphocyte population.

When the cytokines that were assayed in the supernatant taken from day 4 cultures were compared there were some surprising results. In both groups there was no detectable increase in the level of INF-γ a common product of T-helper-cells. There were higher levels of IL-6 in the *H. pylori* negative subjects; this may indicate that in these subjects there is a proportionally higher level of T-helper$_2$-cells in the $CD4^+$ population as compared to the *H. pylori* positive subjects, which would help to confirm the lack of INF-γ detected. However, the level of IL-6 produced was very high in both class of patients.

The expression of TNF-α showed a similar difference between antibody-negative and antibody-positive subjects, although the difference was more significant, $p < 0.001$ as compared to $p < 0.01$. This may relate to the other cytokines released during the 4-day culture period and would be, to some extent, dependent upon the numbers of neutrophils that may be present in the original biopsy. There was a high basal level of serine esterase activity in the two different groups, however, this showed an increase in the antibody-positive group and may indicate that the cytotoxic cells present in the biopsy samples of antibody-positive patients are more activated despite being in lower numbers.

Acknowledgments. The authors would like to thank the Chiles Foundation and the Fredrich Bauer Foundation for their financial assistance.

References

1. Tygat GNJ, Rauws EAJ (1989) The role of *Campylobacter pylori* in gastroduodenal diseases: a believers point of view. Gastrenterol Clin Biol 13: 1186–1216
2. Graham D Y (1989) *Campylobacter pylori* and peptic ulcer disease. Gastroenterology 96: 615–625
3. Bayerdörffer E et al. (1992) Difference in expression of *Helicobacter pylori* gastritis in antrum and body. Gastroenterology (in press)
4. Carrick J et al. (1989) *Campylobacter pylori*, duodenal ulcer and gastric metaplasia: possible role of functional heterotrophic tissue in ulcerogenesis. Gut 30: 790–797
5. Forman D et al. (1991) Association between infection with *Helicobacter pylori* and risk of gastric cancer: evidence from a prospective investigation. B M J 302: 1302–1305
6. Parsonnet J et al. (1991) *Helicobacter pylori* infection in intestinal- and diffuse-type gastric adenocarcinomas. J Natl Cancer Inst 83: 640–643
7. Whitehead R (1984) Mucosal biopsy of the upper gastrointestinal tract, 3rd edn. Saunders, Philadelphia
8. Stolte M, Eidl S (1989) Lymphoid follicles in antral mucosa: immune response to *Campylobacter pylori*. J Clin Pathol 42: 1269–1271
9. Kirchner T et al. (1990) Immunohistological patterns of the local immune response in *Helicobacter pylori* gastritis. In: (eds) Malfertheiner P, Ditshuneit H, *Helicobacter pylori*, gastritis and peptic ulcer. Springer, Berlin Heidelberg New York
10. Schieferdecker HL et al. (1990) the HML-1 antigen of intestinal lymphocytes is an activation antigen. J Immunol 144: 2541–2549

Demonstration of the Major Cytotoxin-Associated Protein of *Helicobacter pylori* in Gastric Biopsies by Western Blotting

N. Figura[1], M. Bugnoli[2], S. Quaranta[3], M. Corsetti[3], D. Armellini[2], M. Matergi[3], L. Di Gregorio[4], L. Abate[4], E. Esposito[4], and P.F. Bayeli[4]

Introduction

Helicobacter pylori (HP) strains differ considerably in their virulence characteristics. Only certains organisms, for example, produce a toxic substance which causes intracytoplasmic vacuolization on cells in vitro [2, 3]. Cytotoxic HP strains (CTHP) can also be considered ulcerogenic because they have been isolated with greater frequency from patients with peptic ulcers than from patients with chronic gastritis only [2]. Thus the vacuolating toxin most probably plays a crucial role in the pathogenic mechanism of the gastric mucosa damage.

The vacuolating activity (VA) is associated with a protein of an approximate mass of 130 kDa (p130) which is most probably also produced in vivo because sera from patients infected by CTHP strains have antibodies to p130 which can be demonstrated by immunoblotting and the neutralization of the in vitro VA of HP broth culture filtrates (BCF) [1]. However, the demonstration of p130 in vivo is still lacking.

This study was carried out to verify whether p130 can be detected directly in gastroduodenal biopsies taken from dyspeptic patients infected by HP organisms.

Material and Methods

Twenty HP infected adult patients were studied. Biopsies were taken from the gastric antrum and examined histologically, smeared for microscopic examination, streaked on plates for culture, and each dipped in 50 μl phosphate-buffered saline, kept at 4°C for 4 h, and centrifuged at 12 500 *g*. Supernatants of biopsy washings (BW) were denatured with Laemmli's solution and run in 6% or 8% sodium dodecylsulfate (SDS) polyacrylamide gel electrophoresis (PAGE) together with concentrated BCF of a CTHP strain (CCUG 17874). Proteins were transferred onto nitrocellulose and incubated with sera diluted 1:2000 from two rabbits: one immunized with a whole cell suspension of the CTHP strain G32, the other with the non CTHP strain G50. Also preimmune sera were tested.

[1] Istituto di Malattie Infettive, University of Siena, Via P.A. Mattioli, 10, 53100 Siena, Italy
[2] Sclavo Research Center, 53100 Siena, Italy
[3] Servizio di Gastroenterologia, Div. Medica 2a, Ospedale di Grosseto, 53100 Siena, Italy
[4] Istituto di Patologia Speciale Medica, University of Siena, 53100 Siena, Italy

Gasbarrini/Pretolani (Eds.)
Basic and Clinical Aspects of H. pylori Infection

The reaction was demonstrated by anti-rabbit IgG serum conjugated with peroxidase, and developed with the enhanced chemiluminescence western blotting detection system (Amersham).

Strains isolated from the 20 patients were tested for cytotoxicity in the following manner: organisms were grown in *Brucella* broth with 5% fetal calf serum, 0.5% Vitox (Oxoid), and the Skirrow's selective supplement. Flasks were incubated in microaerobic environment at 37°C at 150 oscillations per minute for 72 h. After centrifugation at 4°C at 12 500 *g*, supernatants were filtered through 0.22 μm-pore filters and added to HeLa cells at dilutions ranging from 1:2 to 1:20. Cells were inspected for vacuolization after 24 and 48 h. A strain was considered cytotoxic if its BCF induced vacuolization on at least 50% HeLa cells at any dilution.

Serum IgG to p130 were looked for in the 20 patients by western blotting as previously reported [1] with minor modifications: sera were diluted 1:500, and the reaction was demonstrated by an anti-human IgG serum conjugated with alkaline phosphatase.

Results and Discussion

Nineteen patients were infected by in vitro CTHP strains, and one by a non-CTHP organism. Only the latter did not possess serum IgG to p130. The serum from the rabbit immunized with the CTHP strain reacted with proteins of 130,

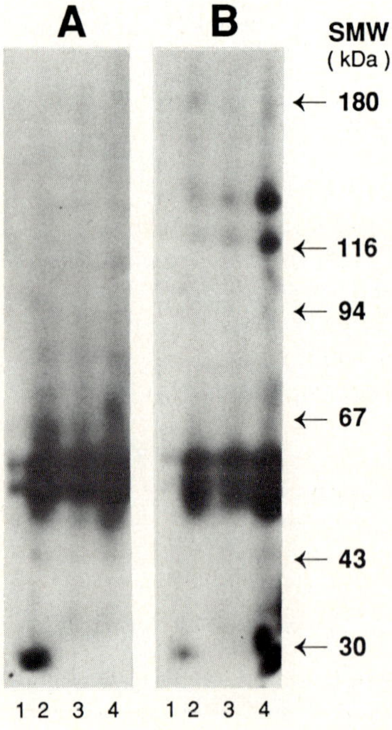

Fig. 1. Immunoblots of washings of biopsies from one patient infected by a non-CTHP organism (*lane 1*) and from three patients infected by CTHP strains (*lanes 2, 3, 4*) with sera from rabbits immunized with a non CTHP strain (*blot A*) and with a CTHP organism (*blot B*)

120, 61, 54, and 29 kDa which were present in all BW with the exception of the one colonized by the non CTHP organism in which 130- and 120-kDa proteins were lacking (Fig. 1). The serum from the rabbit immunized with the non-CTHP organism only reacted with 61-, 54-, and 29-kDa proteins (Fig. 1). Preimmune sera did not react at all.

The detection of p130 in biopsies proved to be more sensitive than the demonstration of a VA on cells in vitro directly exerted by biopsy specimens. In fact, in previous tests we assayed two mucosa samples from each of 40 patients with dyspepsia by putting one biopsy directly on noble agar which had been previously layered on CHO cells and dipping the other in Eagles's medium which after vortexing was added to Vero cells. The vacuolating effect was observed in only one out of 15 cases in which in vitro CTHP organisms were isolated (and only on CHO cells).

The major 130-kDa cytotoxin-associated protein can be easily detected in biopsies colonized by CTHP organisms. The 120-kDa polypeptide probably is a degradation product of the major protein; the 61-, 54-, and 29-kDa proteins most probably represent urease subunits. The in vivo detection of the vacuolating cytotoxin-associated protein strengthens the importance of this toxic factor in the pathogenic mechanism of gastric mucosa damage in type B gastritis.

References

1. Figura N, Bugnoli M, Cusi MG, Pucci AM, Lusini P, Quaranta S, Barberi A, Rossolini A, Di Tommaso AL, De Magistris T, Rappuoli R, Marri L, Musmanno RA, Russi M, Guarna M, Losi M (1990) Pathogenic mechanisms of *Helicobacter pylori*: production of cytotoxin. In: Malfertheiner P, Ditschuneit H (eds) *Helicobacter pylori*, gastritis and peptic ulcer. Springer, Berlin Heidelberg New York, p 86
2. Figura N, Guglielmetti P, Rossolini A, Barberi A, Cusi G, Musmanno RA, Russi M, Quaranta S (1989) Cytotoxin production by *Campylobacter pylori* strains isolated from patients with peptic ulcers and from patients with chronic gastritis only. J Clin Microbiol 27: 225–226
3. Leunk RD, Johnson PT, David BC, Kraft WG, Morgan DR (1988) Cytotoxic activity in broth culture filtrates of *Campylobacter pylori*. J Med Microbiol 26: 93–99

Gastric Functions and *Helicobacter pylori* Infection in Patients with Fundic Atrophic Gastritis

R. Corinaldesi, A. Tucci, V. Stanghellini, C. Tosetti, S. Gasperoni, G.F. Paparo, G. Biasco, S. Siringo, and L. Barbara

Fundic atrophic gastritis (FAG) is a relatively common finding. The pathogenesis of this condition has not yet been defined. Genetic-immunological factors have been claimed to be involved in the pathogenesis of FAG associated with pernicious anaemia (i.e., autoimmune gastritis) [1], while little is known about the possible causes of nonautoimmune FAG.

The aim of the present study was to evaluate *Helicobacter pylori* infection, gastric emptying of solids, and acid secretion in patients with histological evidence of FAG and without pernicious anemia.

Materials and Methods

Subjects. The study group consisted of 33 consecutive outpatients (16 men and 17 women; 53 ± 12 years) with histological evidence of FAG and without pernicious anaemia. Inclusion criteria were: (a) histological evidence of FAG, (b) absence of pernicious anemia (evaluated by means of Shilling test, serum levels of vitamin B_{12}, IgG against intrinsic factor, RBC values), and (c) no intake of antibiotics, bismuth salts, drugs affecting gastric emptying, and/or acid secretion over the past 4 weeks.

Two different groups of healthy controls (HC) were used: 50 subjects (29 men, 21 women; age 38 ± 14 years) for gastric acid secretion and 40 subjects (30 men, 10 women; age 35.1 ± 15.8 years) for gastric emptying.

Endoscopy and Biopsies. Upper GI endoscopy was performed in all the patients after an overnight fast. Six biopsy samples were taken: two from the gastric fundus and two from the gastric antrum for histological examination; one from the gastric fundus and one from the gastric antrum for bacterial culture. Between the procedures, the endoscope (Olympus GIF Q-10) and biopsy forceps (Olympus FB 24-K) were sterilized with 2% glutaraldehyde.

Histology. Biopsies were fixed in formalin, oriented and embedded in paraffin. Sections 2–3 μm thick were stained with hematoxylin and eosin for histological evaluation and with May-Grünwald-Giemsa or Warthin-Starry stains for

Medical Clinic and Gastroenterology, Sant'Orsola Hospital, University of Bologna, Italy

Gasbarrini/Pretolani (Eds.)
Basic and Clinical Aspects of H. pylori Infection

identification of *H. pylori*. The histological evaluation of atrophy was expressed [1–3] as mild, moderate, or severe.

Bacterial Culture. Mucosal biopsies were collected in sterile vials and cultured within 1 h. Blood agar base N.2 (Oxoid, Milan, Italy) supplemented with 7% horse blood and Skirrow's selective supplement (Oxoid, SR 69, Milano, Italy) were used. The cultures were incubated at 37°C in a microaerophilic atmosphere, utilizing Gas Pak jars and Campy Pak II envelopes (BBL Microbiology System, Cockeysville, MD.) for a total of 10 days. Suspected colonies were subjected to morphologic and enzymatic identification. The cultured bacteria were identified as *H. pylori* if they were gram-negative, spiral, and U-shaped bacilli, catalase-, oxidase-, DNAse-, and urease-positive, sensitive to cephalotin (30 μg/disc) and resistant to nalidixic acid (30 μg/disc) [2].

Measurements of Gastric Acid Secretion. We examined, gastric acid secretion in all the patients and in 50 healthy controls. After an overnight fast, a nasogastric tube (16 F) was positioned under fluoroscopic control with the tip in the antrum. After emptying the gastric contents, gastric juice was collected as a 1–4 basal collection in two 30-min samples. Pentagastrin (Merck, Gastrodiagnost, Darmstadt, FRG; 6 μg/kg) was then injected intramuscularly, and secretions were collected for 1 h, in 15-min samples. In each sample, volume and titrable acidity were measured by NaOH 0.1 N to pH 7 (pH-Meter 259, Instrumentation Laboratory). Basal acid output (BAO) and peak acid output (PAO) were then calculated.

Gastric Emptying Test. We studied gastric emptying by a radioisotopic technique in all the patients and in 40 control subjects. At lunchtime, after at least a 5–4 fast, subjects ate a mixed meal (688 kCal; 42% carbohydrate, 37% fat, 21% protein), consisting of 20 g chicken liver, 80 g ground beef, 100 g potatoes, 10 g white bread, and 150 g cream caramel as solid components and 10 g corn oil and 200 cm^3 water, as liquid components. The liver was labeled with 18.5 MBq of ^{99m}Tc-$_{SC}$ as a marker of the solid phase. One-minute counts of the radioactivity leaving the gastric region of interest (ROI) were obtained at 10-min intervals for 240 min on the anterior and posterior walls of the abdomen, with the patient standing in front of the head of a gamma-camera (PHO-Gamma

Table 1. *H. pylori* status (HP +), gastric functions, and histological findings in patients with fundic atrophic gastritis

	HP +	IgG	BAO (mEq/l)	PAO (mEq/l)	Gastrin (pg/ml)	K (%min^{-1})	FAG 1	FAG 2	FAG 3
HC			3.1 ± 1.9	21.4 ± 6.8	48 ± 60	0.7 ± 0.2			
G1	14/14	12/14	1.7 ± 1.9	20.5 ± 9.0	65 ± 78	0.5 ± 0.1**	11	3	0
G2	6/9	6/9	0.1 ± 0.5	1.6 ± 0.5	526 ± 418***	0.3 ± 0.2***	2	5	2
G3	1/10*	6/10	0	0	650 ± 380***	0.3 ± 0.2***	3	2	5

*$p < 0.01$ vs G1, $p < 0.05$ vs G2(χ^2); **$p < 0.01$ vs HC (*t* test); ***$p < 0.001$ vs HC, $p < 0.01$ vs G1 (*t* test).

IV Searle Nuclear, Chicago) interfaced to a digital computer (PDP 11/34). A video monitor allowed selection of a ROI, representing the isotope contained in the stomach. Isotope counts were corrected for radionuclide decay. Geometric means of anterior and posterior counts were fitted using a nonlinear least-square computer program [3] and expressed as emptying rate (K).

Serological Techniques. The basal serum gastrin concentrations were measured by radioimmunoassay in all the patients and in 50 healthy controls, after an overnight fast. Serum IgG antibodies to *H. pylori* were analyzed with an enzyme-linked immunosorbent assay (Helico-G, Porton, Cambridge) in all the patients.

Results and Discussion

On the basis of gastric acid secretion. FAG patients were divided into three subgroups (G): 14 patients with normal gastric acid secretion (G1: 7 men, 7 women; 48 ± 13 years), 9 patients with hypochlorhydria (PAO < m − 2 SD of healthy controls) (G2: 5 men, 4 women; 57 ± 8 years), and 10 with achlorhydria resistant to pentagastrin stimulation (G3: 4 men, 6 women; 56 ± 10 years). The results are reported in the Table 1.

H. pylori infection is a common finding in patients with FAG and still having gastric acid secretion (normohypoclorhydric patients), while it is uncommon in achlorhydric FAG patients. However, serological positivity to *H. pylori* was relatively high in all the three subgroups of FAG patients. Gastric emptying of solids is delayed in FAG patients, particularly in those with hypoachlorhydria.

References

1. Kekki M, Siurala M, Varis K, Sipponen P, Sistonen P, Nevanlinna HR (1987) Classification principles and genetics of chronic gastritis. Scand J Gastroenterol 22 [Suppl 22]: 1–28
2. Langenberg ML, Tytgat GNJ, Shipper MEI, Rietra PJGM, Zanen HC (1984) *Campylobacter*-like organisms in the stomach of patients and healthy individuals. Lancet, i: 1348
3. Elashoff JD, Reedy TJ, Meyer JH (1982) Analysis of gastric emptying data. Gastroenterology 83: 1306–1312

Peptic Ulcer in the Elderly: Not a *Helicobacter*-Related Condition?

J.I. Wyatt, T.M. Shallcross, and R.V. Heatley

Introduction

Recent studies show that most peptic ulceration in adults is associated with *Helicobacter* gastritis and/or the use of non-steroidal anti-inflammatory agents (NSAIDS) [2]. These factors damage the mucosa and impair its defence against acid/peptic attack. The aim of our study was to determine the frequency of these two risk factors for peptic ulceration in elderly patients (aged $\geqslant 70$ years) in comparision with younger adults.

Methods

Forty-nine patients with peptic ulceration diagnosed during 146 consecutive routine endoscopies in patients aged 70 years or older were studied. Use of NSAIDS was recorded from hospital notes and direct questioning, and *H. pylori* status determined by histology of at least two gastric biopsies (antrum and corpus) stained by the modified Giemsa technique. In addition the presence and characteristics of gastritis in these biopsies was recorded, using the Sydney system. All patients studied had established benign peptic ulceration, patients with erosions were not included. For comparision, 36 patients aged 60 years or younger with peptic ulcer, from a series of 161 endoscopies in patients of this age, were studied in the same way. Statistical analysis was by the χ^2 test. The studies were approved by the hospital ethics committee.

Results

There were significantly more gastric ulcers and combined gastric and duodenal ulcers in the elderly patients than in the younger ones (Table 1; $p < 0.005$).

The overall frequency of *H. pylori* infection (by histology) was 81% in the younger group and 51% in the elderly group of ulcer patients. In the younger group duodenal ulcer was more closely associated with *H. pylori* infection, with 18/21 of the patients (86%) positive; the other 3 patients were all taking

St James's University Hospital, Leeds LS9, 7TF, UK

Gasbarrini/Pretolani (Eds.)
Basic and Clinical Aspects of H. pylori Infection

Table 1. Distribution of peptic ulcers in patients aged under 60 years and over 70 years

	Age ⩽ 60			Age ⩾ 70		
	Duodenal ulcer	Gastric ulcer	Both	Duodenal ulcer	Gastric ulcer	Both
n	21	14	1	12	31	6
Hp positive	18	10	1	6	17	3

Table 2. Frequency of *H. pylori* and NSAID use in patients with peptic ulceration

	Age ⩽ 60 years ($n = 36$)	Age ⩾ 70 years ($n = 49$)
Hp positive	29	26
NSAID	12	25
Both factors	7	14
Neither factor	2	12

Table 3. Gastric histology in *H. negative* patients with peptic ulceration

	Normal	Reactive gastritis	chronic gastritis	Lymphocytic gastritis
Age ⩽ 60 ($n = 7$)	1(1)	4(3)	1(1)	1
Age ⩾ 70 ($n = 23$)	6(2)	8(6)	8(3)	1

Number of patients on NSAIDs, in parentheses.

NSAIDS. In the elderly the frequency of *H. pylori* was about 50% irrespective of the site of the ulcer, so that the lower frequency of *H. pylori* in these patients was not accounted for by the high proportion of gastric ulcers in this group.

Table 2 shows the frequency of *H. pylori* and/or NSAID use in the two patient groups. Of the younger group 95% had at least one of these risk factors, compared with 75% of the elderly group. There were duodenal ulcer as well as gastric ulcer patients among the 12 elderly patients with neither risk factor.

All of the *H. pylori* positive patients had gastritis. The histology of the gastric biopsies in the *H. pylori* negative patients is shown in Table 3, with the numbers of patients taking NSAIDS given in parenthesis. Of the 23 elderly *H. pylori* negative patients 17 (74%) had some form of gastritis, but in 6 peptic ulceration developed against a background of histologically normal mucosa.

Discussion

We have found that peptic ulcers differ significantly in elderly patients as compared with younger patients both in terms of their distribution and risk factors. In fact, the prevalence of 51% for *H. pylori* infection in peptic ulcer patients in this age group is identical to the prevalence we have found by histology in elderly patients without ulceration [3]. *H. pylori* does not therefore appear to be a risk factor for ulceration in this age group. Conversely, use of NSAIDS was recorded in 25/49 of the ulcer group compared with 22/82 of a group of elderly patients without ulceration ($p < 0.01$).

It is very unusual to find peptic ulceration in younger adults who are *H. pylori* negative and not taking NSAIDS [1]. In contrast, 12 of our elderly patients had neither risk factor although 8 of them had some form of gastritis on histology. In the light of our other studies in elderly patients [3] at least some of these patients may have had *H. pylori* which were not detected by histology. It is of interest that in 6/49 elderly patients peptic ulceration was not associated with any chronic gastritis, and presumably other aetiological factors not directly related to the gastric mucosa are important in this group.

In conclusion this preliminary study has shown that peptic ulcers in elderly patients differ both in distribution and risk factors from those in younger patients. Further work is required to determine whether other risk factors are important in this age group, and whether the risk of serious complications is higher from ulcers of any particular aetiological group. These results may also be relevant to treatment of peptic ulceration in the elderly.

References

1. Sobala GM, Crabtree JE, Pentith JA et al. (1991) Screening dyspepsia by serology to *H. pylori*. Lancet 338: 94–96
2. Soll A (1990) Pathogenesis of peptic ulcer and implications for therapy. NEJM 3321: 909–915
3. Wyatt JI, Shallcross TM, Crabtree JE, Heatley RV (1992) *H. pylori* gastritis and peptic ulceration in the elderly J Chin Pathol 45: 1070–1074

Serology of *Helicobacter pylori* Infection

Introduction

L.P. Andersen[1], and D.G. Newell[2]

Increasing awareness of the role of *H. pylori* in gastroduodenal diseases has necessitated the rapid development of non-invasive diagnostic techniques. To date the available non-invasive techniques include the urea breath test and serodiagnosis. Serological methods have significant advantages over breath tests, being cheap, simple, and generally available in most routine laboratories. The increased use of these serological tests, for diagnosis, treatment monitoring, and epidemiological studies over the past few years, and the rapidly increasing use of commercially available kits has revealed many potential problems. The aim of this workshop was to highlight and discuss the problems associated with the development and application of the serodiagnosis of *H. pylori* infection. Many of the presentations at this, the IVth European Workshop on *H. pylori* and Gastroduodenal Disease, utilized serology as an investigative tool. A review of these presentations has allowed the identification of both the technical difficulties and those problems associated with the application and interpretation of the results. Such problems can be illustrated as a series of questions.

Problems Associated with Current Serological Technology

- *Test format:* Which serological test should be used – latex agglutination, hemagglutination, enzyme-linked immunosorbent assay (ELISA), immunoblotting, etc?
- *Solid phase immobilisation of antigen:* Are there quantitative or qualitative differences in the antigen-binding capacity of different types of plastic, for example, the microtiter plates used in ELISA?
- *Antigen preparations:* Can crude antigens such as sonicated bacteria or acid/glycin surface extracts give sufficient specificity? Can purified antigens provide sufficient sensitivity? Should different antigens be developed for different purposes? Which antigens should be included in an ideal antigen?
- *Patient blood samples:* Is serum preferable to plasma? What is the stability of serum antibodies during freezing and thawing? How long can serum be stored and what are the optimum conditions for storage?

[1] Department of Clinical Microbiology, Rigshospitalet, and Statens Seruminstitut Copenhagen, Denmark
[2] Central Veterinary Laboratory, Weybridge, Survey, KT15 3BN, UK

Gasbarrini/Pretolani (Eds.)
Basic and Clinical Aspects of H. pylori Infection

- *Cut-off levels:* How should the "gold standard" be defined? Which population should be used to define the cut-off levels, i.e., asymptomatic individuals or patients? Should a population comprise consecutive or selected patients? What should we do about the "gray zone?"
- *Reproducability and standardization:* How great is the variation in results obtained with the same kits in different laboratories or with different kits in the same laboratories? Is it possible to compare results obtained in different laboratories or in different studies, i.e., is it possible to standardize *H. pylori* serology?

Problems Associated with the Application of *H. pylori* Serology

Because the criteria, i.e., cut-off level and sensitivity and specificity, for the serological test is dependent on the intended application, there is some debate on the need for tests dedicated to specific applications. In particular, should the cut-off levels and antigen preparations be different when the test is used for diagnosis or treatment monitoring or epidemiology? Furthermore, should tests used for different populations have dedicated cut-off levels and antigens? For example in children or elderly compared with "normal adults;" or in populations with significantly high or low prevalences of infection with *H. pylori* compared with the "normal;" or in different geographical regions or ethnic groups with a higher or lower prevalence of infection, than "normal," with potentially antigenically cross-reactive bacteria. Many of these problems were considered either in formal presentations or in the active discussion period of the workshop.

The Use of *Helicobacter pylori* Serology in Diagnosis and Treatment Monitoring

L.P. Andersen

The Application of Serology to Diagnosis

The main problem when serology is used for diagnosis of *H. pylori* infection is to define the cut-off level. It is therefore of the greatest importance to define a proper "gold standard" for the presence and absence of *H. pylori* and to define a proper test population for this evaluation. The tests available for diagnosis of *H. pylori* and thus for definition of the "golden standard" are: (a) culture of *H. pylori* from endoscopic biopsies, (b) observation of *Helicobacter*-like organisms (HLO) by microscopy in histological preparation of biopsies, (c) urea breath test (^{14}C and ^{13}C), (d) urease activity in biopsies (the rapid urease test), and (e) polymerase chain reaction (PCR) for detection of *H. pylori* DNA in biopsies. All these tests, except PCR, have no or very few false-positive results whereas, the frequence of false-negative results are more uncertain depending on the intensity of the infection and the patchiness of the bacteria in the stomach allowing sampling errors. PCR has no or extremely few false-negative results, but only very little contamination of the material with *H. pylori* can cause false-positive results. In general it is accepted that at the least culture and preferably also microscopy of sections are necessary for an acceptable "gold standard," but it is clear that the more tests that are included the more reliable is the "gold standard."

A better discrimination between *H. pylori* positive and negative patients is obtained with selected test populations (i.e., ulcer patients versus normal persons) than with consecutive patients. Using different populations may, however, lead to different cut-off levels. Nevertheless most diagnostic *H. pylori* serology will be applied to consecutive patients and the cut-off levels should therefore be defined on consecutive patients.

Even with an optimal "gold standard" and with an adequate population for the evaluation "false-sero positive" results may still occur because of inadequate techniques, sampling errors, cross-reacting antigen preparations, or loss of *H. pylori* infection either due to treatment or natural clearance. On the other hand, "false-sero negative" results may occur in a small proportion, usually about 5% of the *H. pylori* infected patients, who do not produce circulating antibodies against the *H. pylori* infection. For example, Pozuelo et al. (this workshop) found 8% false-negative patients by serology.

[1] Department of Clinical Microbiology, Rigshospitalet, and Statens Seruminstitut Copenhagen, Denmark

Gasbarrini/Pretolani (Eds.)
Basic and Clinical Aspects of H. pylori Infection

The cut-off level that should be chosen may depend on the purpose for, and the consequences, of the serological diagnosis and also on the frequency of *H. pylori* in the population. If the serology is used for screening to eliminate seronegative patients from subsequent endoscopic investigation, it would be preferable to have false-positive results rather than false-negative results (a high sensitivity rather than a high specificity) and thus a low cut-off level should be chosen. Two studies (P.R. Hawtin et al. and M.A. Mendall et al., this workshop) showed that patients aged under 45 years who are not receiving NSAIDs and are without increased *H. pylori* IgG antibodies almost always ($\sim 95\%$) had normal endoscopic results. Thus, about 20% of the endoscopies could be avoided by excluding seronegative patients.

If the serology is used for screening to treat seropositive patients for their *H. pylori* infection as a replacement for endoscopy, false-negative results would be preferable to false-positive results (a high specificity rather than a high sensitivity), and a high cut-off level should be chosen. Such screening should be done only in patients aged under 45 years because of the risk for gastric cancer in older individuals. However, it is not advisable to treat any patients without a prior endoscopy, because endoscopic abnormalities may still be found. It may, however, be realistic in some circumstances because of economic and political reasons.

Results from studies on children have indicated that a lower cut-off value should be chosen for children than for adults. Borderline serological results are often found in young children, which is discussed by S. Cadranel et al. (this workshop). Studies on ethnic groups have indicated that a higher cut-off value should be chosen for Asians and Africans than for Caucasians. Controlled studies that could clarify these questions were not presented at the meeting and are still needed.

Treatment Monitoring

Eradication of *H. pylori* from the stomach of a patient leads to a decrease in the anti-*H. pylori* IgG antibody level over a period of several months. When serology is used for treatment monitoring, it is most important to have a quantitative assay with a high reproducibility. In this case the predictive values are of less importance than when the serology is used for diagnosis. Quantitation of the serology is necessary because it often takens 3–6 months before the IgG antibody level has fallen by half of the level found before treatment, and it may take more than 1 year before the antibody level has reach a stable low level. Nevertheless this antibody level may still be increased compared to *H. pylori* negative patients. However, Di Napoli et al. (this workshop) found a significant decrease in the antibody level after as short a time as 6 weeks. The reproducibility of the assay is of the greatest importance, as a poor reproducability may be mistaken for a fall in the antibody level. It is therefore advisable to test all serum samples from the same patient at the same time. If the ELISA technique is used, sera from one patient should be tested on the same microtiter plate. In this case the storage of the test serum samples is of the greatest importance.

There was some discussion about the sample storage. Also discussed was whether serum samples can be frozen and thawed more than once without major influence on antibody levels. No systematic studies on this subject were presented at this workshop, and such studies need to be carried out. For the moment serum is advised to be stored at −20°C either in small alliquots or in 50% glycerol, which keeps the sample liquid at −20°C.

The IgG antibody level against *H. pylori* thus, seems to be useful for diagnosis of *H. pylori* infection as well as for treatment monitoring, although several problems still need to be solved.

The Use of Serological Detection of *Helicobacter pylori* in Epidemiology

D. Forman

Epidemiological studies of *Helicobacter pylori* have addressed many important public health questions concerning the causes and consequences of infection with this ubiquitous organism. In the 12 months prior to this workshop epidemiological studies were published, for example, on the distribution of *H. pylori* in different social and racial groups [1–2], the mode of bacterial transmission [3] and the relationship to gastric cancer [4–6]. All of these studies were made possible by the use of reliable assays for the detection of anti-*H. pylori* antibodies in serum (or plasma) samples. The non-invasive nature of serology (in comparison with a gastric biopsy) coupled with the relative speed and cheapness of conducting assays on large sample numbers make it the technique of choice for the epidemiological identification of infected individuals.

It may be suggested that, as far as epidemiology is concerned, serology is not only the optimum for the above practical reasons but also that it provides the most reliable routine indication of infection status on theoretical grounds. Thus histopathology or microbiological culture or a urea-CLO test, all based on routine gastric biopsy, may occasionally miss an infection either because of a patchy localisation or because colonisation might have been inhibited in conditions of severe atrophic gastritis with intestinal metaplasia. Similarly the urea breath test misses non-active infections. For a clinician, whose prime interest is whether or not an infection is active, a biopsy-based tested or a breath test may be more relevant. However, an epidemiologist is usually more interested in whether or not an individual has ever been infected and, for this purpose, serology is preferable.

There are, of course, limitations in the use of serological tests. Because these are designed to detect specific antibodies they are obviously dependent on the extent of the immune response to infection. Individuals with an impaired response may therefore produce a false-negative serological test. In this respect there may be a specific problem with loss of immunocompetence in the elderly (Newell, personal communication). Also, results available from antibody tests usually only provide qualitative information, i.e. whether an infection is present or not. Quantification of the titre mainly provides information about the host immune response, and although it has been suggested [5] that the titre may also indicate the degree of inflammation, epidemiological use of serology to date has largely been confined to establishing the presence or absence of infection.

Imperial Cancer Research Fund, Cancer Epidemiology Unit, Radcliffe Infirmary, Oxford OX2 6HE, UK

Gasbarrini/Pretolani (Eds.)
Basic and Clinical Aspects of H. pylori Infection

The use of *H. pylori* serology (or indeed any diagnostic test) in epidemiology is clearly as dependent on good laboratory practice and the validation of the assay as is the use of serology in clinical applications. However, because epidemiology requires the comparison of seroprevalence rates in different patient groups or different populations, the comparability of different serological assays is a particularly critical issue. Even when assays have been extensively internally validated, the use of different antigens and different assays may not be directly comparable. The profligation of both in-house and commercial kit assays has not helped this although the situation is now improving with published comparison studies [7] and inter-laboratory circulation of reference samples (see Feldman et al., this volume).

In epidemiological studies where the intention is to compare seroprevalence of *H. pylori* antibodies in different groups, appropriate matching of samples is absolutely essential. The strong associations between *H. pylori* infection and racial group, socio-economic status, and especially age mean that only with appropriate matching for these criteria can results be interpreted. Other matching criteria are made necessary because of the nature of the assay procedures. Thus, although there are few data which address this point, serum samples are likely to give results that are not directly comparable with plasma samples. Epidemiological studies also frequently make use of blood samples collected years (sometimes decades) previously and stored frozen. Although IgG antibody should be relatively stable, factors such as the temperature and length of storage and the number of freeze-thaw cycles could influence assay results. Where possible, samples should be matched so that these variables do not influence group comparisons. Although there are reports [8] that serum antibody titres do not vary with repeated freeze-thawing and with storage for 3 years at $-20°C$, freeze-thawing may reduce the antibody titre in plasma samples while long-term storage may reduce the titre in serum (Forman, unpublished observations).

References

1. Sitas F, Forman D, Yarnell JWG, Burr MI, Elwood PC, Pedley S, Marks KJ (1991) *Helicobacter pylori* infection rates in relation to age and social class in a population of Welsh men. Gut 32: 25–28
2. Graham DY, Malaty HM, Evans DG, Evans DJ, Klein PD, Adam E (1991) Epidemiology of *Helicobacter pylori* in an asymptomatic population in the United States. Effect of age, race and socioeconomic status. Gastroenterology 100: 1495–1501
3. Perez-Perez GI, Witkin SS, Decker MD, Blaser MJ (1991) Seroprevalence of *Helicobacter pylori* infection in couples. J Clin Microbiol 29: 642–644
4. Forman D, Newell DG, Fullerton F, Yarnell JWG, Stacey AR, Wald N, Sitas F (1991) Association between infection with *Helicobacter pylori* and risk of gastric cancer: evidence from a prospective investigation. Br Med J 302: 1302–1305
5. Nomura A, Stemmermann GN, Chyou P–H, Kato I, Perez-Perez GI, Blaser MJ (1991) *Helicobacter pylori* and gastric carcinoma among Japanese Americans in Hawaii. N Engl J Med 325: 1132–1136
6. Parsonnet J, Friedman GD, Vandersteen DP, Chang Y, Vogelman DEE, Orentreich N, Sibley RK. (1991) *Helicobacter pylori* infection and the risk of gastric carcinoma. N Engl J Med 325: 1127–1131

7. Talley NJ, Newell DG, Ormand JE, Carpenter HE, Wilson WE, Zinsmeister AR, Perez-Perez GI, Blaser MJ (1991) Serodiagnosis of *Helicobacter pylori*: comparison of enzyme linked immunosorbent assays. J Clin Microbiol 29:1635–1639
8. Talley NJ, Zinsmeister AR, Weaver A, DiMagno EP, Carpenter HA, Perez-Perez GI, Blaser MJ (1991) Gastric adenocarcinoma and *Helicobacter pylori* infection. J Natl Cancer Inst 83:1734–1739

Helicobacter pylori Serology: Kit Evaluation and Comparison

E. De Koster, P. Denis, H. Goossens, J.F. Nyst, and M. Deltenre

Numerous abstracts evaluating one or more commercial *Helicobacter pylori* (HP) serology kits have been submitted at this meeting, reflecting the abundance of kits available today in the marketplace. The clinical application of serology is to rule out an ongoing HP infection in dyspeptic patients, family members of an index patients, or after treatment. A positive serology result should lead the patient to endoscopy for confirming the presence of bacteria, determining drug resistance, and evaluating the associated gastrointestinal lesions. This implies that serology kits should be optimized for sensitivity. Practically, this seems to be the case (Tables 1, 2).

There is not agreement concerning what gold standard serology should be tested against. It probably should be a combination of nonserological methods, such as in the Sydney system recommendations: three biopsies in antrum and corpus, one biopsy for culture, and two for histology. Problems with the gold standard arise especially in elderly persons. Age-related atrophic gastritis and immune incompetence lead to discrepancies between urea breath test and serology in elderly patients: 83% of the breath test-negative persons were seronegative, and 68% of the breath test-positive persons were seropositive [10]. In case of atrophic body gastritis the prevalence of HP seropositivity was significantly greater than the prevalence of positive HP staining on histology [5], implying that serological traces of the HP infection persist after the organism can no longer be found with conventional techniques. This could be called a "false-positive serology result." However, the preneoplastic nature of atrophic body gastritis makes identification and endoscopy of these patients important. The histological definition and age range of the studied population are therefore important in evaluating the performance of a particular serology kit. New techniques (in situ immune response [1] monoclonal antibodies, polymerase chain reaction) should clarify these discrepancies and may be included in the gold standard in the future.

Because of differences in the choice and the quality of the tests included in the gold standard as well as population differences the most useful information comes from studies in which several serology kits have been tested using the same sera, eliminating between-centers differences in populations and gold standard. These studies are summarized in Table 1. Loffeld [6] found sensitivities between 81.5% and 95.8%, and specificity ranged from 43.5% to 91.6%. The

Brugmann University Hospital and St. Pieters University Hospital, Free University of Brussels (VUB-ULB), Brussels, Belgium

Gasbarrini/Pretolani (Eds.)
Basic and Clinical Aspects of H. pylori Infection

Table 1. Comparison of serology kits: single-center studies

Test	Sensitivity (%)	Specificity (%)	Positive predictive value (%)	Negative predictive value (%)	Doubtful cases (*n*)
Loffeld et al. [1]					
Malakit 1[a]	90.5	91.6	97.9	68.1	1
Malakit 2[a]	90.5	91.6	97.7	68.7	1
Syn[elisa]	84.3	81.8	95.5	52.9	2
Helico-G	81.5	76.9	88	66.6	5
Roche 1[a]	90.4	84.6	95.9	68.7	2
Roche 2	90.2	84.6	95.8	68.7	3
Whittaker	95.8	91.6	97.8	84.6	7
GAP new 1[a,b]	88.2	88.8	97.8	57.1	7
GAP new 2[a,b]	89.6	75	93.4	64.2	7
Gap old[b]	91.8	43.5	80.4	83.3	4
Schembri et al. [14]					
HEL-p	83	60			
GAP-IeG	78	70			
Pyloriset	79	46			
Helico-G	80	65			
Valeur et al. [15]					
Orion 1st gen.	84	61			
Roche 1st gen[b]	81	70			
Porton-Cambridge	74	78			
Biorad 1st gen.	84	70			
Biometra 1st gen.	94	78			
RH1 1st gen.	97	57			
Roche 2nd gen. beads[b,c]	90	87			
Roche 2nd gen. wells[b,c]	97	83			
Dako 2nd gen.	94	74			
Whittacker 2nd gen.	94	74			
Mégraud et al. [8]					
Roche 1st gen.[b]	51	74			
Roche 2nd gen.[b]	62	90			
GAP IgG	58	77			
Pylostat	48	92			
Pylriset	28	89			
Helico G	47	82			
UBT	72	74			

Loffeld et al. [1]: 67 dyspepsia patients: 54 HP +, 13 HP –. Gold standard: culture, histology. Intra-assay variability: Malakit 0%, Roche 10.7%, Gap 18.2%.
Schembri et al. [14]: 190 dyspeptic patients: 96 HP +, 94 HP –. Gold standard: culture plus at least one of phase contrast microscopy, histopathology, urease.
Valeur et al. [15]: 54 dyspeptic patients: 31 HP +, 23 HP –. Gold standard: culture, histology
Mégraud et al. [8]: 255 asymptomatic adults and 266 children (9 months – 5 years) from Africa (Burkina Faso). Gold standard: immunoblot; part of the subjects: [^{13}C] urea breath test. Figures presented in the table are those for children only: children: 81/266 HP +; by immunoblot. Adults (virtually all HP +) sensitivity of the tested kits: Roche 1G, 83%; Roche 2G, 92%; Pylori-set, 71%; Pylo-stat, 96%; GAP, 90%; Helico G, 88%; UBT, 91%.

[a] These tests were performed more than once: 1, first run; 2, second run.

[b] Two versions of the test have been tested (first- and second-generation kits).

[c] The Roche second-generation test was tested on beads ad in wells.

Table 2. Review of sensitivity and specificity of tests in different centers

Reference	Population	*n*	Age	Gold standard	Sensitivity (%)	Specificity (%)
Biometra (Elisa; crude antigen)						
Valeur [15]	Dyspepsia	HP + :31 HP − :23	6–85(46)	Histology, culture	94	78
Second generation Cobas Core EIA, Roche (ELISA, well or plastic beads; purified antigen)						
Loffeld [6]	Dyspepsia	HP − :54 HP − :13	?	Culture, histology	90.4–90.2	84.6–84.6
Mégraud [8]	Asymptomatic Afrocams	255 adults, 266 children	Adults? Children 9 mo–5 y	Immunoblot	adults: 92 children: 62	children: 90
Valeur [15] (beads)	Dyspepsia	HP + :31 HP − :23	6–85(46)	Histology, culture	90	87
Valeur [15] wells	Dyspepsia	HP + :31 HP − :23	6–85(46)	Histology, culture	97	83
Dako (ELISA, purified antigen)						
Valeur [15]	Dyspepsia	HP + :31 HP − :23	6–85(46)	Histology, culture	84	74
GAP test, BioRad (ELISA, crude antigen)						
Crabtree [2]	Dyspepsia	HP + :82 HP − :54	16–61	Histology	96.3	79.6[a]
Loffeld [6]	Dyspepsia	HP + :54 HP − :13	?	Culture, histology	88.2–89.6	88.8–75
Martelli [7]	Duodenal ulcer	HP + :93 HP − :9	?	Urease, culture	93.5	16.6
Mégraud [8]	Asymptomatic Africans	255 adults, 266 children	Adults? children 9 mo-5 y	Immunoblot	Adults: 90 children 58	Children 77
Schembri [14]	Dyspepsia	HP + :96 HP − :94	?	[b]	83	70
Ventrucci [17]	Dyspepsia	HP + :57 HP − :72	?	Histology corpus, antrum	91	54
Valeur [15]	Dyspepsia	HP + :31 HP − :23	6–85(46)	Histology, culture	84	70
Helico-G, Porton Cambridge (ELISA, crude antigen)						
Loffeld [6]	Dyspepsia	HP + :54 HP − :13	?	Culture, histology	81.5	76.9
Mégraud [8]	Asymptomatic Aricans	255 adults, 266 children	Adults? children 9 mo–5y	Immunoblot	Adults: 88 children 47	Children: 82
Mendall [9]	Dyspepsia	HP + :270 HP − :148	?	Urease, histology	86.7	92.6
Schembri [14]	Dyspepsia	HP + :96 HP − :94	?	– [b]	86	65
Varoli [16]	Dyspepsia	HP + :57 HP − 78	38 + 13 y	Culture, histology	100	80.7
Valeur [15]	Dyspepsia	HP + :31 HP − :23	6–85(46)	Histology, culture	74	78
HEL-p, AMRAD						
Schembri [14]	Dyspepsia	HP + :96 HP − :94	?	– [b]	86	65

(*Cont.*)

Table 2. (*Cont.*)

Reference	Population	*n*	Age	Gold standard	Sensitivity (%)	Specificity (%)
HM-CAP, EPI						
Peacock [11]	Dyspepsia, asymptomatic	HP+:193 HP−:177	?	[^{13}C] urea breath test	98.4	96
Malakit, Biolab (ELISA, purified antigen)						
Denis [3]	Dyspepsia	HP+:59 HP−:35	17–90(49)	Culture + histology	98.3	85.7
Loffeld [6]	Dyspepsia	HP+:54 HP−:13	?	Culture, histology	90.5–90.5	91.6–91.6
Pyloriset, Orion (Latex agglutination; crude antigen)						
Hirschl [4]	Dyspepsia	136	?	Culture + urease + direct examination	90	75.9
Mégraud [8]	Asymptomatic Africans	255 adults, 266 children	Adults? Children 9 mo–5 y	Immunoblot	Adults: 88 children: 47	Children: 89
Riepponen [12]	Dyspepsia	HP+:87 HP−:103	?	Culture, immunoblot	EIA-G: 99 EIA-A: 88	EIA-G: 86 EIA-A: 79
Schembri [14]	Dyspepsia	HP+:96 HP−:94	?	— [b]	92	46
190 Sainz [13]	Dyspepsia	HP+:37 HP−:11	?	Histology, culture, urease	46	82
158 Valeur [15]	Dyspepsia	H+:31 HP−:23	6–85(46)	Histology, culture	84	61
Pyloristat, Whittacker (ELISA, purified antigen)						
Loffeld [6]	Dyspepsia	HP+:54 HP:13	?	Culture, histology	95.8	91.6
Mégraud [8]	Asymptomatic Africans	255 Adults, 266 children	Adults? chindren 9 mo–5 y	Immunoblot	Adults: 96; children: 48	Children: 92
Sainz [13]	Dyspepsia	HP+:37 HP−:11	?	Histology culture, urease	100	82
Valeur [15]	Dyspepsia	HP+:31 HP−:23	6–85(46)	Histology, culture	94	74
RH1 (ELISA, crude antigen)						
Valeur [15]	Dyspepsia	HP+:31 HP−:23	6–85(46)	Histology, culture	97	57
Syn^{elisa}, Elias						
Loffeld [6]	Dyspepsia	HP+:54 HP−:13	?	Culture, histology	84.3	81.8

[a] Two histology negative patients who were positive serologically had a positive immunoblot. Excluding these 83% patients from analysis improves sepcificity to 83%.
[b] Culture plus at least one of phase contrast microscopy, histopathology, urease.

second-generation kits generally obtain better results than first-generation kits. Intra-assay variability is low, especially for the Malakit and Roche tests. In Schembri's study [14], sensitivities vary from 78% to 86%, specificities are low (46%–70%). Valeur's results [15] have been rearranged to permit a clear comparison of first- and second-generation kits. Sensitivity is above 90% for all the tested second generation kits, but only for one-third of the first-generation kits. Specificity is lower, especially for first-generation kits. Again, only one-third of the first-generation kits have a specificity higher than the lowest second-generation kit specificity. In this large batch of tests, no single test was able correctly to diagnose all the patients. All HP positive patients were seropositive in at least one test.

Mégraud [8] gave an interesting approach of the influence of the population on the performance of the tests. He used a series of commercial kits to test African sera. Unfortunately, since these were all asymptomatic individuals, performing endoscopy was judged unethical. The gold standard in this study is therefore immunoblot, which is not optimal. This probably explains the observed low sensitivity and specificity of urea breath test in a subpopulation of the tested children. Nevertheless, it is obvious that the test perform less well in African children than in an adult Western population, underscoring the necessity for calibrating the test to the specific population studies.

An overview of the results in different centers is summarized in Table 2. Remarkable is the dramatic diversity of the performance of the same tests in different centers; if anything, these results prove that it is essentially impossible to compare them, once again stressing the need for standardization of the techniques.

We can conclude that HP serology today is a good test, with generally high sensitivity and good specificity. Although some first-generation kits are excellent, second-generation kits using purfiied antigens usually are more accurate. A positive HP serology is an indication that something is going on in the patient's stomach, which is worthwhile investigating using endoscopy and biopsies. Standardization of the techniques is a key problem that needs to be solved in the near future.

References

1. Crabtree JE, Miller G, Taylor JD et al. (1991) Mucosal and systemic humoral responses to *Helicobacter pylori* in patients with gastric cancer. Ital J Gastroenterol 23 [9, Suppl 2]: 5
2. Crabtree JE, Shalcross TM, Heatley RV, Wyatt JI (1991) Evaluation of Bio-Rad GAP IgG quantitative ELISA for serodiagnosis of *Helicobacter pylori* infection. Ital J Gastroenterol 23 [9, Suppl 2]: 21
3. Denis P, De Koster E, Nyst JF et al. (1991) Evaluation of 'Malakit *Helicobacter pylori*', a new kit for HP serology. Ital J Gastroenterol 23 [9, Suppl 2]: 21–22
4. Hirschl AM, Berger J, Hirschl MM, Rotter ML (1991) The value of the 'Pyloriset' – test for serological diagnosis of *Helicobacter pylori* in treated and untreated patients. Ital J Gastroenterol 23 [9, Suppl 2]: 23
5. Karnes WE Jr, Samloff IM, Siurala M et al. (1991) Positive serum antibody and negative tissue staining for *Helicobacter pylori* in subjects with atrophic body gastritis. Gastroenterology 101: 167–174

6. Loffeld RJLF, Stobberingh E (1991) Comparison of seven commercial assays for detection of IgG antibodies against *Helicobacter pylori*. Ital J Gastroenterol 23 [9, Suppl 2]: 24
7. Martelli P, Modolo ML, Crovatto M et al. (1991) Reliability of ELISA in detecting *Helicobacter pylori* antibodies in duodenal ulcer patients. Ital J Gastroenterol 23 [9, Suppl 2]: 24
8. Mégraud F, Bouchard S, Mayo K, Camou C (1991) Comparison of serodiagnostic kits for *Helicobacter pylori* detection using sera from Africa. Ital J Gastroenterol 23 [9, Suppl 2]: 25
9. Mendall MA, Goggin PM, Bellhouse A et al. (1991) Performance of a commercially available serological test for *H. pylori*. Ital J Gastroenterol 23 [9, Suppl 2]: 25
10. Newell DG, Hawtin PR, Stacey AR et al. (1991) Estimation of prevalence of *Helicobacter pylori* infection in an asymptomatic elderly population comparing [(14)C] urea breath test and serology. J Clin Pathol 44: 385–387
11. Peacock (1991)
12. Riepponen (1991)
13. Sainz S, Navarro F, Monés et al. (1991) Comparative study of two serological techniques (IgG-ELISA and Latex kits) for diagnosing *Helicobacter pylori* infection. Ital J Gastroenterol 23 [9, Suppl 2]: 27
14. Schembri MA, Lambert JR, Lin SK, Nicholson L, Korman MG (1991) Comparison of four serological diagnostic test for *Helicobacter pylori* antibodies. Ital J Gastroenterol 23 [9, Suppl 2]: 27
15. Valeur AK, Andersen LP (1991) Comparison of nine kits for *Helicobacter pylori* antibody detection. Ital J Gastroenterol 23 [9, Suppl 2]: 28
16. Varoli O, Sambri V, Tucci A, Corinaldesi R, Stanghellini V, Paparo GF (1991) Evaluation of 'Helico-G' EIA kit in the serology of *Helicobacter pylori*. Ital J Gastroenterol 23 [9, Suppl 2]: 28
17. Ventrucci (1991)

Standards for Serologic Study of Infection with *Helicobacter pylori*

R. Feldman, S.J.W. Evans, J. Deeks, B. Rathbone, and The *Helicobacter pylori* Serology Study Group

Introduction

Helicobacter pylori serology is now readily available as a result of the development of sero-diagnostic commercial kits. Since adult sera and most frequently tested, it seemed useful to have standards with which to understand adult serogic results. At the meeting of the European Helicobacter Study Group in Toledo, Spain, in 1990, it was suggested that it would be useful to coordinate efforts for standardisation of *H. pylori* serology and to have a cooperative study including those who were involved in antigen production, and the commercial companies.

One of the present authors (B.R.) collected sera from patients coming to a gastroenterology clinic in Leicester in early 1991; he also carried out the clinical investigations. Each patient had three antral biopsies and one body biopsy taken. One antral biopsy was frozen, another was used for a CLO test, and an antral and a body biopsy were sent to one pathologist experienced in identifying *H. pylori* without knowledge of the CLO test. The clinical status is based on the CLO and histology data. All those classified as *H. pylori* negative patients were CLO negative, had normal gastric histology, and had no identifiable *H. pylori* on histology. The patients were selected so that about half were classed as positive and half as negative for *H. pylori*. It was planned to have up to ten patients in each category; in the event a total of 13 were available, seven positive and six negative. Information about patients' age and sex is given in Table 1.

The selection of the laboratories involved in this comparative study was made by identification of individuals interested in participation. Many laboratories were not included because of oversight, because they were not interested, or because they were asked too late in the process. I apologise to any who volunteered but did not receive the sera. The persons and laboratories included in the study is shown in Fig. 3. Individuals participating in the serologic standardisation study, with the names of the antigens used, were the following:

Mr. W. Boteler: Pylostat, FIAX Pylo G, Whittaker
Dr. H. Goossens: Roche Bead
Dr. D. Gassner: Roche MTP, Roche Bead
Dr. D.Y. Graham: E-Z-EM ELISA
Mr. V.M. Haiva: Pylori-set IgG ELISA

London Hospital Medical College, London, UK Leicester Royal Infirmary, Leicester, UK

Gasbarrini/Pretolani (Eds.)
Basic and Clinical Aspects of H. pylori Infection

Table 1. Sera used in the serologic standardisation study

Sample	Status	Sex	Age (years)
1	+	M	53
2	+	M	28
3	+	F	61
4	+	F	56
5	+	F	61
6	+	M	21
7	+	M	49
8	–	F	40
9	–	F	62
10	–	M	37
11	–	F	42
12	–	F	31
13	–	M	44

Dr. M.L. Kiene: Biometra ELISA
Dr. J.C. Sanz-Moreno: Helico G
Dr. G. Sheppard: Helico G
Dr. L.P. Anderson: RH ELISA, DAKO ELISA, RH western blot
Dr. A.M. Hirschl: house ELISA, Roche Bead, Helico G, Pylori-set-Latex-G
Dr. F. Megraud: house ELISA, Roche MTP, Pylostat, Helico G, IBlot
Dr. M.J. Blaser: house ELISA
Dr. M.A. Daw/C. O'Morain: house ELISA
Dr. M. Van Duijn/Pena: house ELISA
Dr. A.F. Mentis: house ELISA
Dr. E. Stobberingh: house ELISA
Dr. T. Wadstrom: house ELISA

Serum Collection and Handling

From each of the 13 patients, sera were separated into ampoules at Leicester and the ampoules stored at $-20°C$. It was neither possible nor economic for each laboratory to receive several replicates of serum from each patient. The amount of serum was sufficient for about 25–30 specimens each.

The design of the study had two aspects: firstly to examine the results of each laboratory on each of a range of patients; secondly to examine the within-laboratory variability of the results for both positive and negative patients. Thus the 17 laboratories received 25 coded ampoules. A single ampoule from each of the 13 patients and two sets of six replicates of two sera, one positive and one negative. The ampoules were coded so that the laboratories did not know which ampoule came from which patient, using a random numbering system.

Shipment of the sera was by courier on dry ice, so that handling and storage problems were minimised, and only one freeze-thaw cycle used.

The reporting of results utilises a code for each participating laboratory, and for each test procedure used. Although there were 17 laboratories, some used only one test while others used up to five.

Statistical Methods

The results from centres and tests are reported in different units and are likely to have systematic differences. To make comparisons between tests and centres using different methods, the results must be standardised. Titre results have a skewed distribution, so we have looked at log values of the results, which have a more symmetrical distribution. The results are expressed in terms of standard deviations above or below the mean titre for the 13 single samples from all patients' sera, calculated separately for each laboratory and test.

Most results, on a log scale, are shown as box plots, where a line in the box indicates the median, with the upper and lower quartiles (75th, 25th per centiles) at the edges of the box, and 'whiskers' drawn to the maximum and minimum values. These diagrams show the centre, spread and shape of the distribution of the results for easy comparison.

Results

This report concerns three aspects of the work done by the participating laboratories: (a) the ability of a laboratory to reproduce results, using replicates of sera, (b) the agreement of centres using the same test, for all 13 sera, and (c) the agreement of results over all centres and tests for each sera.

Examples of the variability of the laboratory reports with replicates, standardised as indicated above, are shown in a series of box plots in Figs. 1–3. In general, although there were some differences, reproducibility was not a problem, either with house ELISAs or commercial kits. No account has been taken of the numbers of tests done on each ampoule. Some laboratories report the mean of two tests for each serum, some report the mean of four tests, and some report an individual result. We are reporting only on the reproducibility of the laboratory results, rather than a test result. The use of replicate measurements reduces random measurement error, and tends to improve the result for a particular laboratory/test. Comparisons should then be made with care as we do not have full details on the number of replicate measurements in all cases.

For a few of the commercial kits were there several users. These results, shown in Fig. 4, although too few to be able to quantify statistically with any precision, did show that there were some differences in reported titres. However, the titre differences by different users of the same test did not affect whether a serum was identified as positive or negative. The agreement on positive or negative results was very high. Further work, with more laboratories using the same kits, is needed to make more meaningful comments from such studies.

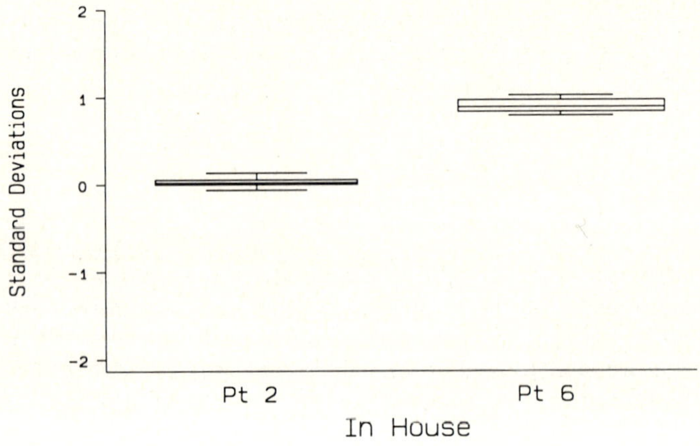

a

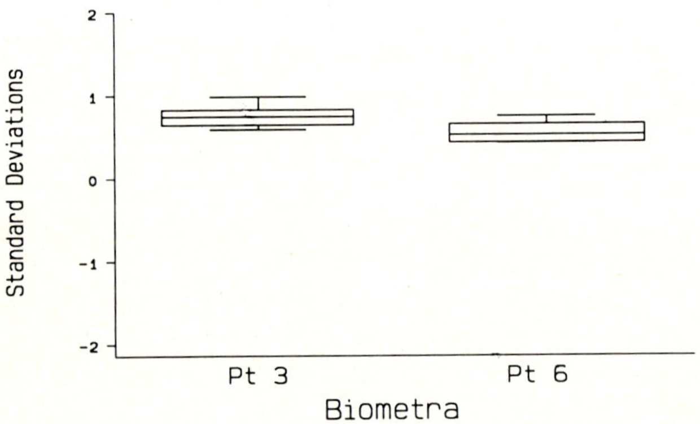

b

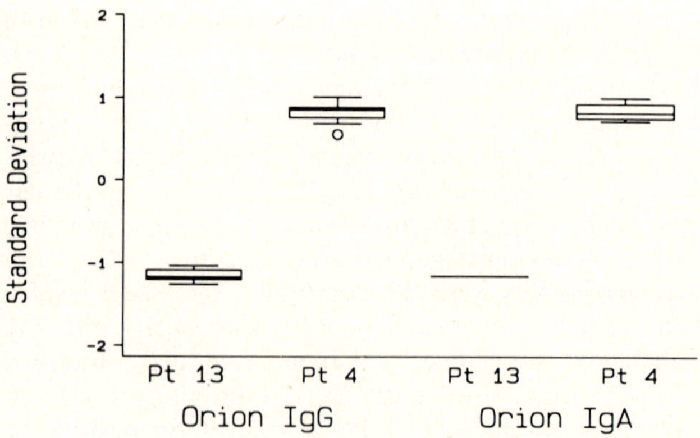

c

Fig. 1a–c. Serum titres with six replicates each, shown as box plots for each patient and test (results were log transformed and standardised). **a** Centre 3. **b** Centre 7. **c** Centre 9

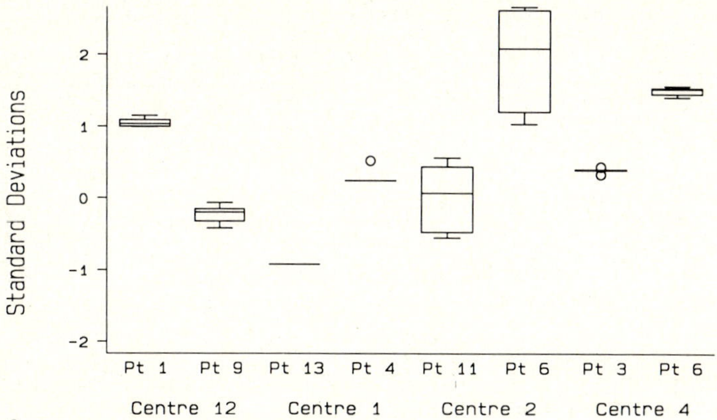

a

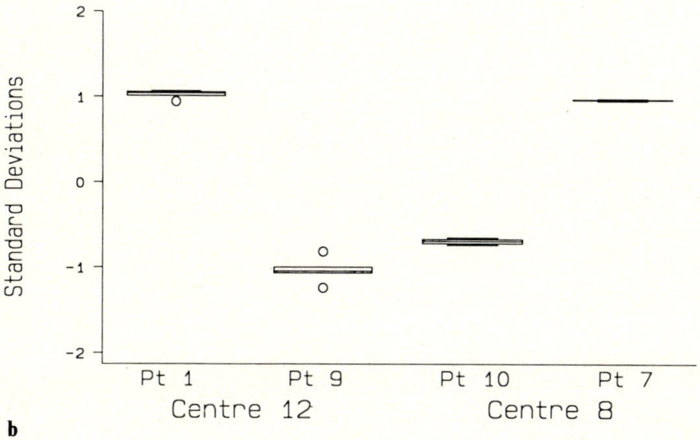

b

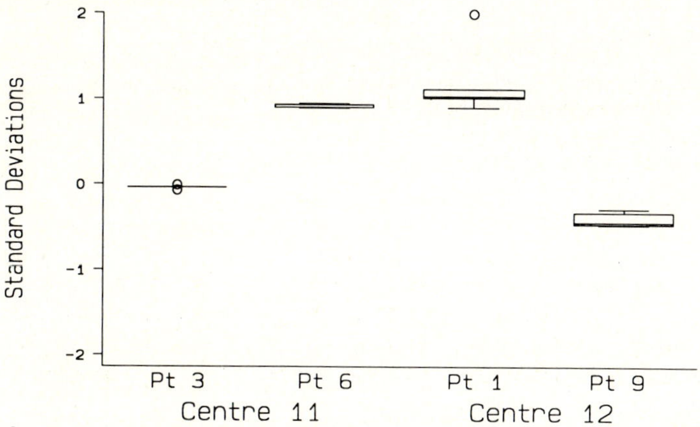

c

Fig. 2a–c. Serum titres with six replicates each, shown as box plots for each patient and centre (results were log transformed and standardised). **a** Helico-G tests. **b** Roche MTP tests. **c** Whittaker tests

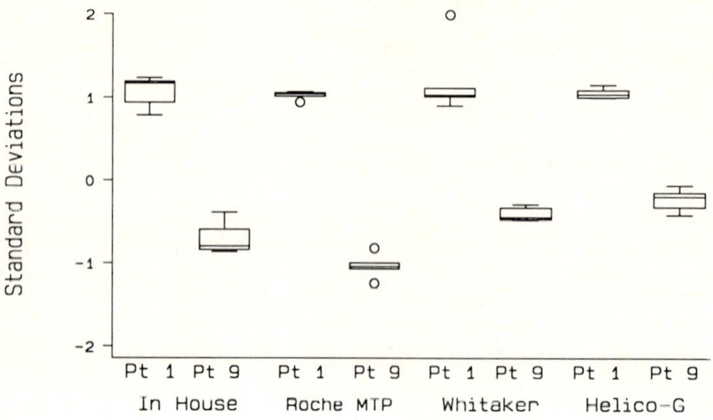

a

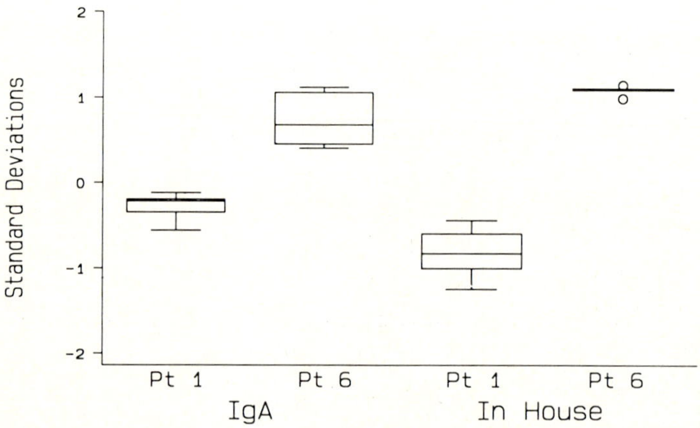

b

Fig. 3a, b. Serum titres with six replicates each, shown as box plots for each patient and test (results were log transformed and standarised). **a** Centre 12. **b** Centre 15

Each test showed several sera with high values, several with low values, and two sera in a very zone. We have selected three patients on the basis of this classification, and show standardised results for each laboratory and test (Fig. 5). The comparability of all antigens in identification of a serum with a high titre and a serum with a low titre was noteworthy. However, the titre in the grey zone was a problem for some tests.

Fig. 4a–c. Serology on sera from 13 patients with different tests. **a** Helico-G ELISA. **b** Roche MTP. **c** Whittaker ELISA

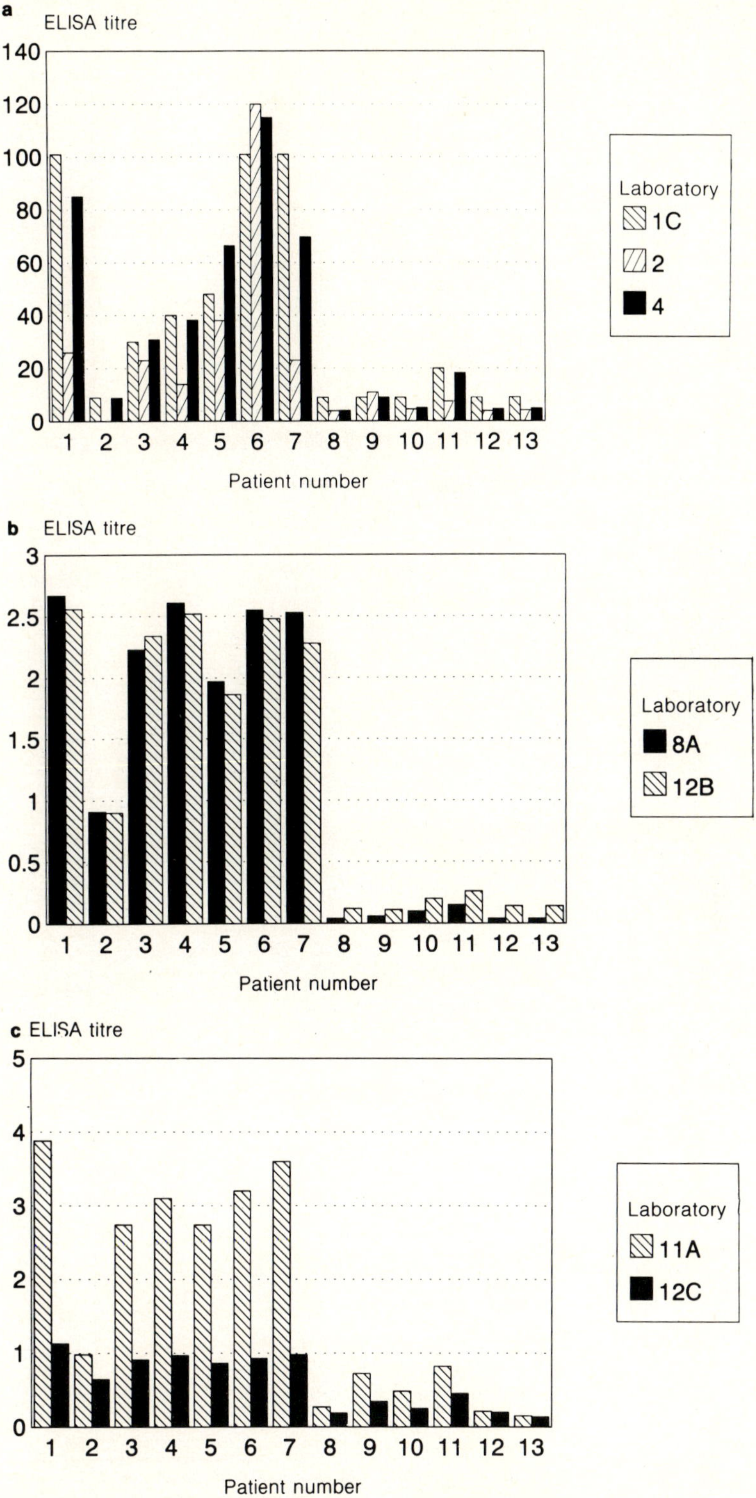
a
ELISA titre
140
120
100
80
60
40
20
0
1 2 3 4 5 6 7 8 9 10 11 12 13
Patient number
Laboratory
1C
2
4
b
ELISA titre
3
2.5
2
1.5
1
0.5
0
1 2 3 4 5 6 7 8 9 10 11 12 13
Patient number
Laboratory
8A
12B
c
ELISA titre
5
4
3
2
1
0
1 2 3 4 5 6 7 8 9 10 11 12 13
Patient number
Laboratory
11A
12C

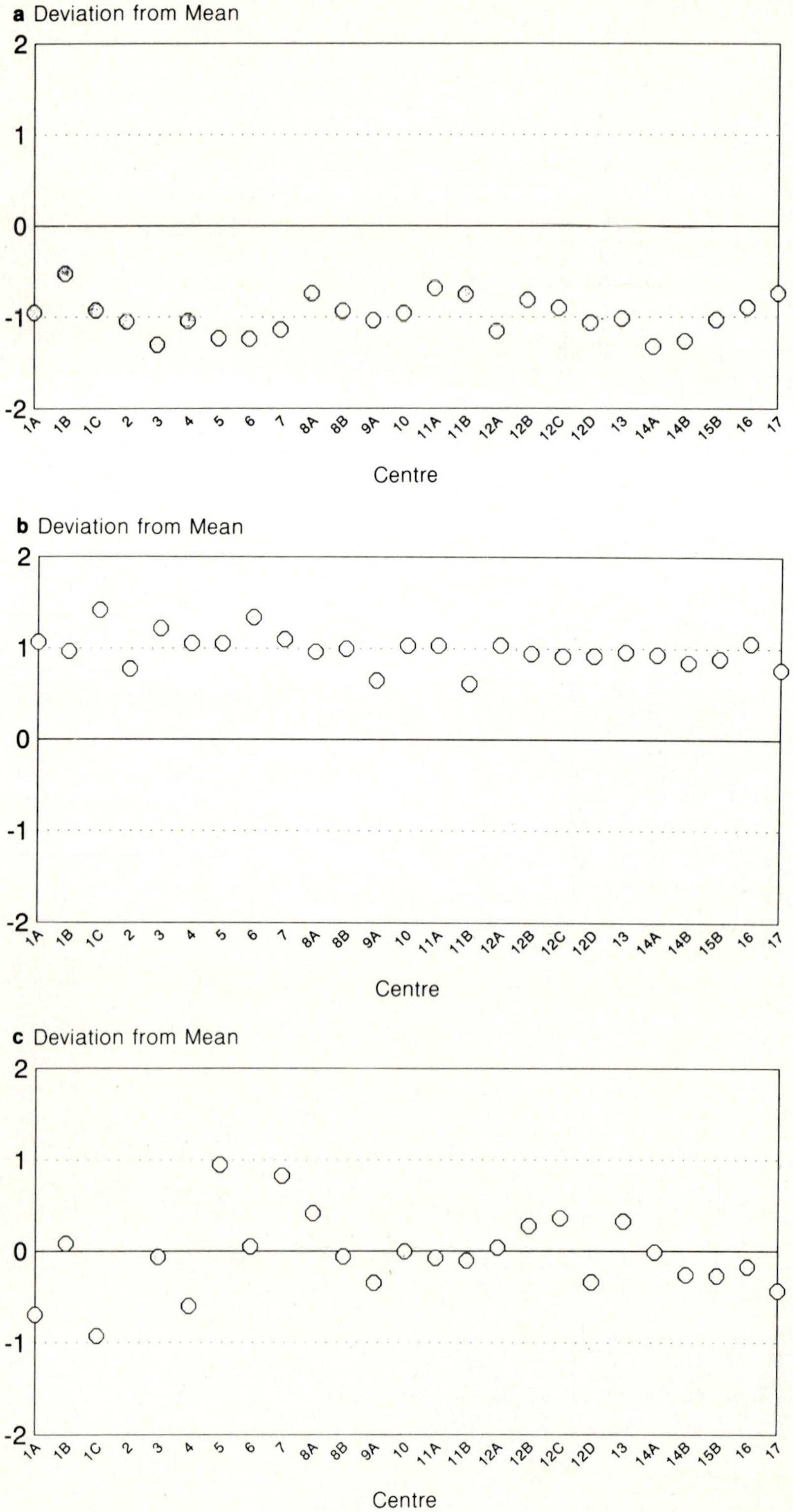
a Deviation from Mean
2
1
0
-1
-2
1A 1B 1C 2 3 4 5 6 7 8A 8B 9A 10 11A 11B 12A 12B 12C 12D 13 14A 14B 15B 16 17
Centre
b Deviation from Mean
2
1
0
-1
-2
1A 1B 1C 2 3 4 5 6 7 8A 8B 9A 10 11A 11B 12A 12B 12C 12D 13 14A 14B 15B 16 17
Centre
c Deviation from Mean
2
1
0
-1
-2
1A 1B 1C 2 3 4 5 6 7 8A 8B 9A 10 11A 11B 12A 12B 12C 12D 13 14A 14B 15B 16 17
Centre

Conclusions

From the results, we conclude that:

- The cooperation of the laboratories was excellent.
- The cooperation of commercial firms is essential.
- All antigens identified high positives and low negatives.
- Some tests were better than others for titres in the grey zone.
- Standardisation to compare tests is possible.
- The European Helicobacter Society could coordinate such developments.
- Standards for children and IgA are also needed.

Acknowledgements. To obtain sufficient fund to pay for serum collection, handling, vialing, statistical advice, and shipment, a letter was sent to many of the commercial companies involved in kit production. From the large number of letters sent, only three companies, Roche, Porton Cambridge, and Orion agreed to send contributions, without which none of the work could have been completed. An additional grant came from the European Helicobacter Study Group itself.

Fig. 5a–c. Variation in standardised serum titres using many different tests. **a** Patient 10. **b** Patient 7. **c** Patient 2.

Helicobacter pylori Antigenic Preparations

A.R. Stacey

Introduction

The ultimate goal of any serodiagnostic assay must be 100% sensitivity and specificity although this is not realistic. To date, commercially available tests reproducibly give figures of greater than 90%. Increased specificity may be achieved by removing cross-reacting proteins from a pool of *H. pylori* antigenic material using a variety of purification techniques. However, as antigens are increasingly purified, a decrease in sensitivity may be observed. When fast protein liquid chromatography (FPLC) purified fractions of *H. pylori* were used as serodiagnostic antigens for a group of 45 patients (22 *H. pylori* positive and 23 *H. pylori* negative patients as determined by culture and [^{14}C] urea breath test) a decrease in sensitivity was observed [16]. However, the sensitivity was restored to 100% when selected fractions were recombined in an pooled antigen (Table 1).

An alternative approach is selectively to enrich an antigen pool with proteins which give a good specificity when used as serodiagnostic antigens. Hirschl et al. [9] found that when proteins eluted from polyacrylamide gel electrophoresis following separation of the denatured crude antigens were used as ELISA antigens, better discrimination between sera from *H. pylori* positive and negative patients was achieved with the higher molecular weight polypeptides. In particular, good discrimination was obtained with protein 8 (106 kDa) and protein 9 (128 kDa, which is probably the 120 kDa species specific protein). In more recent work Hirschl et al. [10] found that the addition of this polypeptide to an acid extract antigen improved the sensitivity and specificity of the both antigens when used individually (Table 2).

Gassner et al. [7] have developed a multi-component antigen with increased levels of urease and reduced levels of potentially cross-reactive flagellin antigens. This antigen now forms the basis of an improved second generation anti-*H. pylori* IgG enzyme immunoassay.

For this type of work to progress further identification of the immunodominant antigens of *H. pylori* and the development of methods for their large-scale production is essential. This is turn requires bulk culture of *H. pylori*. Newell et al. [15] have identified the conditions and regimen for continuous culture of *H. pylori* in a chemostat system. Chemostat-cultured organisms have been shown to be antigenically identical to plate-grown organisms [15]. Having

PHLS Centre for Applied Microbiology and Research, Porton Down, Salisbury SP4 0JG, UK

Gasbarrini/Pretolani (Eds.)
Basic and Clinical Aspects of H. pylori Infection

Table 1. Sensitivity and specificity of *H. pylori* antigenic preparations

	Sensitivity (%)	Specificity (%)
Acid extract	100	100
FPLC fractions 14/15 (urease)	91	91
FPLC fraction 16	87	100
FPLC fractions 17/18 (flagella/catalase)	83	100
FPLC fraction 19	83	100
Pooled FPLC fractions (14–21)	100	82

Table 2. Sensitivity and specificity of *H. pylori* antigen preparations (from [10])

	Sensitivity (%)	Specificity (%)
Acid Extract	70	98
120 kDa polypeptide	84	98
Acid Extract + 120 kDa polypeptide	97	100

established the large-scale production of crude antigenic material, a capability for large-scale downstream processing and purification is also required. The most common purification techniques in use today are chromatography-based using gel filtration and ion-exchange columns. Despite the large array of *H. pylori* proteins and considerable patient-to-patient variation associated with this disease a number of polypeptides are frequently detected. Several *H. pylori* proteins have already been purified, either partially or completely. Some proteins have also been cloned and sequenced, including urease [1], the 120-kDa polypeptide [2] and catalase [14]. Many of these are potentially useful as serodiagnostic antigens and their individual attributes are discussed below.

Urease

H. pylori urease is apparently species specific and consequently must be considered as an important antigen for serodiagnosis. FPLC-purified urease containing material, when used as an ELISA antigen, was found to be both 91% sensitive and specific. Other urease-containing preparations including the high molecular weight cell associated protein HM-CAP antigen [5] also have high sensitivities and specificities. However, these antigens are not pure urease since they contain at least two major proteins. Urease, affinity purified with monoclonal antibodies, was found to be only 83% sensitive. These data show that whilst urease is a specific antigen the sensitivity obtained is often lower than when a complex antigen is used, presumably because not all patients produce anti-urease antibodies.

120-kDa Polypeptide

This antigen is also species specific; however, it is present only in approximately 80% of strains. As mentioned above, enrichment of the proportion of this antigen within a complex antigen increases the specificity and sensitivity of this antigen combination. This antigen is recognised at the mucosal level [3] and may be associated with the severity of disease. Interestingly, antibodies raised against this antigen are long lived, showing very little decrease in staining by western blotting following *H. pylori* eradication by treatment [17].

Cytotoxin

The cytotoxin has received much attention over the past few months. It shares molecular weight with the 120-kDa polypeptide and is produced by up to 80% of strains. However, the methods of detection for these two antigens are quite different, and hence it not possible at this time to say that they are the same protein. The cytotoxin is detectable only in functional vacuolization assays using cell lines such as HeLa [4] or Vero [11]. Anti-cytotoxin antibodies are detected by their ability to inhibit cytotoxin-induced vacuolization or by immunoblotting. Immunostaining of the 120-kDa polypeptide released into broth culture supernatants by toxin-producing strains showed that only 67% of *H. pylori* positive patients had antibodies that recognised this antigen. This test was 96% specific. Interestingly cytotoxin producing strains are associated with more severe disease [4].

Flagella and the Flagella Sheath Material

Very little work has been done on the characterization of the flagella sheath material. It contains the three major polypeptides of 61-, 54- and 29-kDa and is believed to be an extension of the outer membrane. Two of the polypeptides, of 61- and 29-kDa, are the urease polypeptides, whilst the 54-kDa is likely to correspond to the flagellin. Previous work has shown all of these polypeptides to be immunogenic [12], however, some cross-reactions with the flagella of *Campylobacter jejuni* may be observed [13].

56-kDa Polypeptide

This immunogenic polypeptide is closely associated with the urease enzyme; however, it is not necessary for enzyme activity. It is believed to act as a chaperonin in the transport, assembly and stability of the enzyme on the external cell surface. This polypeptide has now been shown to share up to 80% homology with the family of heat-shock proteins. Cross-reactivity between *H. pylori* and antisera raised against the 65-kDa heat-shock protein of *Mycobacterium leprea* has been observed [6], demonstrating the sharing of some antigenic determinants. Consequently this polypeptide has the potential for cross-reactivity and may therefore be unsuitable as a serodiagnostic antigen. However, its presence in the FPLC-derived urease material [16] does not appear adversely to affect the specificity or sensitivity of this urease preparation.

Catalase

H. pylori also produces a catalase enzyme which has been identified with monoclonal antibodies by western blotting as a 54-kDa polypeptide. Recently the enzyme has been cloned and sequenced and been shown be a tetramer with individual units of 54-kDa [14]. Purified native enzyme, courtesy of Hazell et al. [8], when used as an ELISA antigen was 100% specific but only 22% sensitive [14].

15-kDa Polypeptide

This polypeptide forms a prominent band in the total protein profile of *H. pylori* and is immunogenic as revealed by immunoblotting studies. Monoclonal antibodies have been raised against this polypeptide and used to affinity purify for use in an ELISA system. In this assay 83% sensitivity and 93% specificity was obtained (Stacey et al., unpublished data).

Immunoblot analysis of the total anti-*H. pylori* immunoglobulin response confirms the antigenicity of these proteins. However, the antigenic specificity varies with immunoglobulin class and subclass. Stacey et al. [17] observed that IgG1 and IgA antibodies react with the majority of *H. pylori* antigens present in a crude antigenic pool, but fail to react with the lower molecular weight antigens in the range of 15–20 kDa. Conversely, IgG2 antibodies fail to react with the 120-kDa polypeptide. Interestingly, the response to this polypeptide is long-lived and can still be detected in sera from patients up to 1 year following eradication [17]. Evidence such as this suggests that different antigens pools are needed for different uses. Antigens which evoke long-lived responses should not be used to monitor treatment. However, these antigens could be of use for epidemiological studies where evidence of current or previous infection is required.

The use of immunoblotting to study the antigenic specificity suggests that there are several antigenic polypeptides which have not been formally identified. Some of these may be of potential serodiagnostic use, but it must be borne in mind that antigens used in immunoblotting are not in their native three-dimensional state, having been denatured by chemical denaturation and boiling. Equally, there is a large assumption that organisms grown in vitro are antigenically identical to those found in vivo.

However, the information available to date suggests that several antigens should be incorporated into a multi-component antigen which could include the 120-, 61- and 28-kDa polypeptides of the urease enzyme and the 15-kDa polypeptide.

References

1. Clayton CL, Pallen MJ, Kleanthous H, Wren BW, Tabaqcchali S (1989) Molecular cloning and sequencing of *Helicobacter pylori* urease genes and detection of *H. pylori* using the polymerase chain reaction technique. In: Malfertheiner P, Ditschnuneit H (eds) *Helicobacter pylori*, gastritis and peptic ulcer. Springer, Berlin Heidelberg New York, pp 74–80
2. Clayton CL, Kleanthous H, Herrmann J, Jacobs E, Kist M, Tabaqcchali S (1989) Molecular cloning of immunodominant antigen epitopes of *Helicobacter pylori* for development of a specific ELISA to diagnose *H. pylori* infection. In: Malfertheiner P, Ditschuneit H (eds) *Helicobacter pylori*, Gastritis and peptic ulcer. Springer, Berlin Heidelberg New York, pp 167–171
3. Crabtree JE, Taylor JD, Wyatt JI, Heatley RV, Shallcross TM, Tompkins DS, Rathbone BJ (1991) Mucosal IgA Recognition of *Helicobacter pylori* 120 kDa protein, peptic ulceration and gastric pathology. Lancet 338: 332–335
4. Cover TL, Dooley CP, Blaser MJ (1990) Characterization of and human serologic responses to proteins in *Helicobacter pylori* broth culture supernatants with vacuolizing cytotoxin activity. Infect Immun 58: 603–610
5. Evans DJ, Evans DG, Graham DY, Klein PD (1989) A sensitive and specific serologic test for detection of *Camplyobacter pylori* infection. Gastroenterology 96: 1004–1008
6. Evans DJ, Evans DG, Engstrand L, Graham DY (1991) The 62 K urease-associated protein of *Helicobacter pylori* is a heat-shock protein. Ital J Gastroenterol 23 [Suppl 2]: 30
7. Gassner D, Dreismann H (1991) Second generation antigen-based enzyme immunoassays for serodiagnosis of *Helicobacter pylori* – a fast and reliable alternative to invasive methods. Ital J Gastroenterol 23 [Suppl 2]: 22
8. Hazell SL, Evans DJ Jr, Graham DY (1991) *Helicobacter pylori* catalase. J Gen Microbiol 137(1): 57–61
9. Hirschl AM, Pletschette M, Hirschi MH, Berger J, Stanek G, Rotter ML (1988) Comparison of different antigen preparations in an evaluation of the immune responses to *Campylobacter pylori*. Eur J Clin Microbiol Infect Dis 7: 570–575
10. Hirschl AM, Rathbone BJ, Wyatt JI, Berger J, Rotter ML (1990) Comparison of ELISA antigen preparations alone or in combination for serodiagnosing *Helicobacter pylori* infections. J Clin Pathol 43: 511–513
11. Leunk RD, Ferguson MA, Morgan DR, Low DE, Simor AE (1990) Antibody to cytotoxin in infection by *Helicobacter pylori*. J Clin Microbiol 28: 1181–1184
12. Newell DG (1987) Human serum antibody responses to the surface protein antigens of *Campylobacter pyloridis*. Serodiag Immunother 1: 209–217
13. Newell DG (1987) Identification of the outer membrane proteins of *Campylobacter pyloridis* and antigenic cross-reactivity between *C. pyloridis* and *C. jejuni*. J Gen Microbiol 133: 163–170
14. Newell DG, Nuijten P, Stacey AR, Hazell SL (1991) The cloning, sequencing and antigenicity of *Helicobacter pylori* catalase. Italian J Gastroenterol 23 [Suppl 2]: 7
15. Newell DG, Lee FK, Hudson MJ (1991) The continuous culture of *Helicobacter pylori*: expression of surface antigen and use for serodiagnosis. Ital J Gastroenterol 23 [Suppl 2]: 44
16. Stacey AR, Hawtin PR, Newell DG (1990) Antigenicity of fractions of *Helicobacter pylori* prepared by fast protein liquid chromatography and urease captured by monoclonal antibodies. Eur J Clin Microbiol Infect Dis 9: 732–737
17. Stacey AR, Bell GD, Newell DG (1991) The value of class and subclass ELISA's and antibody specificity in monitoring treatment of *Helicobacter pylori*. Ital J Gastroenterol 23 [Suppl 2]: 9

The Value of Class and Subclass ELISAs and Antibody Specificity in Monitoring Treatment of *Helicobacter pylori*

A.R. Stacey[1], G.D. Bell[2], and D.G. Newell[3]

Serology has been proposed as a non-invasive test for the monitoring of treatment to eradicate *Helicobacter pylori* infection. However, the total IgG response associated with this chronic mucosal infection is generally long lived. Preliminary data [3] suggested that certain IgG subclasses had a shorter life and were better indicators of successful treatment. Moreover, some antigens would be expected preferentially to induce antibody responses with shorter half-lives. Therefore the persistence of patient serum anti-*H. pylori* class and subclass responses was investigated in sequential samples from both successfully and unsuccessfully treated patients followed over a 12-month period. In addition, the antigen specificity of these antibodies was studied using western blotting techniques.

Materials and Methods

Sixty patients were diagnosed as being *H. pylori* positive on the basis of culture, rapid urease test and/or histology of antral biopsy specimens. Patients were then treated with antimicrobial agents. [^{14}C] urea breath tests [1] were performed pre-treatment and at 1, 3, 6 and 12 months post-treatment to monitor *H. pylori* status on 32 successfully and 28 unsuccessfully treated patients. Matching serum samples were taken and stored at $-20°C$ until assayed for total circulating anti-*H. pylori* immunoglobulin concentration using the method of Stacey et al. [4]. The levels of IgA antibodies were assessed using the same techniques substituting goat anti-human IgA heavy-chain peroxidase conjugate (Dako 1:1000) as the detection antisera. The levels of the IgG subclasses IgG1, IgG2 and IgG4 were assessed by incubation with monoclonal anti-subclass reagents followed by incubation with sheep anti-mouse Ig peroxidase conjugate as previously described [5].

Western blots were performed using acid-extractable material [2] separated by SDS-PAGE and blotted onto nitrocellulose. Bound antibodies were detected using the same detection systems as for the ELISAs.

[1] PHLS Centre for Applied Microbiology and Research, Porton Down, Salisbury SP4 0JG, UK
[2] Department of Medicine, Ipswich Hospital, Ipswich IP4 5PD, UK
[3] Central Veterinary Laboratory, Weybridge KT15 3NB, UK

Gasbarrini/Pretolani (Eds.)
Basic and Clinical Aspects of H. pylori Infection

Results

By 1 month post-treatment the median total immunoglobulin level had fallen by 50% in the successfully treated patients (Fig. 1a). This median level decreased still further during the following 11 months of the study. By 12 months after successful treatment the median immunoglobulin level had fallen from 65.3 to 5.8 μg/ml. This trend was also seen in the IgG1 subclass levels. The median IgG2 and IgG4 antibodies levels suggest very little change, however, in patients in whom an IgG2 or IgG4 response was detected prior to treatment the response to treatment was rapid falling by over 200% in the first month post-treatment. The decrease in IgA levels was less rapid and less marked, falling by less than 50% over the 12-month study period.

In the unsuccessfully treated group a slight reduction in the median total immunoglobulin, IgG2 and IgG4 antibody levels occurred 1 month following treatment, but this effect was reversed during the following 5 months (Fig. 1b). By the end of the study period no significant decrease in median antibody levels of all the classes and subclasses was observed, with the possible exception of IgG2, where the median levels were slightly lower 6 months post-treatment than pre-treatment. The median IgA antibody level increased during the course of this study.

The variations in the patterns of antibody staining for *H. pylori* antigens following successful and unsuccessful treatment was studied by western blotting (Fig. 2). Sequential sera from successfully treated patients showed a gradual decrease in the intensity of staining for a large number of polypeptides, parti-

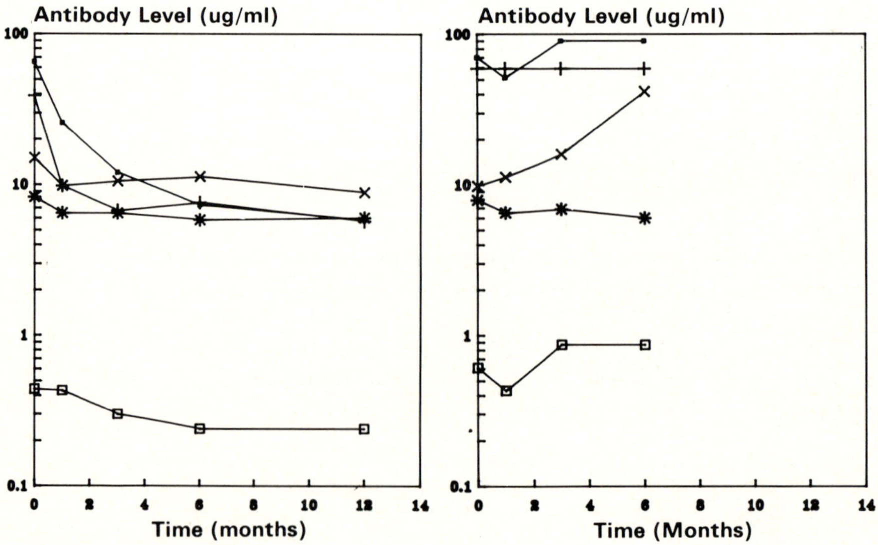

Fig. 1. Median levels (expressed as μg/ml) of total immunoglobulin (—●—), and IgG1 (—|—), IgG2 (—*—), IgG4 (—□—) and IgA (—*—) antibodies in 32 successfully treated (**a**) and unsuccessfully treated (**b**) patients

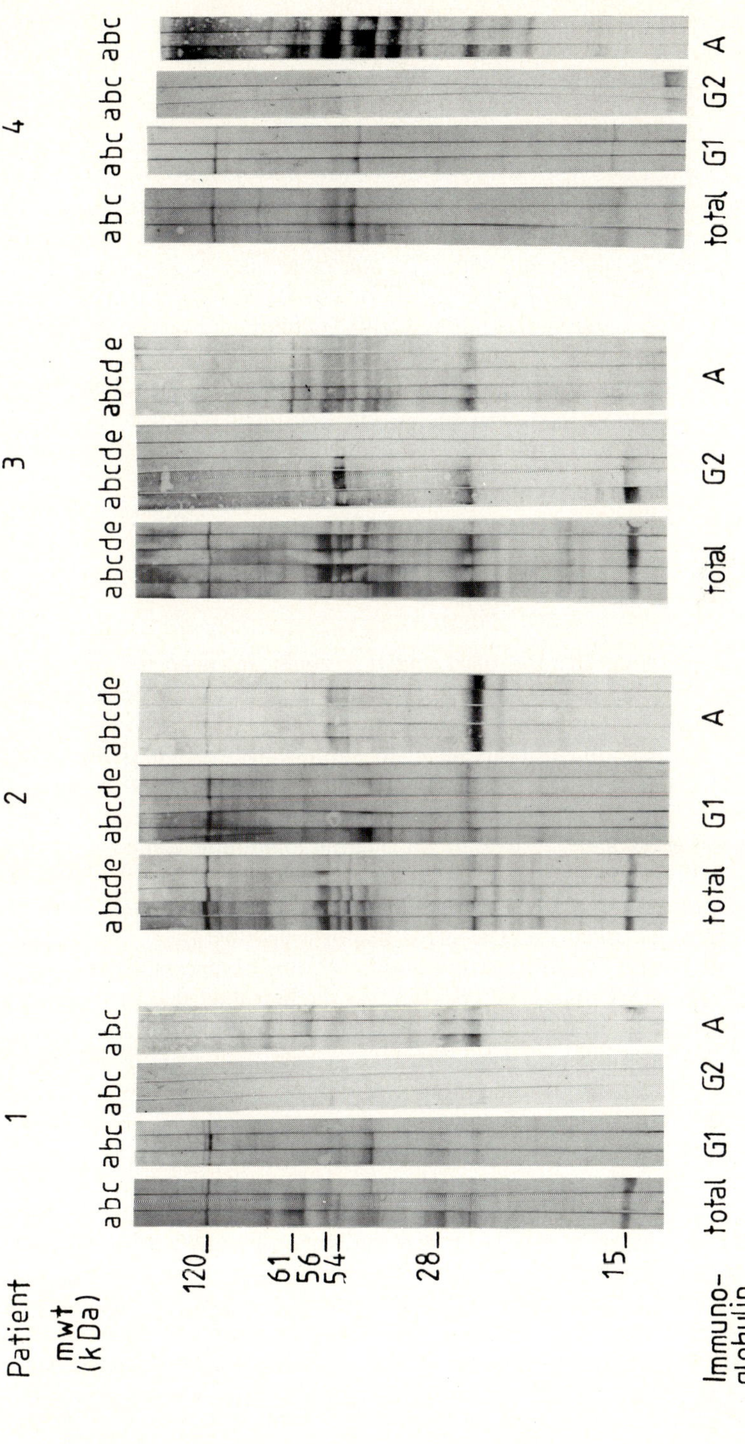

Fig. 2. Antigenic specificity of sequential sera from four successfully treated patients showing variations in staining patterns with immunoglobulin class and subclass. Sera were taken pre-treatment **(a)**, and 1 month **(b)**, 3 months **(c)**, 6 months **(d)** and 12 months **(e)** post-treatment

cularly in the range of 50–61 kDa, including the urease, flagellin and catalase antigens. However, some polypeptides including the 120- and 15-kDa polypeptides, were detected even after 6 and 12 months post-treatment (patients 2 and 4).

Differences in the staining patterns with respect to subclass were observed. IgG2 antibodies did not react with the high molecular weight 120-kDa polypeptide (patient 3). In contrast IgG1 antibodies in general failed to react with the low molecular weight polypeptides, such as the 15-kDa (patients 1, 2 and 4). IgA antibodies also failed to react with the lower molecular weight polypeptides in the range of 15–20 kDa (patients 2 and 3). Interestingly, some patients whose total immunoglobulin staining was reduced with treatment showed no equivalent reduction in the staining of IgA antibodies.

Similar variations in staining of polypeptides with class and subclass was observed for the group of patients for whom treatment was not successful, although no reduction in the intensity of staining following treatment was seen (data not shown).

Discussion

Following successful eradication of *H. pylori* a significant decrease in specific anti-*H. pylori* antibodies was observed. Conversely, patients who were unsuccessfully treated, despite a temporary decrease in median antibody level, showed no long-term decrease in antibody titre. In successfully treated patients the decrease in the levels of IgG1, IgG2 and IgG4 antibodies reflected the decrease in the total immunoglobulin levels. The most rapid reduction in antibody level occurred in the IgG1 and the overall total immunoglobulin responses. Since IgG1 is the major subclass in the circulating immune response, it might be expected that the anti-*H. pylori* IgG1 response would reflect the total immune response against the organism. The rapid response to treatment of the IgG1 antibodies implies that this subclass is a good indicator of successful treatment. However, a preliminary study [3] reported that the best indicator of successful treatment appeared to be IgG4. In this study IgG4 responses did fall quickly; however, very few patients had a detectable IgG4 response prior to treatment.

Whilst the reduction in the total immunoglobulin was reflected by decreased levels of the IgG subclasses, a reduction in IgA antibodies was less marked. The percentage of antibody-positive patients 1 year post-treatment showed only a slight decrease, suggesting that anti-*H. pylori* IgA antibodies are long lived and therefore may be of use in epidemiology where evidence of previous or current infection is required. However, like IgG4 specific IgA antibodies were not detectable in all patients.

The decrease in immunoglobulin levels in successfully treated patients was accompanied by a reduction in the intensity of staining observed by western blotting, particularly in the range of 50–61 kDa. Interestingly despite the general decrease in intensity of antibody staining some polypeptides, including the 120- and 15-kDa polypeptides, were consistently detected upto 6 and 12 months following successful eradication. Since the responses to these polypeptides are long lived, they may not be suitable for inclusion in a composite antigen used for the monitoring of treatment.

The variations in antigenic specificity with immunoglobulin class and subclass may reflect the complementary immunological roles that these types of antibodies have in the overall humoral immune response. IgG1 antibodies are complement fixing, IgG2 antibodies are particularly associated with chronic bacterial infections, and IgA antibodies prevent adherence of pathogens primarily to mucosal surfaces.

The overall results from this study suggest that the use of IgA for monitoring treatment would not be practical since the IgA response is slow to respond to treatment. Moreover, some patients cleared of infection are sero-positive 1 year post treatment. Although the IgG2 and IgG4 response fell quickly after successful treatment not all patients had detectable responses prior to treatment. The IgG1 response reflected very closely the total immunoglobulin levels involved in the anti-*H. pylori* antibody response; however, assaying for IgG1 antibodies may be of little additional benefit to the measuring of total immunoglobulin levels. However, in the future the differences in the antigenic specificity and the immunoglobulin responses to treatment may be exploited in the designing of a variety of kits for different purposes including initial diagnosis, monitoring of treatment and epidemiology.

References

1. Bell GD, Weil J, Harrison G, Morden A, Jones PH, Gant PW, Trowell JE, Yoong AK, Daneshemnd TK, Logan RFA (1987) ^{14}C-Urea breath test analysis, a non-invasive test for *Campylobacter pylori* in the stomach. Lancet 1: 1367–1368
2. Newell DG (1987) Human serum antibody responses to the surface protein antigens of *Campylobacter pyloridis*. Serodiag Immunother 1: 209–217
3. Newell DG, Bell GD, Weil J, Jones P, Grant P, Harrison G (1989) The effect of treatment on circulating anti-*Helicobacter pylori* antibodies – a two-year follow-up study. In: Malfertheiner P, Ditschuneit H (eds) *Helicobacter pylori*, gastritis and peptic ulcer. Springer, Berlin Heidelberg New York, pp 172–175
4. Stacey AR, Hawtin PR, Newell DG (1990) Antigenicity of fractions of *Helicobacter pylori* prepared by fast liquid protein chromatography and urease captured by monoclonal antibodies. Eur J Clin Microbiol Infect Dis 9: 732–737
5. Steer HW, Hawtin PR, Newell DG (1987) ELISA for serodiagnosis of *Campylobacter pyloridis* infection in patients with gastritis and benign peptic ulceration. Serodiag Immunother 1: 253–259

Future Prospects for *Helicobacter pylori* Serology

D.G. Newell

The immunological detection of *H. pylori* infection is now well established, and its major advantages of simplicity, cost and speed make this the most acceptable of the non-invasive diagnostic tests. The original serological tests devised were based on relatively low technology, and although these provided adequate results for much of the current epidemiological information, it is evident that improvements are justified. The major areas for future improvements will involve the introduction of new formats, new antigens and novel detections systems. To a large degree the extent of such changes will be determined by the test application.

The Relationship Between Application and Serological Test Parameters

Few significant changes are forseen to the current applications of the serological tests for *H. pylori*, i.e., epidemiological studies, diagnosis and treatment monitoring. There is increasingly evidence, however, that the application predetermines the test parameters, in particular the relative importance of sensitivity specificity, cost, user friendliness and the desirability of quantification.

The criteria of sensitivity and specificity are the major test of the efficiency of the test measured against a "gold standard". For microbiological infections the only true "gold standard" is culture, but where the organism is fastidious and the sampling unreliable, a serological test could provide a better indicator of true infection than culture. This is particularly true for *H. pylori* serology. The validity of the methods of determining the sensitivity and specificity must therefore be questioned for such tests.

In addition, sensitivity and specificity, in this test may be antagonistic. The variability of circulating host antibody responses to this organism clearly shows that single antigens do not provide adequate sensitivity (Stacey, this volume). However, many of the immunodominant antigens, including the urease, flagellins and the 56-kDa heat-shock protein, have cross-reacting epitopes with other bacteria thus reducing the specificity. Currently, therefore, sensitivity and specificity in *H. pylori* serology are to some extent mutually exclusive.

Central Veterinary Laboratory, Weybridge, Surrey KT15 3BN, UK

Gasbarrini/Pretolani (Eds.)
Basic and Clinical Aspects of H. pylori Infection

The efficiency of a serological test is largely dependent on the cut-off, or threshold, established in populations of "known" *H. pylori* status. It is now obvious that the majority of the tests developed to date are based on supposedly "normal" populations, i.e., Caucasians from the developed world and aged between 20 and 55 years. Moreover, symptomatic individuals, recruited from endoscopy clinics, and therefore having an abnormally high prevalence of infection have been used. The worth of these tests in assessing infection in populations outside of these "normal" criteria, particularly in asymptomatic individuals, in the young or the elderly, must therefore be questioned.

Seroepidemiological Tests

For epidemiological studies specificity generally has a greater importance than sensitivity, while speed and cost are additional major factors when thousands of samples are anticipated. To this end the introduction of test systems which can be automated would be a significant advantage. Moreover, epidemiologists prefer quantitative rather than qualitative, data for statistical analysis. In addition, tests for epidemiological purposes should take into account increased prevalence of infections with antigenically cross-reacting organisms and geographical differences in strain antigenicity. Serological tests dedicated to geographical regions and even ethnic populations may need to be developed in the future.

Serodiagnosis

Serodiagnosis is the most demanding application for these tests. The administration of antimicrobial treatment on the basis of seropositivity alone in symptomatic individuals cannot at this time be recommended. Nevertheless, the development of improved treatment regimens and recognition of the increased risk of gastric cancer with *H. pylori* infection may result in widespread treatment of both symptomatic and asymptomatic individuals on the basis of seropositivity alone. In the mean time seropositivity usually indicates the need for further clinical investigation by endoscopy. In this case sensitivity is far more important than specificity while cost and time, are relatively less important than accuracy. At present such serological diagnosis is done in laboratories by skilled staff, so that test performance can be monitored; however, it seems likely that diagnostic kits for bedside or general practitioner surgery use will become available in the future presumably marketed on the basis of cost benefit. Such tests must be easy to interpret and to monitor against standardized laboratory tests. Furthermore, any test designed for diagnostic purposes must accommodate already observed differences in serological response with age. For example, many elderly patients have impaired immune responses to *H. pylori* infection reflected in poor circulating antibodies, suggesting that serology in the elderly is generally unreliable. On the other hand, children, anecdotally have generally low antibody concentrations but with low background levels, indicating that the threshold for seropositivity should be different from the adult. Thus it seems that age-specific tests or at least strict age limitations for such tests may become necessary.

Treatment Monitoring

Sensitivity also has a greater importance than specificity in serological tests designed for monitoring treatment. Most importantly such tests require quantitative results for comparison of pre- and post-treatment antibody levels. Tests which require serial antibody dilutions to obtain a quantitative value are therefore unlikely to be useful for treatment monitoring. Another problem largely overlooked and particularly relevant to treatment monitoring is the method of quantifying results. In ELISA the relationship between optical density and immunologloblin bound to the plate is logarithmic not linear. This needs to be taken into account when interpreting results given as optical densities. In addition, the selection of antigens and possibly detection systems may need to be tailored to reflect the rapid reduction in antigen load. The development of tests specifically for treatment monitoring would seem to be a high priority.

Alternative ELISA Formats

ELISA has been to date the technique of choice for *H. pylori* serology. It has the major advantages over alternative systems of cost, speed, simplicity and sensitivity. However, the standard plate-based ELISA is likely to be replaced with alternative formats in the future. The need for cheap and rapid bedside tests will require adaptation for low skill base use. Such tests will require individual solid phase units instead of the multiple well plates currently produced. The introduction of dip-stick tests, perhaps utilizing whole blood instead of serum, is an the obvious potential improvement. The adaptation of the test to alternative antibody sources like saliva or urine would also have a number of advantages. Such tests, perhaps detecting secretory IgA, be totally non-invasive and would reflect mucosal immunity rather than circulating antibodies thus overcoming the problem of that group of infected individuals (about 5%) who do not produce a detectable circulating antibody response.

Most currently available ELISA's are peroxidase-based, but new conjugate/enzyme/substrate complexes are constantly being developed with greater stability and reproducibility and shorter reaction times. Competition ELISAs, based on the ultimate specificity of monoclonal antibodies, are unlikely to be useful as they are generally difficult to control and tend to have a poor sensitivity, reliant as they are on only a few epitopes.

Alternative Technologies

Other serological assay systems are currently being developed. Latex-based serological techniques, in particular, are extremely user friendly. Problems of sensitivity and specificity with currently available latex tests will almost certainly be solved with the introduction of more suitable antigens. Techniques are also available which could utilize whole blood in an homologous red cell agglutination system so that the patient's own red cells would be the indicator.

New Antigens

Despite current sensitivities and specificities of over 90% in this increasingly commercially competitive environment new and improved antigens are a major marketing asset. Accepting the recognized phenomena of host variation and bacterial antigen conservation no test will ever be 100% sensitive and specific. Compromise will always be essential. Moreover, such phenomena mean that sensitivity and specificity will always be to some extent mutually exclusive. Nevertheless, many research groups are still seeking a single native pure antigen. There is no evidence that such an antigen will be possible without producing severe sensitivity problems. Complex native antigens will therefore be required. However, potentially cross-reactive antigens need to be excluded either by selective removal of undesirable components or by selective recovery and recombination of desirable components to produce antigen cocktails. Thus currently chromatographic purification with recombination to include the most useful antigens seems to be the optimum approach. The question of which antigens and in what proportion will no doubt be discussed at length for many years to come.

Which ever antigen is the final choice the bulk growth of *H. pylori* will be required. To date static culture either in broth or on plates has been necessary. This may have several disadvantages. In particular, it is likely that antigen expression under such culture conditions does not reflect the in vivo situation. The recent introduction of techniques for continuous culture could provide significant quantities of cell mass potentially in the same condition as could be anticipated in vivo.

An alternative to native antigen production and purification is the synthesis of recombinant antigens in *Escherichia coli*. Some of the major antigens, including urease and the 120-kDa protein have already been cloned. This will eventually enable the construction of synthetic cocktails of suitable antigens using by genetic engineering techniques. Such techniques would also allow species specific epitopes of other, currently less suitable antigens like the flagellins, to be included in the cocktail without the inherent problems of antigenic cross-reactivity.

In conclusion, the value of serology in the non-invasive diagnosis of *H. pylori* infection is now well established. The development and distribution of second-generation tests with improved antigens allowing greater accuracy is now well advanced. However, claims of "near perfection" in such tests should be treated with some sceptism. Given the nature of the disease and inherent biological variability it seems unlikely that further significant improvements in sensitivity and specificity will occur in the future. Nevertheless, future developments will almost certainly involve improvements in the presentation of kits to reduce the time and cost and to allow use by personnel with a lower skill base.

The *Helicobacter pylori*-San Marino Study: Seroepidemiology of *Helicobacter pylori* Infection in the Republic of San Marino

G. Gasbarrini[1], S. Pretolani[1], G.C. Ghironzi[2], G. Giulianelli[2], E. Tonelli[3], M.R.A. Gatto[3], S. Ferrari[3], F. Mégraud[4], M. Baraldini[1], D. Cilla[1], S. Baldinelli[1], E. Bazzocchi[1] and F. Bonvicini[1]

Introduction

Helicobacter pylori infection is now recognized as one of the most common gastrointestinal bacterial infections in man [1]. During the last decade *H. pylori* has been indicated as a commensal bacterium of the gastric mucosa [2] but recently it has been considered the main etiological factor for chronic gastritis [3] and its presence appears to be an essential condition for the recurrence of peptic ulcer disease [4]. Moreover, case control studies indicate that people with *H. pylori* infection have a high risk for development gastric adenocarcinoma, in both eastern [5] and western countries [6].

Epidemiologic studies on selected populations have demonstrated that the prevalence of *H. pylori* increases with age [7, 8]. Race, ethnic origin (black and hispanic Americans), low socioeconomic conditions [9] and residence in custodial institutions [10] have been demonstrated to be associated with *H. pylori* infection. Person-to-person spread of the organism is supported by the evidence for intrafamilial clustering of *H. pylori* infection [11] and by a higher prevalence of infection in physicians and nurses of endoscopic gastroenterological units [12]. Polluted water supply has been suggested as a transmission route [13].

However, detailed information on the epidemiology of *H. pylori* infection in randomly selected populations is scanty and only recent studies have confirmed the previous hypothesis on an association with low socioeconomic status [14, 15].

We therefore undertook an epidemiologic study of *H. pylori* infection in the Republic of San Marino. This small independent country is the oldest republic of the world and is situated in the north central part of the Italian peninsula (Fig. 1). The Republic of San Marino was chosen for the *H. pylori* study because it presents several advantages for our purposes: (a) it is possible to sample randomly the adult population of the whole country where different social classes, jobs, alimentary and lifestyle habits are represented (b) the sociodemographic conditions of the inhabitants are very similar to ones of largest western European countries, the population is now very stable and the immigrating act is highly restrictive; (c) the national health system provides excellent statistical

[1] Department of Internal Medicine, University of Bologna, Policlinico S. Orsola, Via Massarenti 9, 40138 Bologna, Italy
[2] Department of Internal Medicine, Institute for Social Security, Via La Toscana 3, Republic of San Marino
[3] Institute of Hygiene, University of Bologna, Via S. Giacom. 12, Bologna, Italy
[4] Bactériologie–Einfants, USN Tastet, Université de Bordeaux, Place Amélie Raba Léon 1, 33076 Bordeaux, France

Gasbarrini/Pretolani (Eds.)
Basic and Clinical Aspects of H. pylori Infection

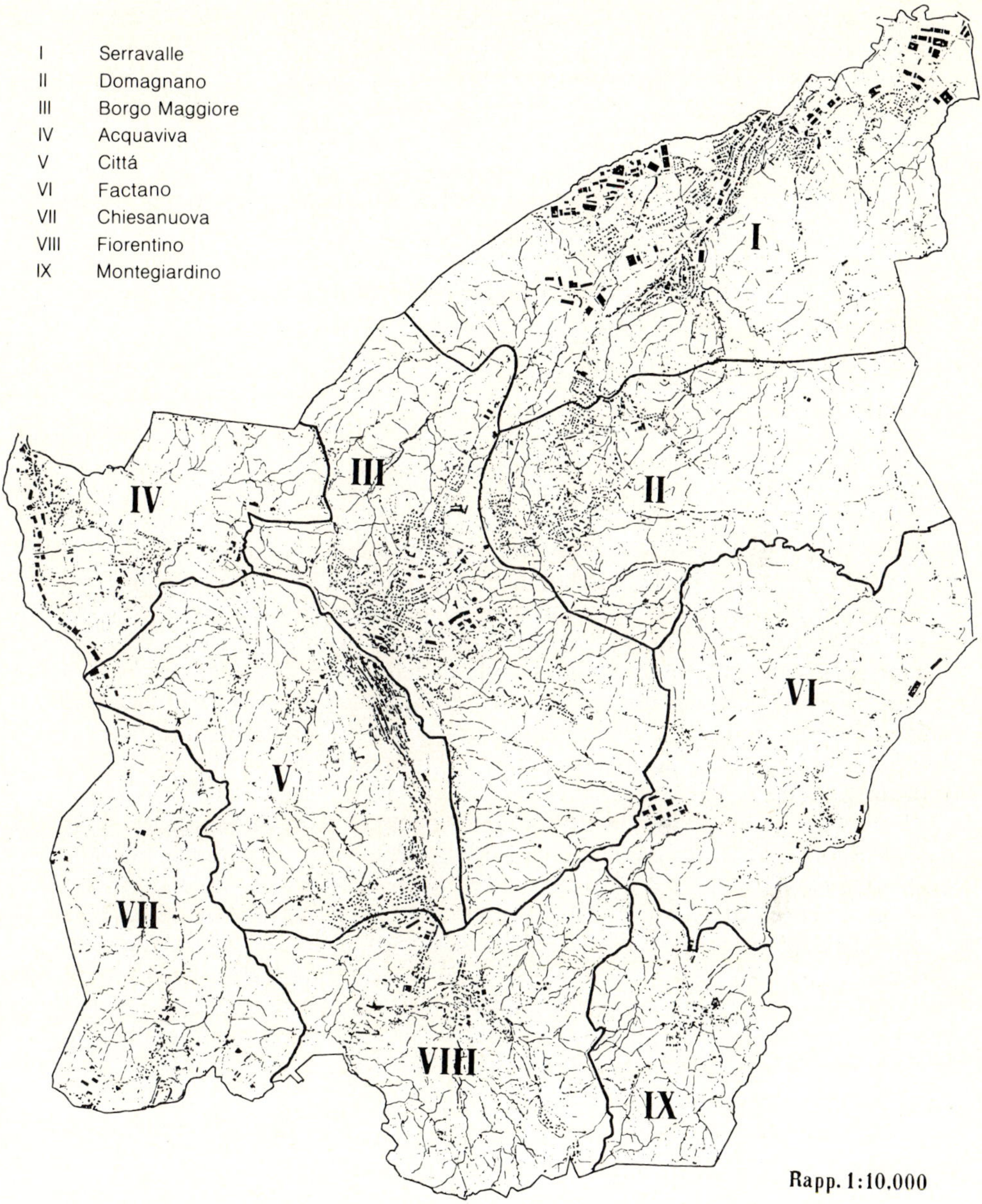

Fig. 1. The Republic of San Marino: geographical division of the nine districts

records and it is easy to obtain a capillary recruitment of the population; and (d) in San Marino there is a high incidence of clinically relevant gastroduodenal diseases such as gastritis, peptic ulcer and gastric cancer. In paticular, there was an incidence of gastric carcinoma of 6.3 cases per 10000 per year in 1990, and this figure has not shown any tendency to decline in the last 10 years [16].

The present study was designed to examine: (a) the prevalence the age distribution of *H. pylori* infection in the general population of the whole country; (b) the possible relationships between *H. pylori* infection and factors such gender, place of birth, socioeconomic status, occupation, life style habits (smoking, alcohol consumption, use of nonsteroidal anti-inflammatory drugs (NSAIDs), H_2 antagonists or antacids, dietary practices) contact with dogs, cats or with farm animals, environmental level of sanitation and history of gastritis, peptic ulcer or gastric cancer in subjects and in parents.

A secondary attempt was to provide a well-defined sample of the population which could represent the basis for future prospective epidemiological studies in the same geographical area.

Methods

Study Population

Between June 1990 and July 1991 we performed a cross-sectional study on the adult (18 years and over) population of the Republic of San Marino (17000 inhabitants). A random stratified proportional sampling by age, sex and district was made. Estimated prevalence of antibodies by age reported in a previous paper [7] were used to determine sample dimension [17]. The sample was of 2904 subjects. The response rate was of 77% and the final sample studied was of 2237 subjects. Table 1 shows the age and sex distribution of the sample.

Six months before starting the study, the mass media were utilized to inform the population of San Marino about the object of the study. A letter containing the purposes of the study was sent to all the subjects enrolled. Moreover, short explanatory calls were given to the subjects before the appointment for the inverview and the blood drawing. A consent form was signed by each individual before participating in the study. The same trained physician interviewed 2237 subjects, 1048 males (46.8%) and 1189 females (53.2%). A standardized questionnaire was administered to each subject and a blood sample was taken for the detection of *H. pylori*-specific antibodies. The questionnaire included items concerning sociodemographic informations (age, gender, occupation, place of birth and present district of residence in San Marino, proximity to civil or

Table 1. Study population by age and sex (San Marino study, 1990–91, $n = 2237$)

Age group (years)	Men (n)	Women (n)	Total (n)	Percentage
20–29	228	233	461	20.6
30–39	230	232	462	20.7
40–49	218	224	442	19.8
50–59	170	189	359	16.0
60–69	140	168	308	13.0
70–79	82	97	179	8.0
> 80	11	14	26	1.2
	1,079	1,157	2237	100

industrial sewage and breeding places as well, contact with pets or farm animals, travel, attendance of swimming pools). The history of gastrointestinal diseases in parents, siblings, and partners was also recorded. Detailed information was obtained on smoking habits, alcohol and drugs use, dietary practices and water source supplies.

A personal history was also taken, paying particular attention to gastrointestinal diseases.

Serologic Methods

Serum samples obtained from each subject at time of interviewing were stored at − 70°C. Later on, all sera were tested by a sensitive enzyme-linked immunosorbent assay (ELISA) for evaluation of immunoglobulin G (IgG) antibody to *H. pylori* proteins. The antigen was a centrifuged sonic extract of two strains of serogroups 1 and 3 by the Lior schema. [7]. A dilution of 1:100 of each serum was tested in duplicate. The optical density obtained was transformed in ELISA units using a regression curve made by progressively diluting a strongly positive serum according to the method described by Goodwin [18]. The threshold of 0.350 gave a sensitivity of 95%. All positive sera were checked by immunoblotting, in order to obtain exquisite specificity.

Statistical Analysis

H. pylori infection was defined as positive ELISA and immunoblot results. The data were analyzed using the SPSS-X program and the Mantel Haentzel or Pearson χ^2 test were used to examine the relationships with *H. pylori* infection in all the considered variables. The analyses were done on the whole population and for each district separately. We divided subjects into seven age groups (20–29, 30–39, 40–49, 50–59, 60–69, 70–79, > 80).

Results

H. pylori infection was present in 1137 or 50.8% of the population studied. The male to female ratio was 1:0.88 (Table 2). The prevalence of the infection increases with age from 22.6% (age 20–29) to 68.2% (age 70–79), particularly after the

Table 2. Seropositivity by sex

	H. pylori positive		*H. pylori* negative		
	(*n*)	(%)	(*n*)	(%)	Total
Males	533	50.9	515	49.1	1048
Females	604	50.8	585	49.2	1189
Total	1137	50.8	1100	49.2	2237

χ^2 Pearson = 0.0008

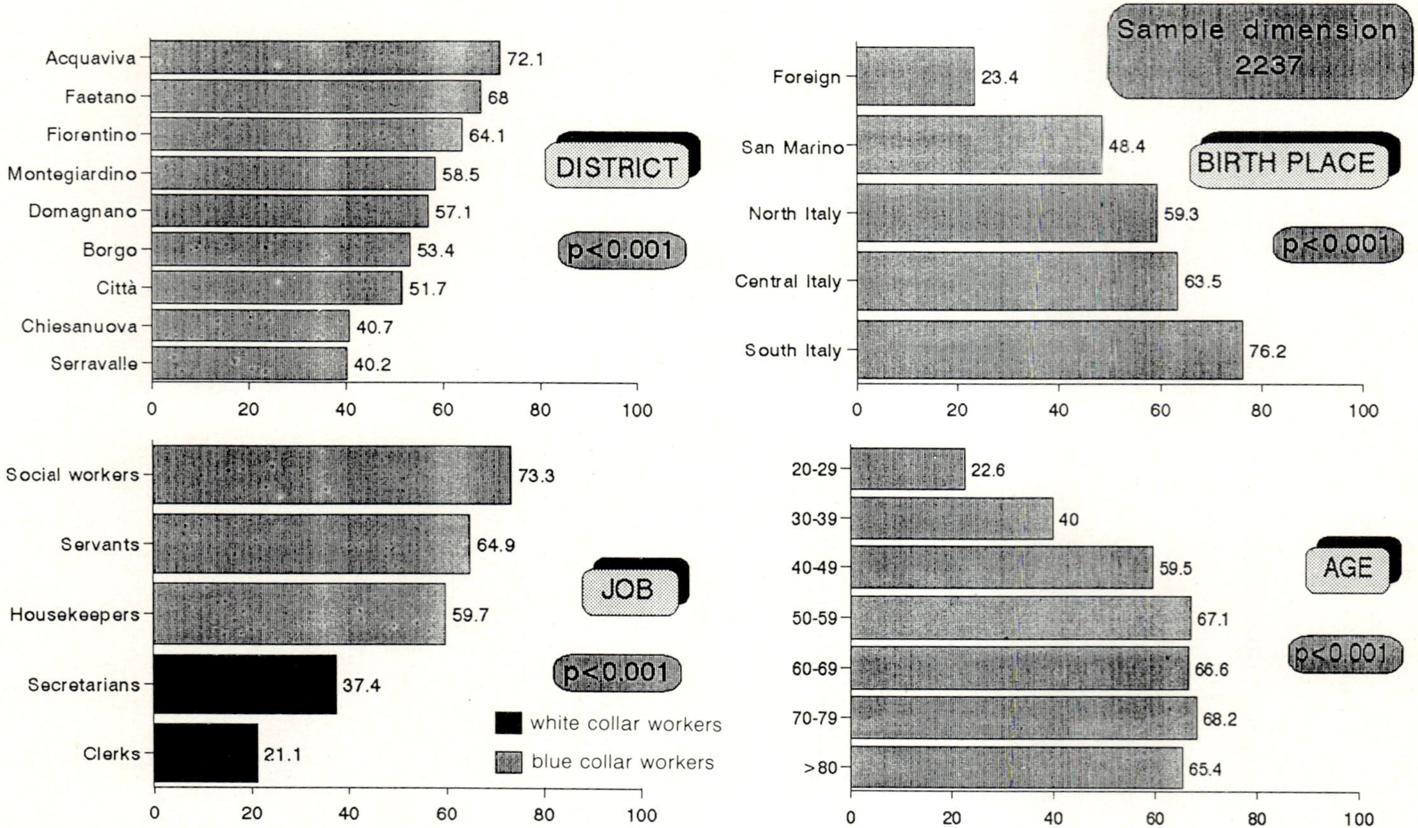

Fig. 2. Seropositivity for *Helicobacter pylori* by sociodemographic data in the Republic of San Marino

third decade ($\chi^2 = 276$, $p < 0.0000$) (Fig. 2). Higher positivity rates of infection were found in subjects living in less industrialized districts ($\chi^2 = 82.8$, $p < 0.0000$) and in subjects born in southern regions of Italy ($\chi^2 = 85.5$, $p < 0.0000$) (Fig. 2). Manual labor was also associated with a higher prevalence of the infection ($\chi^2 = 183.7$, $p < 0.0000$).

Contact with farm animals was associated with a higher prevalence of infection ($\chi^2 = 15.6$, $p < 0.001$), while contact with dogs or cats and living in the neighborhood of animal breeding places or sewage treatment plants was not associated (Fig. 3).

Analyzing the dietary practices, a lower prevalence was found in mineral water drinkers ($\chi^2 = 32.2$, $p < 0.0000$) and in vegetarians, even if in the latter the difference did not reach the level of significance (Fig. 3).

As concerns alcohol consumption, a higher prevalence of infection was found in drinkers ($\chi^2 = 31.2$, $p < 0.0000$). Smoking was associated with lower prevalence of *H. pylori* antibodies ($\chi^2 = 4$, $p < 0.04$) (Fig. 4). No difference was found in subjects taking NSAIDs, but people with previous treatment with H_2 antagonists had a statistically significant higher prevalence of *H. pylori* antibodies $\chi^2 = 37.2$, $p < 0.0000$) (Fig. 4).

The presence of dental prostheses was associated with the infection ($\chi^2 = 26.1$, $p < 0.0000$), while having had dental therapy was associated with lower seropositivity ($\chi^2 = 8$, $p < 0.005$). Subjects who had previous diagnosis of gastritis ($\chi^2 = 10$,

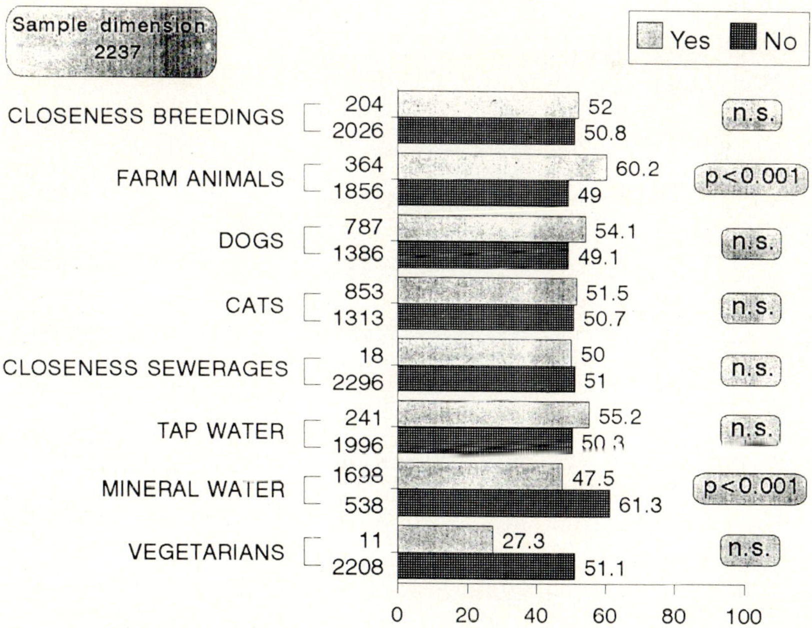

Fig. 3. Seropositivity for *Helicobacter pylori* by environmental factors and lifestyle habits in the Republic of San Marino

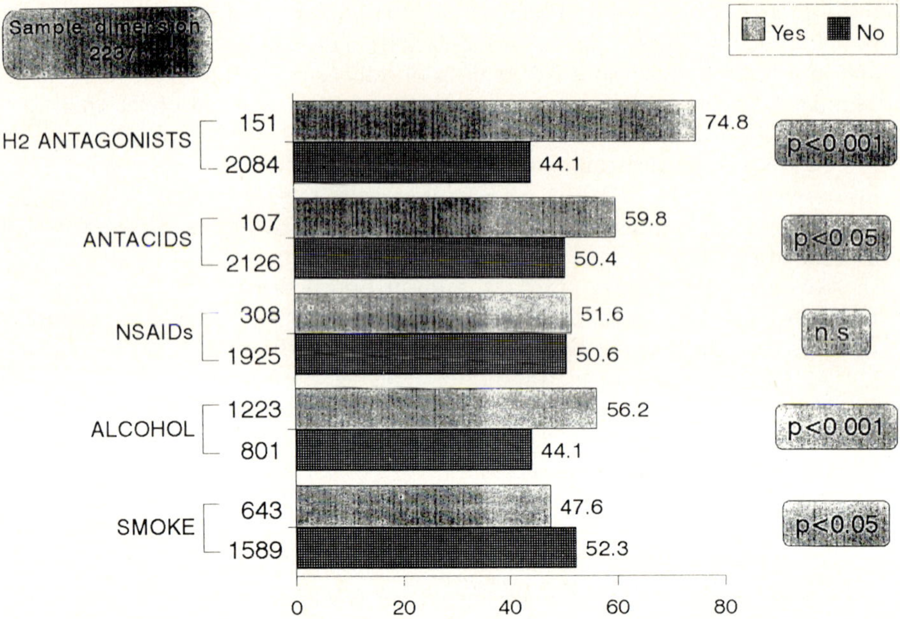

Fig. 4. Seropositivity for *Helicobacter pylori* by smoking habits and alcohol and drugs use

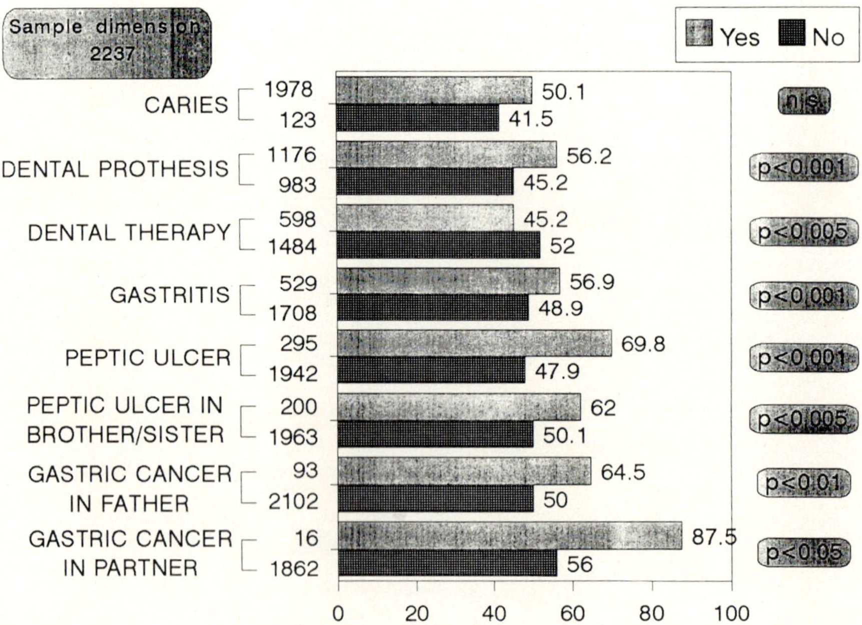

Fig. 5. Seropositivity for *Helicobacter pylori* by associated disease in the Republic of San Marino

$p < 0.001$) or peptic ulcer ($\chi^2 = 49$, $p < 0.0000$) showed a high seropositivity (Fig. 5). When seropositivity was matched with a positive history for gastrointestinal diseases in relatives a significant association was found if peptic ulcer had been diagnosed in a sibling. Presence of gastric adenocarcinoma in the father (Pearson $\chi^2 = 9.6$, $p < 0.008$) or in the partner (Pearson $\chi^2 = 6.7$, $p < 0.03$) was also associated with higher seropositivity.

Discussion

The presence of *H. pylori* infection is widely diffuse in both western and eastern countries, but the available epidemiologic data are obtained from studies on blood donors or volunteers. These studies can be affected by bias errors and they may not be representative of the true picture in the general population. There is only one published study based on a large random sample of population [15], but it was retrospectively conducted on sera obtained by two previous epidemiologic studies realized in a single Welsh town.

The clinical interest in large epidemiological surveys is reinforced by the recently described association of *H. pylori* infection and gastric cancer. If the hypothesis that *H. pylori* infection represents a risk factor for gastric carcinogenesis is confirmed [19, 20], eradicating the organism in high risk subjects could be an effective program of primary prevention of gastric cancer and this policy will modify the clinical approach to patients with *H. pylori* infection.

We report here the results of the first cross-sectional study performed during a year in a random sample of the adult population of an entire country, the Republic of San Marino. The study was specifically planned in order to characterize the epidemiology of *H. pylori* infection and to identify possible associations of seropositivity with environmental factors and gastroduodenal diseases such as chronic gastritis and gastric cancer. Our data indicate that in San Marino there is a higher prevalence of *H. pylori* infection with respect to Italy and other European countries [7, 8, 15]. *H. pylori* seropositivity increases with age and the hypothesis of a cohort effect is supported by the similar trend of increase observed in the last 20 years for other indicators of economic and sanitation conditions in San Marino.

The association of the infection with manual labor, place of birth in the south and in a less developed district confirm the importance of low socioeconomic conditions. A positive history for alcohol use and previous H_2 antagonist treatment is associated with *H. pylori* infection. This association remains to be confirmed by prospective studies, but it suggests that these factors may facilitate the colonization of gastroduodenal mucosa by *H. pylori*.

The presence of high infection rates in subjects with dental prostheses (and lower seropositivity in those who had dental therapy) suggests the hypothesis of a reservoir of infection in the mouth and support the oral–oral route for the transmission of the organism.

As in San Marino there is a higher prevalence of gastric cancer and its incidence has not been reduced over the past years [16], the high infection rate found in subjects with a positive history for gastric cancer in father or partner suggest an association between *H. pylori* and the risk for developing gastric cancer.

Prospective studies of *H. pylori* positive subjects and of their relatives will be necessary to confirm the above reported data and to evaluate the relevance of the *H. pylori* infection in the natural history of chronic gastritis and gastric cancer.

References

1. Peterson WL (1991) *Helicobacter pylori* and peptic ulcer disease. N Engl J Med 324:1043–1048
2. Bartlett JG (1988) *Campylobacter pylori*: fact or fancy? Gastroenterology 94:229–238
3. Blaser MJ (1990) *Helicobacter pylori* and the pathogenesis of gastroduodenal inflammation. J Infect Dis 161:623–633
4. Rauws EAJ, Tytgat GNJ (1990) Cure of duodenal ulcer associated with eradication of *Helicobacter pylori*. Lancet 335:1233–1235
5. Nomura A, Stemmermann GN, Chyou PH, Kato I, Perez–Perez GI, Blaser MJ (1991) *Helicobacter pylori* infection and gastric carcinoma among Japanese Americans in Hawaii. N Engl J Med 325:1132–1136
6. Parsonnet J, Friedman GD, Vandersteen DP, Chang Y, Vogelman JH, Orentreich N, Sibley RK (1991) *Helicobacter pylori* infection and the risk of gastric carcinoma. N Engl J Med 325:1127–1131
7. Mégraud F, Brassens-Rabbé MP, Denis F, Belbouri A, Quynh Hoa D (1989) Seroepidemiology of *Campylobacter pylori* infection in various populations. J Clin Microbiol 27:1870–1873
8. Dooley CP, Cohen H, Fitzgibbons PL et al (1989) Prevalence of *Helicobacter pylori* infection and histologic gastritis in asymptomatic persons. N Engl J Med 321:1562–1566
9. Correa P, Fox J, Fontham E et al (1990) *Helicobacter pylori* and gastric carcinoma. Serum antibody prevalence in populations with contrasting cancer risks. Cancer 66:2569–2574
10. Lambert JR, Lin SK, Nicholson L et al (1990) High prevalence of *H. pylori* antibodies in institutionalized adults. Gastroenterology [Suppl] 98:A74
11. Drumm B, Perez–Perez GI, Blaser MJ, Sherman PM (1990) Intrafamilial clustering of *Helicobacter pylori* infection. N Engl J Med 322:359–363
12. Mitchell HM, Lee A, Carrick J (1989) Increased incidence of *Campylobacter pylori* infection in gastroenterologists: further evidence to support person to person transmission of *C. pylori*. Scand J Gastroenterol 24:396–400
13. Klein PD, Graham DY, Gaillour A, Opekum AR, Smith EO (1991) Water source as risk factor for *Helicobacter pylori* infection in Peruvian children. Gastrointestinal Physiology Working Group. Lancet 337:1503–1506
14. Graham DJ, Malathy HM, Evans DG, Evans DJ Jr, Klein PD, Adam (1991) Epidemiology of *Helicobacter pylori* in an asymptomatic population in the United States. Gastroenterology 100:1495–501
15. Sitas F, Forman D, Yarnell JW, Burr ML, Elwood PC, Pedley S, Marks KJ (1991) *Helicobacter pylori* infection rates in relation to age and social class in a population of Welsh men. 32:25–28
16. Statistiche sanitarie della Repubblica di San Marino 1987–1990 (1991) Centro Eleborazione Dati e Statistica Repubblica di San Marino
17. Cochran WG (1977) Sampling Techniques, 3rd edn. Wiley, New York
18. Goodwin CS, Blincow E, Peterson G, Sanderson C, Cheng W, Marshall B, Warren JR, McCulloch R (1987) Enzyme-linked immunosorbent assay for Campylobacter pyloridis: correlation with presence of C. pyloridis in the gastric mucosa. J Infect Dis 155:488–494
19. Correa P (1991) Is gastric carcinoma an infectious disease? N Engl J Med 324:1170–1171
20. Sipponen P (1991) Helicobacter pylori and gastric premalignant conditions. Acta Gastroenterol Belg 54:340–344

Molecular Biology of *Helicobacter pylori*

Construction of Isogenic Mutants of *Helicobacter pylori* Deficient in Urease Activity

R.L. Ferrero, V. Cussac, P. Courcoux, and A. Labigne

Introduction

Isolates of *Helicobacter pylori* that do not express urease activity appear to arise spontaneously in vitro [1]. Unlike changes in phenotype, the genotypic change(s) present in these spontaneous mutants cannot be easily defined. Therefore the use of spontaneous mutants, or those created by chemical mutagenesis, in studies aimed at resolving the contribution of urease to pathogenesis remains problematic. The solution to this problem would be to genetically engineer *H. pylori* mutants modified in a single determinant but otherwise genotypically identical to the parent strain. These isogenic mutants might then be tested in appropriate in vitro and/or in vivo models. It was with this rationale in mind that isogenic *H. pylori* urease-negative mutants were constructed. To achieve this goal, genetic exchange systems allowing the introduction of foreign DNA into *H. pylori* cells, first needed to be developed.

H. pylori mutants were created using a shuttle mutagenesis approach involving several steps. Firstly, recombinant plasmids harboring the urease operon of *H. pylori* (comprising nine genes designated *ureA* to *ureI* [2]) were disrupted by the insertion of a MiniTn3 kanamycin transposon [5], *H. pylori* cells were then electrotransformed with the kanamycin *ure* gene disrupted derivative plasmids. Finally, kanamycin-resistant *H. pylori* transformants were selected on antibiotic-supplemented media. Two of the kanamycin-resistant *H. pylori* transformants, transformed with derivative plasmids disrupted in a structural gene (*ureB*), were further studied and were shown to be urease-negative. Southern hybridization analyses demonstrated that the urease-negative mutants had been constructed by allelic exchange involving the simultaneous gene replacement of the *ureB* gene with the kanamycin *ureB* disrupted copy and the loss of the vector. *H. pylori* mutants with disruptions in the accessory *ureG* and *ureI* genes have also been constructed and should permit the investigation of the functions of the accessory urease genes in enzyme expression.

Transposon Mutagenesis of Cloned *H. pylori* Urease Genes

The restriction map of plasmid pILL753, containing the nine *H. pylori* urease genes shown to be necessary for the expression of urease activity in *Escherichia coli* [2], is shown in Fig.1. A MiniTn3 transposable element carrying the *Campylo-*

Unité des Entérobactéries, INSERM U199, Institut Pasteur, 75724 Paris Cedex 15, France

Gasbarrini/Pretolani (Eds.)
Basic and Clinical Aspects of H. pylori Infection

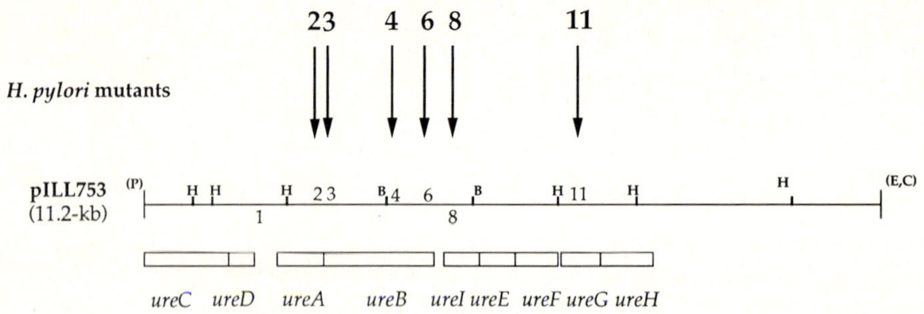

H. pylori mutants	2	3	4	6	8	11
Gene disrupted	*ureA*	*ureB*	*ureB*	*ureB*	*ureI*	*ureG*
Urease phenotype of HP mutants	-	-	-	-	-	-

Fig. 1. Linear restriction map of the *H. pylori* (strain 85P) cloned DNA fragment present in plasmid pILL753. Numbers located along the length of the restriction map correspond to the sites of insertion of the MiniTn3-Km transposon into pILL753 [2]. *Vertical arrows* (*numbered 2, 3, 4, 6, 8, 11*) refer to *H. pylori* mutants created by shuttle mutagenesis. Numbers in parentheses, to the size in kilobases (kb) of the cloned *H. pylori* DNA fragment. *Boxes*, the nine urease genes previously identified [2]; *ureA* and *ureB* being the structural genes. The lengths of these boxes correspond to the lengths of DNA required to encode the polypeptides. B, *Bam*HI; E, *Eco*RI; P, *Pst*I; H, *Hind*III; C, *Cla*I; Sm, *Sma*I. Letters in parentheses indicate that the restriction sites belong to the vector

bacter kanamycin-resistance gene (MiniTn3-Km) was inserted randomly into pILL753 using the delivery system described in detail elsewhere [5]. The derivatives were designated pILL753::x, where "x" refers to the site of MiniTn3-Km insertion which was assigned following restriction analyses of the corresponding disrupted plasmids. Based on this transposon insertional mapping, mutants designated 3, 4, and 6 were shown to map to one of the two urease subunit-encoding genes (*ureB*); while mutants numbered 2, 8 and 11 were disrupted in *ureA*, *ureI*, and *ureG*, respectively.

The Introduction of Disrupted Plasmids into *H. pylori* Cells via Electrotransformation

H. pylori bacteria were electrotransformed using the following procedure. Briefly, *H. pylori* cells (10^{10} bacteria/ml) were harvested from blood agar plates, washed in 15% glycerol/9% sucrose solution, and suspended in a final volume of 50 μl glycerol/sucrose at 4°C. One microliter (500 mg/ml) of supercoiled plasmid DNA, harboring the MiniTn3-Km transposon, was freshly dialysed against distilled water and added to the cells for 1 min on ice. The cells and DNA were transferred to a prechilled (kept at -20°C) 0.2 cm electroporation cuvette (BioRad), and placed in the Gene Pulser apparatus (BioRad). Pulses were achieved with the following settings: 25 F, 2.5 kV, and 200 ohms, giving a time constant ranging from 4 to 5 ms. The cells were suspended in 100 μl SOC buffer (2% Bacto-tryptone, 0.5% Bacto yeast extract, 10 m*M* NaCl, 2.5 m*M* KCl, 10 m*M* $MgCl_2$, 10 m*M* $MgSO_4$, 20 m*M* glucose) and spread on blood agar plates. The plates were incubated at 37°C under microaerobic conditions for 48 h. The bacteria were harvested and resuspended in 0.5 ml *Brucella* broth, and aliquots of 100 μl were plated onto blood agar plates containing (20 mg/1) kanamycin.

Attempts to electrotransform the *H. pylori* isolate (85P), used in the original cloning procedure, were unsuccessful. However, out of ten randomly chosen *H. pylori* isolates, one strain (N6) was found to be electrotransformable and appeared to readily acquire kanamycin resistance from the purified derivative disrupted pILL753 plasmids. Kanamycin-resistant transformants were obtained with a low frequency (up to 50 transformants/μg DNA). These isolates showed the typical *Helicobacter* morphology, were oxidase and catalase positive and were strictly microaerophilic.

Characterization of Isogenic Mutants of *H. pylori* Disrupted in *ureB*

Several kanamycin-resistant *H. pylori* transformants arising from the electro-transformation of *H. pylori* strain N6 were found to be urease-negative when tested by a quantitative urease assay [3] (the limit of detection was < 5 nmol urea $min^{-1} mg^{-1}$ protein). In contrast, the parent strain exhibited an urease activity of 24.6 ± 5.4 μmol urea $min^{-1} mg^{-1}$ protein.

To demonstrate that the creation of an urease-negative phenotype in *H. pylori* bacteria resulted from simultaneous gene replacement of the chromosomal copy of a given *ure* gene with the kanamycin-disrupted homologue, total DNA was extracted from transformants N6::TnKm-3 and N6::TnKm-4 and analyzed by the Southern hybridization technique. After digestion with *Hin*dIII, and *Bam*HI, the generated restriction fragments were transferred from agarose gels to nitrocellulose and probed with the three following randomly ^{32}P-labeled fragments : the kanamycin sequence (*Cla*I 1.4-kilobase fragment from pILL600 [6], the urease-overlapping DNA region (8.1-kb*Eco*RI-*Pst*I fragment of pILL590 [6], and the pILL570 plasmid vector. The result of the analyses cofiirmed the replacement of the chromosome-borne *ureB* gene with that of the kanamycin gene-disrupted sequence carried on pILL753 [4].

Construction of *H. pylori* Mutants Disrupted in the Accessory Urease Genes

H. pylori mutants with disruptions in the accessory (nonstructural) urease genes have been subsequently created using the procedure described above. Isogenic mutants disrupted in *ureA*, *ureI*, and *ureG* (Fig. 1), like those disrupted in *ureB*, have an urease-negative phenotype. This demonstrates that these genes play a role in urease expression in *H. pylori*. By comparison, *ureI* is not essential for the expression of *H. pylori* urease in *E. coli* [2]. The significance of this observation awaits further investigation.

Conclusion

The results of this study demonstrated that it was possible to construct isogenic mutants of *H. pylori* in which a chromosomal copy of a specific *H. pylori* urease gene was replaced with a kanamycin gene-disrupted allele carried on a plasmid. We have shown: (a) that electrotransformation of *H. pylori* strains is feasible although restricted to certain isolates; (b) that the *Campylobacter* kanamycin-resistance gene {aph(3')-III} could be expressed in *H. pylori*, and (c) that the creation of a stable and precise mutation in an *H. pylori* gene of interest was possible by virtue of allelic exchange. With the cloning of other putative virulence factors, it will be possible to create mutants with disruptions in other structural genes. These developments should result in a better understanding of the contribution of each putative determinant to the pathogenic process.

References

1. Cox DM, McLaren A, Snowden, MA (1990) The isolation and characteristics of urease-negative variants of *Helicobacter pylori*. Rev Esp Enferm Dig 78(S1): 29
2. Cussac V, Ferrero RL, Labigne A (1992) Expression of *Helicobacter pylori* urease genes in *Escherichia coli* grown under nitrogen-limiting conditions. J Bacteriol 174: 2466–2473
3. Ferrero RL, Lee A (1991) The importance of urease in acid protection for the gastric-colonising bacteria *Helicobacter pylori* and *Helicobacter felis* sp. nov. Microb Ecol Hlth Dis 4: 121–134
4. Ferrero RL, Cussac V, Courcoux P, Labigne A (1992) Construction of isogenic urease-negative mutants of *Helicobacter pylori* by allelic exchange. J Bacteriol 174: 4212–4217
5. Labigne A, Courcoux P, Tompkins L Cloning of *Campylobacter jejuni* genes required for leucine biosynthesis, and construction of *leu* negative mutant of *C. jejuni* by shuttle transposon mutagenesis. Res Microb 143: 15–26
6. Labigne A, Cussac V, Courcoux P (1991) Shuttle cloning and nucleotide sequences of *Helicobacter pylori* génes responsible for urease activity. J Bacteriol 173: 1920–1931

Cloning of a *Helicobacter pylori* Flagellin Gene and Construction of a Non-flagellated Mutant by Transformation-Mediated Allelic Exchange

R. Haas[1], H. Leying[1], J.P.M. van Putten[1], T.F. Meyer[1], G. Geis[2], S. Suerbaum[2], and W. Opferkuch[2]

Introduction

Helicobacter pylori produces four to six polar flagella consisting of a central filament of flagellin subunits and a flagellar sheath, a membrane-like structure containing specific proteins and lipopolysaccharide (Geis et al., in preparation). Flagella confer active movement upon the bacteria, a function which has been shown to be important for virulence in bacteria causing gastrointestinal disease [1, 19].

The penetration of the viscous layer of mucous coating the gastric mucosa seems to be a prerequisite for *H. pylori* to colonize the human stomach and establish an infection. Active movement of the bacteria due to flagellar rotation in combination with a curved, or S-shaped, morphology seems to allow this pathogen to overcome the natural protective barrier of mucous and therefore to colonize a unique ecological niche, the gastric epithelial surface. Expression of tissue-specific adhesins allows the bacteria to bind and colonize certain gastric epithelial cells, a property that might result in long-lasting infection of the human host.

Infection of gnotobiotic piglets by Eaton et al. [2] indicated that low motility of *H. pylori* correlates with a diminished ability to colonize the animals. The isolates compared by Eaton et al. were, however, not isogenic. This makes a comparison difficult since the strains might differ in other virulence functions.

In this study we cloned a *H. pylori* flagellin gene on a multicopy plasmid in *Escherichia coli.* A *H. pylori* mutant deficient in the production of flagella was constructed. This approach allows us to obtain insight into the molecular organization of *H. pylori* flagellin genes, as well as the complex structure of *H. pylori* flagella and sheath. Furthermore, the role of flagella can be more precisely defined by comparing the *H. pylori* wild type and isogenic mutant for their abilities to colonize and cause disease in an animal model.

[1] Max-Planck-Institut für Biologie, Abteilung Infektionsbiologie, Spemannstrasse 34, 72076 Tübingen, FRG

[2] Ruhr-Universität Bochum, Abteilung Medizinische Mikrobiologie und Immunologie, Universitätsstrasse 150, 44801 Bochum 1, FRG

Gasbarrini/Pretolani (Eds.)
Basic and Clinical Aspects of H. pylori Infection

Results and Discussion

Cloning of the H. pylori flagellin gene flaA. The 51-kDa flagellin of *H. pylori* strain 898-1 was purified as described by Geis et al. [4]. The N-terminal amino acid sequence was determined and used as a basis for the synthesis of oligonucleotide HL001. Southern hybridizations of the *H. pylori* chromosome with HL001 demonstrated a specific reaction of the probe with a single fragment in different digests of chromosomal DNA (data not shown). Probe HL001 was used to screen a plasmid library of *H. pylori* chromosomal DNA established in *E. coli* HB101. A recombinant clone, pHL305-4, was isolated (Fig. 1), which contained the complete putative flagellin gene, designated *flaA*, on a 9.3 kb *Bgl*II fragment in the multicopy plasmid pIC20R2 [12] (Fig. 1). The insert of pHL305-4 was subcloned in the same vector, resulting in plasmid pHL319-2-4 (Fig. 1). A comparative Southern hybridization of *H. pylori* chromosomal DNA and plasmid pHL319-2-4 indicated that no gross rearrangements in the cloned fragment had

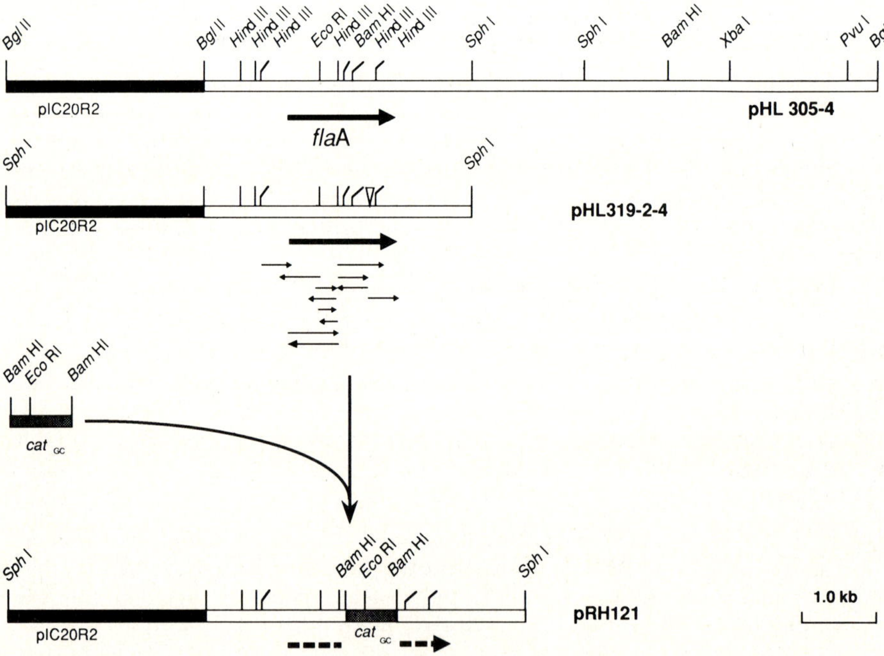

Fig. 1. Linear restriction map of recombinant plasmids harbouring the *flaA* gene. Plasmid pHL305-4 consists of the vector pIC20R2 [12], which carries a 9.3 kb *Bgl*II fragment with the complete *flaA* gene and downstream sequences. Plasmid pHL319-2-4 represents a *Bgl*II-*Sph*I subclone of pHL305-4. The location of the *flaA* gene is indicated (*thick arrow*). *Thin arrows* reveal the sequencing strategy for the *flaA* gene corresponding in length to the size of the fragments sequenced. The open triangle in pHL319-2-4 indicates the insertion of mini-Tn1721 transposon Tn*Max1* [20]. Insertion of the cat_{GC} marker in the *Bam*HI site of pHL319-2-4 gave rise to plasmid pRH121, carrying a defect *flaA* gene. *Hind*III restriction sites are mapped only for the sequenced region and the region immediately upstream

occurred. Appropriate restriction fragments were subcloned in M13 vectors according to the sequencing strategy shown in Fig. 1, and the complete *flaA* gene was sequenced by the dideoxy chain termination method [17].

Features of flaA. The nucleotide sequence of *flaA* reveals a single open reading frame of 1530 nucleotides, coding for a protein of 510 amino acids with a molecular weight of 53.2 kDa [22]. The deduced thirteen N-terminal amino acids were identical with the flagellin sequence obtained by analysis of the mature protein. Furthermore, the predicted molecular weight of the protein was consistent with the data obtained for the purified protein in SDS-PAGE [4].

Upstream of *flaA* a well-conserved ribosome binding site [18] as well as a σ^{28}-like promoter sequence [13] were identified. A stem-loop structure consistent with a rho-independent transcription terminator [16] is located downstream of the *flaA* gene.

Mapping of restriction sites in plasmid pHL319-2-4 revealed the presence of three *Hin*dIII recognition sequences in the region 300–700 nucleotides upstream of the *flaA* gene (Fig. 1). In the chromosome of strain 898-1-, however, only one of the three sites was cleavable by the enzyme, indicating a protection of the other two sites by a specific modification event in this area of the chromosome. A possible role for this specific DNA modification in regulation of *flaA* promoter activity is under investigation.

Homologies of FlaA with Other Bacterial Flagellins. Comparison of the deduced amino acid sequence of *H. pylori* FlaA with other bacterial flagellins revealed the best homology with *Campylobacter* species, reflecting the close phylogenetic relationship between the genus *Helicobacter* and *Campylobacter*, which have only recently been seperated [5, 15]. Homology was highest between the N-terminal and C-terminal domains of the compared flagellins, but rather low in the central region. The overall identity of amino acids between *H. pylori* FlaA and *C. coli* FlaA [11] or *Salmonella typhimurium* phase-1 flagellin [7] was 56% and 29% respectively.

Construction of an Isogenic flaA Mutant by Transformation-Mediated Allelic Exchange. Based on the phenomenon of natural competence for transformation [14], we established a method for mutagenesis of *H. pylori*. The chloramphenicol-acetyltransferase (cat_{GC}) resistance marker [6, 8] was introduced into the *Bam*HI site of plasmid pHL319-2-4, in order to interrupt and mutate *flaA*, giving rise to plasmid pRH121 (Fig. 1).Transformation of *H. pylori* strain 69A with plasmid pRH121 resulted in chloramphenicol-resistant *H. pylori* transformants, which could be isolated at an average frequency of 1×10^{-5}. Since the pIC20R2 vector did not replicate in *H. pylori*, all transformants had rescued the marker by replacement of the intact chromosomal *flaA* locus by the defective plasmid-borne *flaA* gene via homologous recombination. Southern hybridization experiments confirmed the incorporation of the *cat* marker in the chromosomal *flaA* gene by allelic replacement [21].

Electron microscopy of the obtained flagellin mutants revealed the absence of flagella (Fig. 2; top left), which was consistent with the nonmotile phenotype of the mutants as compared with the strongly flagellated wild type strain (Fig. 2;

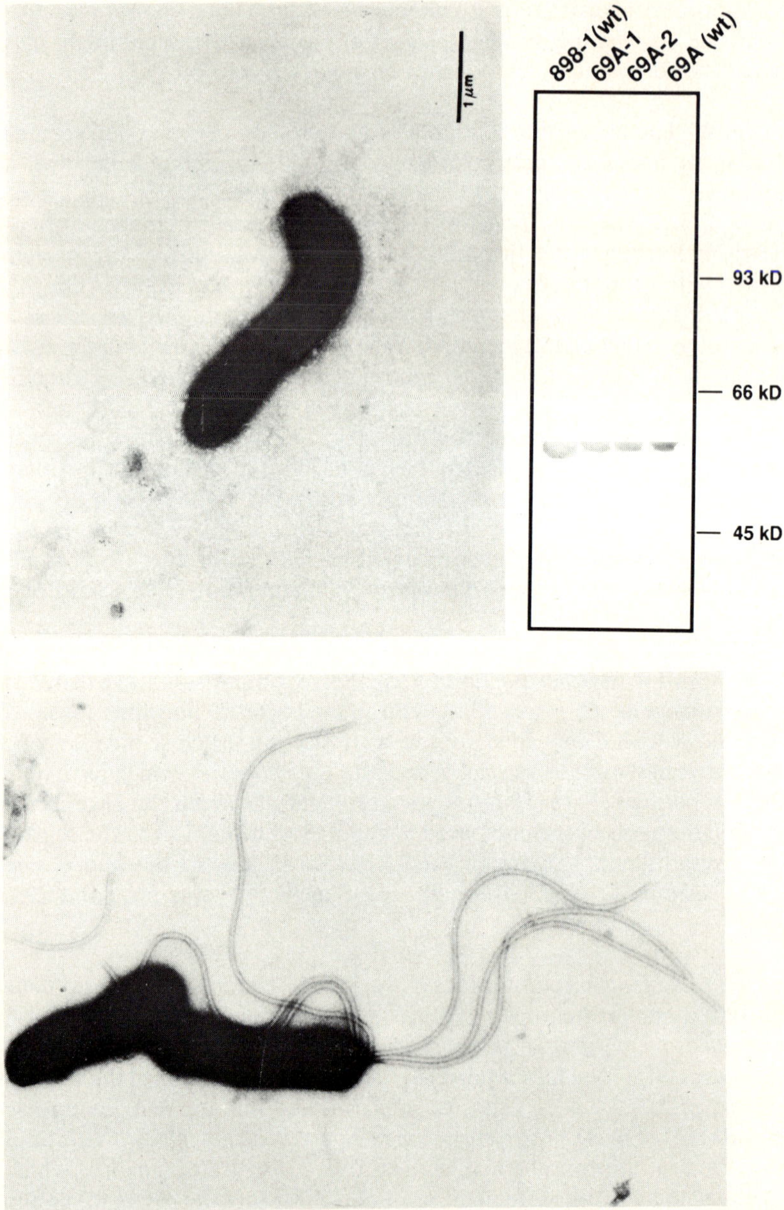

Fig. 2. Comparison of *H. pylori* 69A mutant and wild type by electron microscopy and immunoblotting. *H. pylori* strain 69A produces multiple polar flagella (*bottom*). An isogenic mutant of 69A does not produce flagella as seen in electron microscopy (*top left*; see text for mutant construction). Immunoblot showing whole cell lysates of *H. pylori* 898-1 and 69A wild type strains (*wt*) and two independent 69A mutant isolates (69A-1; 69A-2) reacted with a rabbit antiserum raised against purified *H. pylori* flagellin. Bar, 1 µm (for both micrographs)

bottom). Immunoblotting of the mutants and wild type with a polyclonal rabbit antiserum raised against purified *H. pylori* flagellin (Fig. 2; top right) revealed that the mutants, unable to synthesize FlaA, produced a flagellin molecule cross-reacting with the antiserum. These data suggest that, in addition to *flaA*, at least one further flagellin gene is present in *H. pylori*. Without expression of *flaA*, however, the second flagellin is unable to produce significant amounts of flagella visible by electron microscopy. Recently Kostrzynska et al. [9] have purified two distinct flagellin species from *H. pylori*, a major and minor flagellin. The N-terminal sequence of their major flagellin is identical with FlaA, whereas their minor flagellin is markedly different in amino acid sequence. The flagellin band seen in the immunoblot of the mutants might be identical with the minor flagellin described by Kostrzynska et al.

Future Prospects

With our approach of cloning *H. pylori* flagellin gene in *E. coli* we are now able to study the organization of chromosomal *fla* genes and their regulation in *H. pylori*. *C. jejuni* has been used as host for functional expression of *H. pylori* urease [10] and is a promising system for expression of *H. pylori* genes and complementation studies. Expression of *H. pylori* FlaA and reconstitution of complete *H. pylori* flagella in a *C. jejuni* flagellin mutant might be one possible approach to identify the genes involved in expression and assembly of the flagellar sheath complex. A further important question concerns the role of the flagella for colonization of the host. In future studies *H. pylori* 69A wild type strain and the isogenic mutant will be compared for their abilities to colonize in the piglet model [2, 3]. This approach should clarify the role of flagella and motility as virulence factors for this important pathogen.

References

1. Attridge SR, Rowley D (1983) The role of the flagellum in the adherence of *Vibrio cholerae*. J Infect Dis 147: 864–872
2. Eaton KA, Morgan DR, Krakowka S (1989) *Campylobacter pylori* virulence factors in gnotobiotic piglets. Infect Immun 57: 1119–1125
3. Engstrand L, Gustavsson S, Jörgensen A, Schwan A, Scheynius A (1990) Inoculation of barrier-born pigs with *Helicobacter pylori*: a useful animal model for gastritis type B. Infect Immun 58: 1763–1768
4. Geis G, Leying H, Suerbaum S, Mai U, Opferkuch W (1989) Ultrastructure and chemical analysis of *Campylobacter pylori* flagella. J Clin Microbiol 27: 436–441
5. Goodwin CS, Armstrong JA, Chilvers T, Peters M, Colins MD, Sly L, McConnell W, Harper WES (1989) Transfer of *Campylobacter pylori* and *Campylobacter mustelae* to *Helicobacter* gen. nov. as *Helicobacter pylori* comb. nov. and *Helicobacter mustelae* comb. nov., respectively. Int J Syst Bact 39: 397–405
6. Haas R, Facius D, Gibbs CP, Rudel T, van Putten JPM, Meyer TF (1990) Pilin variation in *Neisseria gonorrhoeae* and modulation of cellular adherence. In: Achtman M, Kohl P, Marchal C.

(eds) *Neisseria* 1990:Proceedings of the 7th international pathogenic *Neisseria* conference. De Gruyter, Berlin; pp 585–590

7. Joys TM (1985) The covalent structure of the phase-1 flagellar filament protein of *Salmonella typhimurium* and its comparison with other flagellins. J Biol Chem 260: 15758–15761
8. Kirby N, Vapnek D (1979) Nucleotide sequence analysis of the chloramphenicol resistance transposon Tn9. Nature 282: 864–869
9. Kostrzynska M, Betts JD, Austin JW, Trust TJ (1991) Identification, characterization, and spatial localization of two flagellin species in *Helicobacter pylori* flagella. J Bacteriol 173: 937–946
10. Labigne A, Cussac V, Courcoux P (1991) Shuttle cloning of genes responsible for urease activity from *Helicobacter pylori* and nucleotide sequence determination. J Bacteriol 173: 1920–1931
11. Logan SM, Trust TJ, Guerry P (1989) Evidence for posttranslational modification and gene duplication of *Campylobacter* flagellin. J Bacteriol 171: 3031–3038
12. Marsh JL, Erfle M, Wykes EJ (1984) The pIC plasmid and phage vectors with versatile cloning sites for recombinant selection by insertional inactivation. Gene 32: 481–485
13. Mirel DB, Chamberlin MJ (1989) The *Bacillus subtilis* flagellin gene (*hag*) is transcribed by the σ^{28} form of RNA polymerase. J Bacteriol 171: 3095–3101
14. Nedenskov-Sørensen P, Bukholm G, Bøvre K (1989) Natural competence for genetic transformation in *Campylobacter pylori*. J Infect Dis 161: 365–366
15. Romaniuk PJ, Zoltowska B, Trust TJ, Lane DJ, Olsen GJ, Pace NR, Stahl DA (1987) *Campylobacter pylori*, the spiral bacterium associated with human gastritis, is not a true *Campylobacter* sp. J Bacteriol 169: 2137–2141
16. Rosenberg M, Court D (1979) Regulatory sequences involved in the promotion and termination of RNA transcription. Annu Rev Microbiol 13: 319–353
17. Sanger F, Nicklen S, Coulson AR (1977) DNA sequencing with chain-terminating inhibitors. Proc Natl Acad Sci USA 74: 5463–5467
18. Shine J, Dalgarno L (1974) The 3′-terminal sequence of *Escherichia coli* 16S ribosomal RNA: complementarity to nonsense triplets and ribosome binding sites. Proc Natl Acad Sci USA 71: 1342–1346
19. Wassenaar TM, Bleumink-Pluym MC, van der Zeijst BAM (1991) Inactivation of *Campylobacter jejuni* flagellin genes by homologous recombination demonstrates that *flaA* but not *flaB* is required for invasion. EMBO J 10: 2055–2061
20. Haas R, Kahrs AF, Facius D, Allmeier H, Schmitt R, Meyer TF (1993) Tn*Max* – a versatile mini-transposon for the analysis of cloned genes and shuttle mutagenesis. Gene, in press
21. Haas R, Meyer TF, van Putten JPM (1993) Aflagellated mutants of *Helicobacter pylori* generated by genetic transformation of naturally competent strains using transposon shuttle mutagenesis. Molec Microbiol 8: 753–760
22. Leying H, Suerbaum S, Geis G, Haas R (1992) Cloning and genetic characterization of a *Helicobacter pylori* flagellin gene. Molec Microbiol 6: 2863–2874

Identification and Characterization of an Adhesin Gene of *Helicobacter pylori* by Cloning

D.G. Evans[1], T.K. Karjalainen[2], D.J. Evans, Jr.,[1], D.Y. Graham[1], and C.H. Lee[2]

Introduction

Helicobacter pylori colonizes gastric epithelial cells; in 1988 [8] we described the fibrillar NLBH as the putative colonization factor for this organism. Recently, Saitoh et al. [16] demonstrated that *H. pylori* binds to *N*-acetylneuraminyl-lactose-ceramide isolated from human gastric mucosa. The work reported here represents the first step in elucidating the molecular composition of the NLBH, i.e., cloning of the adhesin subunit of the NLBH. Subsequent work will be required to clone and identify additional gene products which are involved in expression of the native structure on the surface of *H. pylori.*

Methods

Construction of H. pylori Genomic Library. The *H. pylori* expression library was constructed in lambda Zap II, obtained from Stratagene (La Jolla, CA) following the methods of Sambrook et al. [17]. Following in vitro packaging, XL1-blue host cells were used to amplify the library and to screen for expression of gene product(s) identifiable with specific anti-NLBH antibody. In vivo excision of pBluescript containing insert DNA from lambda Zap II was carried out by coinfecting XL1-blue cells with lambda Zap II, with insert DNA, and helper phage R408, according to Short et al. [21].

Plasmid Constructs. An antibody-positive lambda Zap II clone was used to construct pHPA, a pBluscript SK(+) phagemid containing a 2.8-kb *Hin*DIII-*Eco*RI fragment of *H. pylori* genomic DNA containing the gene for the 20-K adhesin subunit. pHPA was digested with *Sma*I, resulting in deletion of a 1.8-kb fragment which was isolated and cloned into pBluescript SK(+); this subclone was named pHPA23. The remaining vector and the 1.0-kb insert DNA was religated; this subclone was named pHPA22. Additional restriction enzymes were employed to contruct other subclones for mapping.

[1] Department of Medicine, Baylor College of Medicine and Veterans Affairs Medical Center, Houston, Texas, USA
[2] Department of Pathology, Indiana University School of Medicine, Indianapolis, Indiana, USA

Gasbarrini/Pretolani (Eds.)
Basic and Clinical Aspects of H. pylori Infection

DNA Manipulations and Sequencing. Plasmid DNA was isolated by the alkaline lysis method of Birnboim and Doly [3]; purification was by CsCl–ethidium bromide gradient centrifugation. Transformations were carried out by the PEG method of Chung et al. [5]. Labeling of DNA probe and Southern hybridization were carried out by standard methods. DNA fragments cloned into either pBluescript of pTZ phagemid (U.S. Biochemical, Cleveland, OH) vectors were sequenced. Single-stranded DNA templates were prepared by the PEG method of Sanger et al. [18]. The dideoxynucleotide chain termination method according to Sanger et al. [18] was applied using a Sequenase kit (U.S. Biochemical). Portions of the cloned DNA were sequenced using synthetic oligonucleotide primers with double-stranded DNA as template, according to Zhang et al. [23].

In Vivo Expression of Cloned H. pylori proteins. T7 RNA polymerase-induced transcriptions and translation of cloned DNA was carried out using the in vivo expression system of Tabor and Richardson [22], with pBluescript or pTZ19R containing inserts downstream from the T7 promoter transformed into *Escherichia coli* K38 carrying pGP1 encoding the RNA polymerase under control of lambda PL promoter.

Results

Cloning of the 20-K NLBH Adhesin Gene of H. pylori. In previous work we prepared a polyclonal rabbit serum containing antibodies specific for the 20-K adhesin subuint of the *H. pylori* NLBH, demonstrable by its specificity in detecting the 20-K protein in extracts and whole cell lysates (WCL) of *H. pylori* in western immunoblots following SDS-PAGE; this serum also blocked hemagglutination by *H. pylori* cells and detected the NLBH in a receptor-binding assay, the fetuin ELISA [8, 9]. This anti-adhesin antibody was used to screen a *H. pylori* genomic library constructed in lambda Zap II. Analysis of DNA obtained by in vivo excision of pBluescript from ten different antibody-positive plaques revealed that these clones contained DNA inserts ranging from 2.8 to 4.5 kb. All reacted with a 159-bp *Sma*I-*Bgl*II DNA probe derived from the 2.8-kb DNA insert, as did native *H. pylori* chromosomal DNA but not pBluescript vector DNA.

Table 1. Immunodetection of the *H. pylori* 20-K adhesin subunit in WCL of *E. coli* hosting pHPA or its subclones by Western immunoblot following SDS-PAGE

WCL source	DNA	20-K adhesin detected?
E. coli HB101	No *H. pylori* DNA	No
E. coli HB101	pHPA; 2.8-kb DNA insert	Yes
E. coli HB101	pHPA22; 1.0-kb DNA insert	Yes
E. coli HB101	pHPA23; 1.8-kb DNA insert	No
H. pylori	Native, chromosomal	Yes
+ Control, purified 20-K adhesin protein		Yes
− Control, pure, unrelated *H. pylori* protein		No

The plasmid containing the 2.8-kb DNA insert, which was named pHPA, was selected for further study. Restriction mapping of the insert in pHPA was carried out; one (each) *Sma*I, *Bgl*II, *Sac*I, and *Kpn*I restriction sites were found within the insert. These were used to clone restriction fragments for sequencing the adhesin region; also, subclones containing 1.0 kb of the pHPA insert (called pHPA22) and the remaining 1.8 kb (called pHPA23) were constructed.

Analysis of pHPA and Its Subclones for Expression of the H. pylori NLBH 20-K Adhesion Subunit Using Specific Antibody. WCL preparations of pHPA and its subclones were analyzed by SDS-PAGE and western immunoblots for the 20-K adhesin subunit, as summarized in Table 1. These results show that the genetic determinant for the 20-K adhesin subunit is located within the 1.0-kb DNA framgment in pHPA22 derived from the clone pHPA.

Since the specific anti-NLBH antibody used for the immunoblots is directed against the fetuin-binding subunit, the previously described fetuin ELISA [9] was used to ascertain whether or not the cloned 20-K protein possessed receptor-binding activity. As indicated in Table 2, a correlation between antigenic identity with the NLBH 20-K protein and fetuin-binding activity was confirmed.

Nucleotide Sequence of the Adhesin Region. Another subclone of pHPA, pHPA26, contained a 1.4-kb *Hin*DIII-*Kpn*I fragment which included the DNA region encoding the 20-K protein. This fragment was sequenced and the three potential

Table 2. Immunodetection of the *H. pylori* 20-K adhesin (fctuin-binding protein) in WCL of *E. coli* hosting pHPA or its subclones by fetuin ELISA employing specific anti-NLBH antibody

WLC source	DNA	20-K adhesin detected?
E. coli HB101	No *H. pylori* DNA	No
E. coli HB101	pHPA; with 2.8-kb insert	Yes
E. coli HB101	pHPA; with 1.0-kb insert	Yes
E. coli HB101	pHPA24; with 1.8-kb insert	No
H. pylori	Native, chromosomal	Yes
+ Control, purified 20-K adhesin protein		Yes
Controls using plates coated with asialofetuin in place of fetuin		No

Table 3. Important features of three potential ORFs found within the adhesin region of pHPA26

	ORF1	ORF2	ORF3
Size	357 bp	549 bp	876 bp
Starting position	1	576	1177
SD Sequence[a]	No	Yes	No
PC Sequence[b]	No	Yes	No
Termination motif	No	Yes	No
Coding potential, MW	14.5 K	20.5 K	5 K

[a] Shine Dalgarno (AGGA) sequence.

[b] *E. coli*-like promoter consensus sequences (TTGACA, −35, and TATAAT, −10).

Table 4. Expression of peptides by pHPA and its subclones in the T7-RNA polymerase system

Plasmid	ORF(s)	Expressed peptides
pHPA	1, 2, 3	15 K, 20 K
pHPA22	1, 2	15 K, 20 K
pHPA23	3	None
pHPA24	2	20 K

All in pBluescript; pHPA and pHPA22 also gave the same results in the vector pTZ18u.

open reading frames (ORFs) were found encoded on the same DNA strand; their features are noted in Table 3. It can be seen that only one of these, ORF2, has all of the required features for spontaneous expression in *E. coli.*

Table 4 lists the subclones of pHPA and an analysis of the peptides expressed by these, as determined with the T7-RNA polymerase system. It was confirmed that only two cloned proteins could be expressed and of these only the ORF2-encoded protein has the properties which define the 20-K NLBH adhesin subunit.

Sequence Homology Between the Cloned 20 K NLBH Adhesin of H. pylori and Other Fimbrial/Fibrillar Adhesin Proteins. Data bank searches failed to find other proteins identical or homologous with the deduced amino acid sequence of the *H. pylori* 20-K adhesin. However, by using a technique which allows gaps in the sequences to account for addition/deletion mutations it became clear that the cloned receptor-binding adhesin subunit of NLBH has a sequence which is related to a variety of other fimbrial/fibrillar proteins. The *H. pylori* 20-K adhesin shares identity with enterotoxigenic *E. coli* K99 [15] and 987P [7], Pap A of uropathogenic *E. coli* [2], pilin of *Haemophilus influenzae* strain M37 [6] and fimB, fimC and fimD of *Bacteroides nodosus* [11]. No such homology or identity could be found between the *H. pylori* 20-K adhesin and the enterotoxigenic *E. coli* adhesins K88 [10], F41 [1], CS3 [4] or CFA/I [12] or with the type 4 pilins of *Vibrio cholerae*, tcpA [20], *Neisseria gonorrheae* MS11 [14], *Pseudomonas aeruginosa* PAK pili [19], Moraxella bovis pili [13], or *B. nodosus* fimA or fimZ [11].

In common with other adhesins, the *H. pylori* adhesin has two cysteines, one of which is conserved in location, the carboxy-terminal end is hydrophobic, and there is a penultimate aromatic amino acid residue. Altogether, these findings further substantiate our conclusion that the NLBH of *H. pylori* is a fibrillar structure.

Discussion

The gene encoding the 20-K adhesin subunit of *H. pylori* NLBH has been cloned and has been expressed in *E. coli.* The gene product was identified on the basis of its antigenic identity with that expressed by *H. pylori*, its molecular weight and its fetuin-binding properties. Also, the deduced amino acid sequence of the cloned protein places it in the K99-987P-PapA family of related adhesin proteins.

The protein expressed by the cloned gene *hpaA* was detectable only in whole cell lysates of *E. coli* and is apparently not exported to the surface, as evidenced by the failure of the host cells to hemagglutinate. However, this is not totally unexpected even if this binding subunit is also the major structural subunit of *H. pylori* fibrillae. It would be highly unusual if surface expression of *H. pylori* fibrillae did not require expression of other related gene products, i.e., proteins involved in the transport and assembly of functional fibrillae as well as gene products involved in regulation of expression. Therefore, cloning and expression of the binding subunit of the NLBH is only the first step in elucidating the entire NLBH expression system and work is in progress to clone and/or identify the other components of the *H. pylori* adhesion system.

References

1. Anderson DG, Moseley SL (1988) *Escherichia coli* F41 adhesin: genetic organization, nucleotide sequence, and homology with the K88 determinant. J Bacteriol 170: 4890–4896
2. Baga M, Normark S, Hardy J, O'Hanley P, Lark D, Olsson O, Schoolnik G, Falkow S (1984) Nucleotide sequence of the *pap*A gene encoding the Pap pilus subunit of human uropathogenic *Escherichia coli*. J Bacteriol 157: 330–333
3. Birnboim HC, Doly J (1979) A rapid alkaline extraction procedure for screening recombinant plasmid DNA. Nucleic Acids Res 7: 1513–1523
4. Boylan M, Smyth CJ, Scott JR (1988) Nucleotide sequence of the gene encoding the major subunit of CS3 fimbriae of enterotoxigenic *Escherichia coli*. Infect Immun 56: 3297–3300
5. Chung CT, Niemela S, Miler RH (1989) One-step preparation of competent *Escherichia coli*: transformation and storage of bacterial cells in the same solution. Proc Natl Acad Sci USA 86: 2172–2175
6. Coleman T, Grass S, Munson R Jr (1991) Molecular cloning, expression, and sequence of the pilin gene from nontypeable *Haemophilus influenzae* M37. Infect Immun 59: 1716–1722
7. De Graaf FK, Klaasen P (1987) Nucleotide sequence of the gene encoding the 987P fimbrial subunit of *Escherichia coli*. FEMS Microbiol Lett 42: 253–258
8. Evans DG, Evans DJ Jr, Moulds JJ, Graham DY (1988) *N*-acetylneuraminyllactose-binding fibrillar hemagglutinin of *Campylobacter pylori*: a putative colonization factor antigen. Infect Immun 56: 2896–2906
9. Evans DJ Jr, Evans DG, Smith KE, Graham DY (1989) Serum antibody responses to the *N*-acetylneuraminyllactose-binding hemagglutinin of *Campylobacter pylori*. Infect Immun 57: 664–667
10. Gaastra W, Mooi F, Stuitje A, de Graaf F (1981) The nucleotide sequence of the gene encoding the K88ab protein subunit of porcine enterotoxigenic *Escherichia coli*. FEMS Microbiol Lett 12: 41–46
11. Hobbs M, Dalrymple BP, Cox PT, Livingstone SP, Delaney SF, Mattick JS (1991) Organization of the fimbrial gene region of *Bacteroides nodosus*: class I and class II strains. Molec Microbiol 5: 543–560
12. Karjalainen TK, Evans DG, So M, Lee C-H (1989) Molecular cloning and nucleotide sequence of the colonization factor antigen I of *Escherichia coli*. Infect Immun 57: 1126–1130
13. Marrs CFG, Schoolnik G, Koomey JM, Hardy J, Rothbard J, Falkow S (1985) Cloning and sequencing of a *Moraxella bovis* pilin gene. J Bacteriol 163: 132–139
14. Meyer TF, Billyard E, Haas R, Storzbach S, So M (1984) Pilus genes of *Neisseria gonorrheae*: chromosomal organization and DNA sequence. Proc Natl Acad Sci USA 81: 6110–6114
15. Roosendaal B, Gaastra W, de Graaf FK (1984) The nucleotide sequence of the gene encoding the K99 subunit of enterotoxigenic *Escherichia coli*. FEMS Microbiol Lett 22: 253–258

16. Saitoh T, Natomi H, Zhao W, Okuzumi K, Sugano K, Iwamori M, Nagai Y (1991) Identification of glycolipid receptors for *Helicobacter pylori* by TLC-immunostaining. FEBS Lett 282: 385–387
17. Sambrook J, Fritsch EF, Maniatis T (1989) Molecular cloning: a laboratory manual. Cold Spring Harbor Laboratory Press, Cold Spring Harbor
18. Sanger F, Nicklen S, Coulson AR (1977) DNA sequencing with chain-terminating inhibitors. Proc Natl Acad Sci USA 74: 5463–5467
19. Sastry PA, Pearlstone JR, Smillie LB, Paranchych W (1983) Amino acid sequence of pilin isolated from *Pseudomonas aeruginose* PAK. FEMS Microbiol Lett 151: 253–256
20. Shaw CE, Taylor RK (1990) *Vibrio cholerae* 0395 *tcp*A pilin gene sequence and comparison of predicted protein structural features to those of type 4 pilins. Infect Immun 58: 3042–3049
21. Short JM, Fernandez JM, Sorge JA, Huse WD (1988) Lambda ZAP: a bacteriophage lambda expression vector with in vivo excision propreties. Nucleic Acids Res 15: 7583–7600
22. Tabor S, Richardson CC (1985) A bacteriophage T7 RNA polymerase/promoter system for controlled exclusive expression of specific genes. Proc Natl Acad Sci USA 82: 1074–1078
23. Zhang H, Scholl R, Browse J, Somerville C (1988) Double-stranded DNA sequencing as a choice for DNA sequencing. Nucleic Acids Res 16: 1220–1226

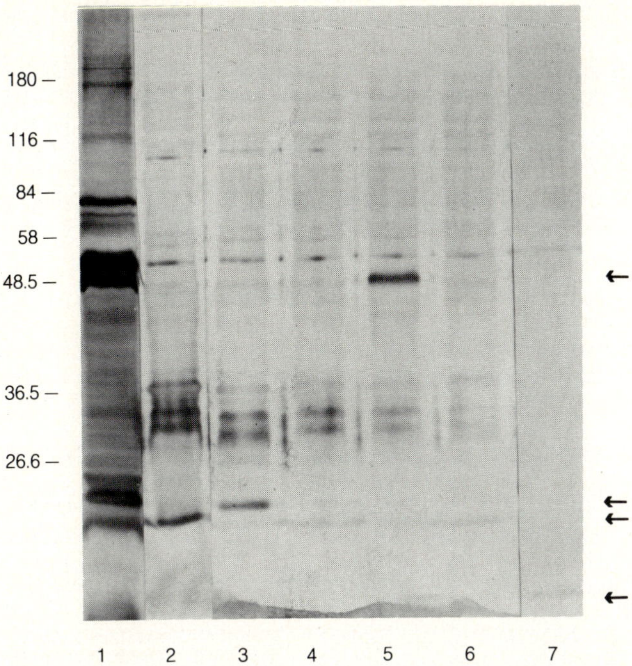

Fig. 1. Immunoblot of λ EMBL 3 plate lysates of recombinant phage reacted with the membrane antibody. Crude membrane preparation (*lane 1*), λ E5 (*lane 2*), λ E9 (*lane 3*), λ E14 (*lane 4*), λ E16 (*lane 5*), λ E24 (negative control, *lane 6*) and λ E10 (*lane 7*)

these recombinants, with the membrane antibody, identified three recombinant phage to express proteins of 17, 19 and 48 kDa (Fig. 1). We were able to clone and express the 48-kDa antigen in *E. coli* and had shown *lac* promotor dependency in pUC by IPTG induction. A bulk plasmid preparation of one such pUC recombinant clone, termed E16/12, was digested with *Bam*H1 liberating an insert of approximately 12 kb. Subcloning of this 12-kb fragment identified expression of this protein from a 1.4-kb *Hin*dIII fragment.

Nucleotide Sequence Analysis of the Gene Encoding the 48-kDa Antigen. Computer analysis of the nucleotide sequence of the 1.4-kb subclone (designated E16/185) revealed an open reading frame (ORF) of 451 residues. It spanned virtually the complete insert and did not appear to contain any promotor sequences or a recognisable Shine-Dalgarno sequence. The molecular weight of the polypeptide predicted from this ORF is 48.9 kDa and corresponds roughly to that seen following electrophoresis on SDS-PAGE. Figure 2 shows the results of a database search of the 451 residues and which revealed 48% identity in a 320 amino acid overlap with the similar-sized product of *htr*A from *Salmonella typhimurium* and 46% identity with the equivalent protein from *E. coli*. All three deduced proteins possess the characteristic catalytic triad of histidine, aspartic acid and serine, residues associated with members of the trypsin-like serine proteases. A putative leader sequence of 30 residues exists at the N terminus, typical of those proteins

```
Hp                      MPKVKERVSVPSKDDTIYSYHDSIKDSIKAVVNISTEKKIKN
                                   :          :       :
St    MKKTTLAMSALALSLGLALSPLSATAAETSSSAMTAQQMPSLAPMLEKVMPSVVSINVEG
Lc    MKKTTLALSRLALSLGLALSPLSATAAETSS-ATTAQQMPSLAPMLEKVMPSVVSINVEG

Hp    NFISGGVFNDPFFQQFFGD---------------------LGGMIPKERMEHALGSGVII
                  :::::::                      ::         ::::::::
St    STTVNTPRMPRNFQQFFGDDSPFCQDGSPFQNSPFCQGGGNGGNGGQQQKFMALGSGVII
Ec    STTVNTPRMPRNFQQFFGDDSPFCQEGSPFQSSPFCQGGQGGNGGQQQKFMALGSGVII

                 *                              *
Hp    SKD-GYIVTNNHVIDGADKIKVTIPGSNKEYSATLVGTDSESDLAVIRITK-DNLPTYKF
        : :: :::::: : :  :::      :   :  :: :  :: : : :    ::   :
St    DAAKGYVVTNNHVVDNASVIKVQLSDGRK-FDAKVVGKDPRSDIALIQIQNPKNLTAIKL
Ec    DADKGYVVTNNHVVDNATVIKVQLSDGRK-FDAKMVGKDPRSDIALIQIQNPKNLTAIKM

                                                               *
Hp    SDSNDISVGDLVFAIGNPFGVGESVTQGIVSALNKSGIGINSYENFIQTDASINPGNSGG
       ::    :::   ::::::: :: :: ::::::  ::     ::::::::: :: :::::
St    ADSDALRVGDYTVAIGNPFGLGETVTSGIVSALGRSGLNVENYENFIQTDAAINRGNSGG
Ec    ADSDALRVGDYTVGIGNPFGLGETVTSGIVSALGRSGLNAENYENFIQTDAAINRGNSGG

Hp    ALIDSRGGLVGINTAIISKTGGNHGIGFAIPSNMVKDIVTQLIKTGKIERGYLGVGLQDL
      ::    : : ::::::    ::: ::::::::::::    :    :   :: ::     :
St    ALVNLNGELIGINTAILAPDGGNIGIGFAIPSNMVKNLTSQMVEYGQVKRGELGIMGTEL
Ec    ALVNLNGELIGINTAILAPDGGNIGIGFAIPSNMVKNLTSQMVEYGQVKRGELGIMGTEL

Hp    SGDLQNS--YDNKEGAVVISVEKDSPAKKAGILVWDLITEVNGKKVKNTNELRNLIGSML
         :      :   :: :  :   : : ::::   : ::  :::       ::   : :
St    NSELAKAMKVDAQRGAFVSQVMPNSSAAKAGIKAGDVITSLNGKPISSFAALRAQVGTMP
Ec    NSELAKAMKVDAQRGAFVSQVLPNSSAAKAGIKAGDVITSLNGKPISSFAALRAQVGTMP

Hp    PNQRVTLKVIRDKKERTFTLTLAERKNPNKKETISAQNGAQGQLNGLQVEDLTQKTKRSM
            :   :  :  :  : :                    :                :
St    VGSKISLGLLREGKAITVNLEL----------------QQSSQSQVDSSTIFSGIEGAEM
Ec    VGSKLTLGLLRDGKQVNVNLEL----------------QQSSQNQVDSSSIFNGIEGAEM

Hp    RLSDDVQGVLVSQVNENSPAEQAGFRQGNIITKIEEVEVKSVADFNHALEKYKGKPKRFL
            ::: :: :  :::: : :   :  :       ::  :     :     ::   :
St    SNKGQDKGVVVSSVKANSPAAQIGLKKGDVIIGANQQPVKNIAELRKILDS---KPSV-L
Ec    SNKGKDQGVVVNNVKTGTPAAQIGLKKGDVIIGANQQAVKNIAELRKVLDS---KPSV-L

Hp    VLDLNQGYRIILVK
       :    :   :
St    ALNIQRGDSSIYLLMQ
Ec    ALNIQRGDRHLPVNAVISLNPFLKTGRGSPYNL
```

Fig. 2. Multiple alignment of *htr*A from *H. pylori, S. typhimurium* and *E. coli. Double dots* indicate, identical residues; *boxed residues*, positions from where oligonucleotide primers were designed for PCR; *asterisks*, residues showing the characteristic catalytic triad of a classical serine protease; *underlined sequence* (N terminus), the putative leader sequence for *H. pylori*

that are targeted through a cell membrane. We are currently sequencing upstream to identify promoter sequences in order to determine this genes RNA polymerase dependency.

PCR of htr*A Gene Fragments from H. pylori.* To determine the frequency of this gene in *H. pylori* strains, we performed PCR on purified DNA using *H. pylori* specific sequencing primers in conventional PCR, and conserved internal primers to the *htr*A gene in nested PCR. Figure 3 (above) shows PCR using the *H. pylori* specific sequencing primers (48/1 and 48/2) to amplify a 1.14-kb product. Figure 3 (below) shows the use of the internal primers in a nested PCR to amplify a 471-bp fragment, confirming amplification of the correct gene sequence. We have been able to amplify the 1.14-kb fragment from the purified DNA of 50 clinical isolates studied.

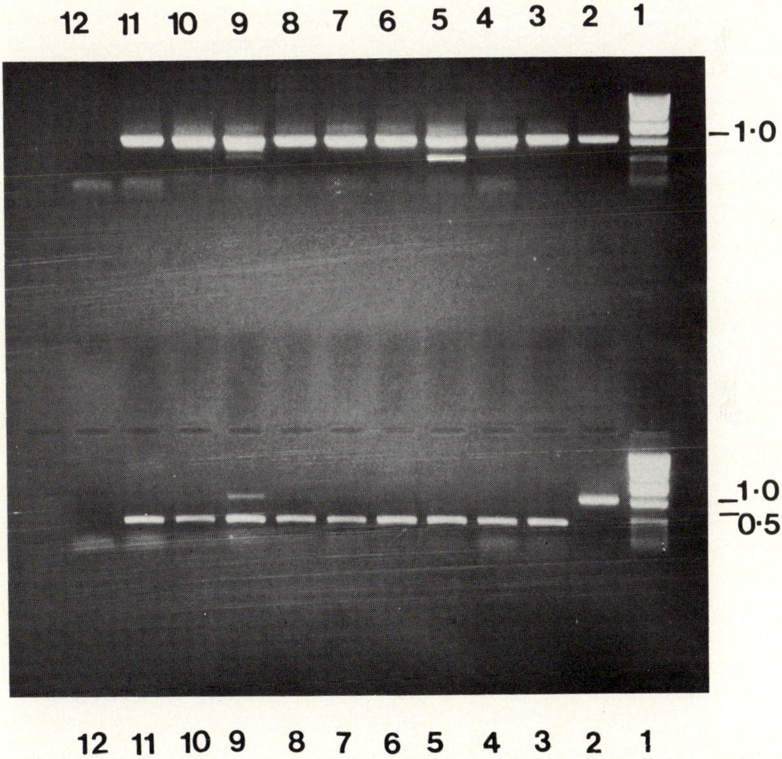

Fig. 3. *Above*, 1% w/v agarose gel showing PCR analysis of *H. pylori* total DNA using *H. pylori* specific sequencing primers 48/1 and 48/2 to amplify a 1.14-kb product. 1-kb ladder (*lane 1*), HPG126 (*lane 2*), HPM388 (*lane 3*), HPM698 (*lane 4*), HPM450 (*lane 5*), HPG255 (*lane 6*), HPM049 (*lane 7*), HPM585 (*lane 8*), HPM707 (*lane 9*), HPM257 (*lane 10*), HPM711 (*lane 11*) and a no-DNA negative control (*lane 12*). *Below*, 1% w/v agarose gel showing a nested PCR of *H. pylori* total DNA using primers 48/1 and 48/2 initially for 20 cycles, then the internal primers 48/3 and 48/4 for a further 20 cycles to amplify a 471-bp fragment. Lanes as above, except for *lane 2* showing HPG126 using primers 48/1 and 48/2 only

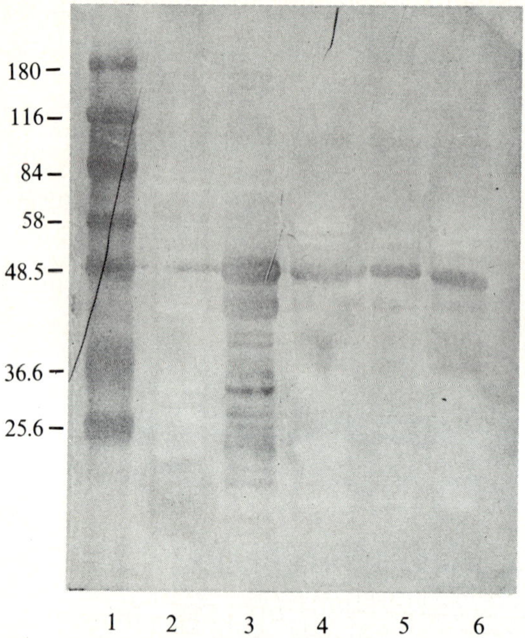

Fig. 4. Immunoblot of *H. pylori* whole cells reacted with adsorbed monospecific antibody to the IPTG-induced 48-kDa antigen. Prestained mol. wt. marker (*lane 1*), E16/185 *E. coli* subclone (*lane 2*), HPG126 (*lane 3*), HPM630 (*lane 4*) and HPM585 (*lane 5*)

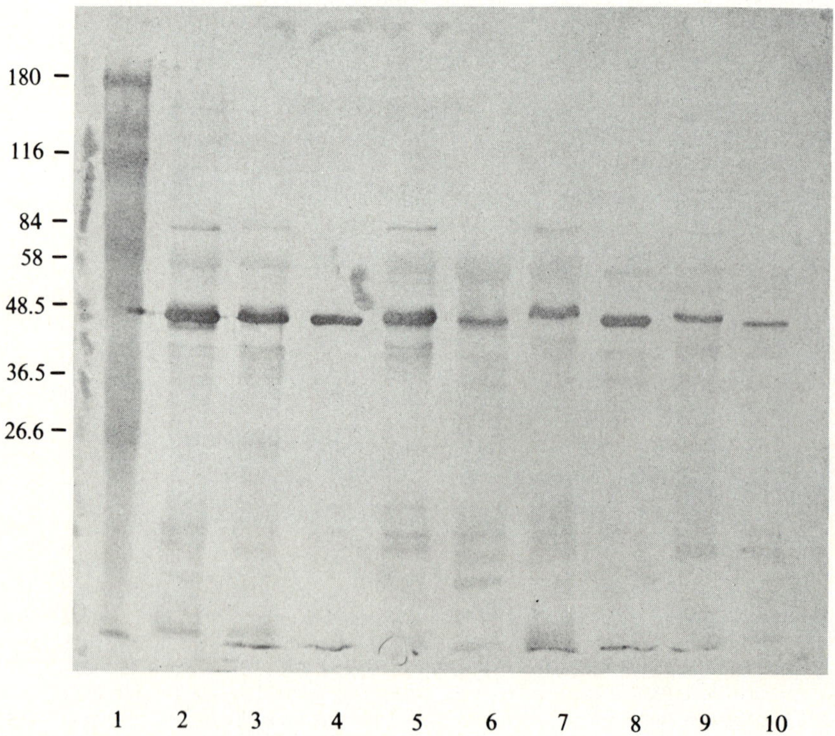

Fig. 5. Immunoblot of sarkosyl insoluble fractions of outer membrane preparations from *H. pylori* reacted with adsorbed anti-whole-cell antibody. Prestained mol. wt. marker (*lane 1*), HPG126 (*lane 2*), HPM388 (*lane 3*), HPM698 (*lane 4*), HPM450 (*lane 5*), HPG255 (*lane 6*), HPM049 (*lane 7*), HPM585 (*lane 8*), HPM707 (*lane 9*) and HPM257 (*lane 10*)

Immunolabelling of the 48-kDa Antigen. Having determined that the gene is present in all strains studied, we then wanted to demonstrate expression. By preparing a monospecific antibody to the IPTG-induced E16/185 subclone and reacting the adsorbed antibody with *H. pylori* whole cell protein preparations, we demonstrated expression from all strains. Figure 4 shows reaction of the 48-kDa antigen with the monospecific antibody from a few of those *H. pylori* strains tested.

By reacting anti-whole-cell antibody with the sarkosyl insoluble outer membrane fractions from *H. pylori* strains, we are able to demonstrate the presence of the 48-kDa antigen in all preparations (Fig. 5). This implies a membrane association, as has been shown for the product of *htr*A in *E. coli* [5].

Discussion

We have cloned and shown expression in *E. coli* of a 48-kDa antigen from *H. pylori.* Sequence analysis identified this protein to have identity with the product of *htr*A, a stress-response gene isolated from *E. coli* and *S. typhimurium.* In *E. coli,* the *htr*A gene product is essential for bacterial survival at temperatures above 42°C and has been localised to the periplasm [5]. It acts as an endopeptidase during aberrant protein production at the elevated temperatures. In *S. typhimurium, htr*A mutants were found to be more susceptible to oxidative stress, suggesting that they may be less able to withstand oxidative killing within macrophages [3]. The stress required, if any, for expression and the action of this gene product in *H. pylori* are unknown. HtrA in *H. pylori* possesses the characteristic catalytic triad of serine proteases. The regions around the catalytic residues are highly conserved, showing similarity with distantly related proteases, such as the V8 protease of *Staphylococcus aureus.* There is a putative signal sequence at the N terminus of the *H. pylori* polypeptide. A similar feature is found in both the *E. coli* and *S. typhimurium* proteins. In *E. coli* HtrA is synthesized as a precursor which undergoes post-translational modification of approximately 3 kDa from the N terminus [4]. Such a modification in *H. pylori* would result in a mature product of 46 kDa and would more closely resemble the observed molecular weight following SDS-PAGE. Having also shown by immunoblotting a membrane association in *H. pylori,* these facts indicate that the leader peptide is necessary for protein transport. We are currently attempting to mutagenise this gene and reintroduce the defective gene back into *H. pylori.* Stress responses upon the isogenic strains will then be investigated.

Acknowledgement. This work was supported by a grant from the British Medical Research Council.

References

1. Barlow AK, Heckels JE, Clarke IN (1987) Molecular cloning and expression of *Neisseria meningitidis* Class 1 outer membrane protein in *E. coli* K12. Infect Immun 55:2734–2740
2. Czinn Z, Carr H, Sheffler L, Aronoff S (1989) Serum IgG Antibody to the outer membrane proteins of *Campylobacter pylori* in children with gastroduodenal disease. J Infect Dis 159:586–589

3. Johnson K, Charles I, Dougan G, Pickard D, O'Gaora P, Costa G, Ali T, Miller I, Hormaeche C (1991) The role of a stress-response protein in *Salmonella typhimurium* virulence. Mol Microbiol 5: 401–407
4. Lipinska B, Fayet O, Baird L, Georgopoulos C (1989) Identification, characterisation, and mapping of the *E. coli htr*A gene, whose product is essential for bacterial growth only at elevated temperatures. J Bacteriol 171: 1574–1584
5. Lipinska B, Zylicz M, Georgopoulos C (1990) The HtrA (Deg P) protein, essential for *E. coli* survival at high temperatures, is an endopeptidase. J Bacteriol 172: 1791–1797
6. Newell DG (1987) Identification of the outer membrane proteins of *Campylobacter pyloridis* and antigenic cross-reactivity between *C. pyloridis* and *C. jejuni*. J Gen Microbiol 133: 163–170
7. Owen RJ, Bickley J, Costas M, Morgan DR (1991) Genomic variation in *Helicobacter pylori*: application to identification of strains. Scand J Gastroenterol 26: 43–50
8. Perez-Perez GI, Blaser MJ (1987) Conservation and diversity of *Campylobacter pyloridis* major antigens. Infect Immun 55: 1256–1263
9. Sanger F, Nicklen S, Coulson AR (1977) DNA sequencing with chain terminating inhibitors. Proc Natl Acad Sci USA 74: 5463–5467

Diagnosis of *Helicobacter pylori* in Gastric Juice Aspirates Using Polymerase Chain Reaction

T.U. Westblom[1], S. Phadnis[2], S. Normark[2], and S.J. Czinn[3]

Introduction

Polymerase chain reaction (PCR) is a sensitive molecular method that can detect very small amounts of DNA. DNA is a highly stable molecule that can survive in the environment even when the host organism is no longer viable. PCR therefore promises to be a powerful tool for diagnosis of *H. pylori* infection.

Current methods of *H. pylori* diagnosis rely heavily on biopsies collected during gastroduodenoscopy. Indirect evidence of infection can be obtained with ELISA assays [1], latex agglutination tests for serum antibodies [2], and urea breath tests [3]. Still, definitive diagnosis requires a positive culture from biopsy material or visualization by histologic examination [4]. Some investigators have suggested that *H. pylori* also can be found in gastric juice aspirates, but recovery rates using traditional culture techniques have been low [5–7]. We have therefore evaluated PCR as a way of identifying *H. pylori* in gastric juice aspirates.

Materials and Methods

We have adapted the PCR technique to *H. pylori* by using a segment of the ureA gene as target DNA. We have previously described how primers from this gene can identify *H. pylori* without the need for prior DNA extraction [8]. The sensitivity and specificity of the primer sequences were both 100% when tested on 23 stock isolates of *H. pylori*. Twelve strains of other urease positive bacteria were used as negative controls, including *H. mustelae*, *P. mirabilis*, and *M. morganii*. Using an annealing temperature of 60°C and an extension temperature of 72°C for 30 cycles, we have shown that PCR can detect the presence of *H. pylori* when as few as 30 CFU of bacteria are present in the samples [9].

We now compared this method with a modified protocol using additional cycles but a lower denaturation temperature as described by Yap and McGee [10]. A hot start procedure was used for all samples. The denaturation tempera-

[1] Division of Infectious Diseases and Immunology, St. Louis University School of Medicine, St. Louis, Missouri, USA
[2] Department of Molecular Microbiology, Washington University School of Medicine, St. Louis, Missouri, USA
[3] Department of Pediatrics, Case Western Reserve University, Claveland, Ohio, USA

Gasbarrini/Pretolani (Eds.)
Basic and Clinical Aspects of H. pylori Infection

ture was kept at 95°C for the first 10 cycles, but then lowered to 89°C for an additional 40 cycles. All 50 cycles used an annealing temperature of 60°C and an extension temperature of 72°C. Target samples consisted of gastric juice aspirates from patients who had undergone gastroduodenoscopy with biopsies for culture and histology. Five milliliters of gastric juice had been buffered to a neutral pH before being concentrated by ultracentrifugation at 10 000 g for 20 min. Pellets had been resuspended in 50 μl sterile distilled water and then heat inactivated at 98°C for 10 min before amplification. Amplified DNA fragments were visualized in a 4% TAE gel by staining with ethidium bromide.

Results

First we ran five samples of gastric juice aspirates at 30 cycles using a conventional denaturation temperature. One sample showed a positive band of the expected 360 bp size. Four juice samples were negative in spite of positive biopsy cultures and histology. When the same samples were run with 50 cycles instead, four of the five juice aspirates were positive. In this first pilot study PCR had a sensitivity of 80% and a specificity of 100% for detection of clinical infection with *H. pylori.*

Discussion

Current diagnostic modalities often require gastric biopsies obtained by gastroduodenoscopy. We analyzed gastric juice aspirates with PCR since such specimens can be obtained without the need for endoscopy. *H. pylori* has only rarely been grown from gastric juice. Our first experiment also had a low yield of only 20% positive specimens. By increasing the number of cycles to 50 we could identify 80% of the infected patients. This suggests that *H. pylori* is present in the gastric juice, but only in low numbers compared to mucosal biopsies [8]. Still, it may be possible to increase the sensitivity even further. One of the limiting factors of the PCR assay is the half life of the polymerase enzyme at high temperatures. This is not crucial when 30 or fewer cycles are used, but the Taq polymerase (Perkin Elmer) can lose much of its activity if utilized through higher number of cycles. Recently other polymerases have become available that are much less sensitive to high temperatures than Taq. Next we intend to explore these enzymes in hopes of increasing the sensitivity of our assay further. Preliminary tests in our laboratory have shown that sensitivity can be increased to at least 93% with such enzymes while maintaining a specificity of 100%.

We conclude that it is possible to accurately diagnose *H. pylori* infection from gastric juice specimens alone. Since such samples can be obtained by passing a soft nasogastric tube into the stomach, it may be possible in the future to diagnose *H. pylori* infection without endoscopy.

References

1. Czinn SJ, Carr HS, Speck WT (1991) Diagnosis of gastritis caused by *Helicobacter pylori* in children by means of an ELISA. Rev Infect Dis 13 [Suppl 8]: S700–S703
2. Westblom TU, Madan E, Gudipati S, Midkiff BR, Czinn SJ (1992) Diagnosis of *Helicobacter pylori* infection in adult and pediatric patients using pyloriset, a rapid latex agglutination test. J Clin Microbiol 30: 96–98
3. Marshall BJ, Surveyor I (1988) Carbon-14 urea breath test for the diagnosis of *Campylobacter pylori* associated gastritis. J Nucl Med 29: 11–16
4. Westblom TU (1991) Laboratory diagnosis and handling of *Helicobacter pylori*. In: Marshall BJ, McCallum RW, Guerrant RL (eds) *Helicobacter pylori* in peptic ulceration and gastritis. Blackwell Scientific, Cambridge, pp 81–91
5. Delmee M, Debongnie JC, Warzee P, Mainguet P (1987) Une methode originale de prelevement bacteriologique pour l'etude de *Campylobacter pylori* dans l'ulcere duodenal. Gastroenterol Clin Biol 11: 550–553
6. Debongnie JC, Delmee M, Mainguet P (1989) *Campylobacter pylori* in gastric, duodenal and jejunal juices and mucosae of patients with duodenal ulcer. Acta Gastroenterol Belg 52: 3–8
7. Bazhenov LG, Saidkhanov BA, Khodzhaeva NU (1990) The determination of *C. pylori* in patients with gastroduodenal diseases. Lab Delo (10): 71–73
8. Westblom TU, Phadnis S, Normark S (1991) Polymerase chain reaction (PCR) for diagnosis of *Helicobacter pylori* infection. Gastroenterology 100: A625
9. Westblom TU, Phadnis S, Normark S (1991) Sensitivity of an assay for detection of *Helicobacter pylori* in human saliva using polymerase chain reaction (PCR). Microbial Ecol Hlth Dis 4(S): S156
10. Yap EPH, McGee JOD (1991) Short PCR product yields improved by lower denaturation temperatures. Nucleic Acids Res 19: 1713

Molecular Fingerprinting of *Helicobacter pylori*: An Evaluation of Methods

D.D. Morgan[1], C. Clayton[1], H. Kleanthous[1], C. McNulty[2], and S. Tabaqchali[1]

Introduction

In order to fully investigate the role of *Helicobacter pylori* in the aetiology and pathogenesis of peptic ulcer disease sensitive methods of identifying and fingerprinting isolates of this organism are required. Conventional typing methods for bacteria, such as phage typing and serotyping have proven largely ineffective in typing *H. pylori*. Limited success has been achieved using systems based upon preformed enzymes such as the API-Zym system; however, the biotypes defined by such systems are limited and a large proportion of isolates fall into one biotype [1]. The more successful methods of identifying and fingerprinting *H. pylori* make use of molecular biological methods such as sodium dodecyl sulphate polyacrylamide gel electrophoresis (SDS-PAGE), restriction endonuclease digestion of genomic DNA and ribosomal RNA gene hybridisation patterns [2, 3].

A number of the existing molecular fingerprinting methods examining both genotypic and phenotypic characteristics have been evaluated in our laboratory. The methods examined are SDS-PAGE of whole cell proteins; SDS-PAGE of [S35] methionine-labelled proteins, immunoblot analysis of whole cell proteins, restriction endonuclease analysis of genomic DNA, and restriction endonuclease analysis of polymerase chain reaction (PCR) products.

Materials and Methods

Bacterial Strains. The isolates of *H. pylori* used in this study were comprised of a number of pre- and post-treatment isolates taken from patients undergoing an erythromycin treatment clinical trial. These strains were kindly provided by Dr. C. McNulty. A number of single isolates of *H. pylori* from patients attending gastroenterology clinics at St. Bartholomew's Hospital were also studied. All isolates were cultured on Columbia agar supplemented with 5% defibrinated horse blood for 2–3 days at 37°C under microaerobic conditions.

[1] Department of Medical Microbiology, St. Bartholomew's Hospital Medical College, West Smithfield, London, UK
[2] Gloucester Public Health Laboratory, Gloucester Royal Hospital, Gloucester, UK

Gasbarrini/Pretolani (Eds.)
Basic and Clinical Aspects of H. pylori Infection

SDS-PAGE of Whole Cell Proteins. All isolates were cultured as described above. Sample were prepared and polyacrylamide gels were run according to previously described protocols [2].

SDS-PAGE of [^{35}S] Methionine-Labelled Proteins. Isolates were grown microaerobically for 48 h at 37°C in brain heart infusion broth (Oxoid) supplemented with 5% foetal calf serum and 50 μCi [^{35}S]methionine (Amersham International). SDS-PAGE samples and gels were run as previously [2]. After electrophoresis the gels were fixed, dried and exposed to autoradiography film for 2–3 days according to previously described protocols [4].

Immunoblot Analysis of Whole Cell Proteins. SDS-PAGE gels were electrophoresed and proteins transferred to nitrocellulose membranes according to standard protocols. The transferred proteins were then reacted with rabbit antisera raised against sonicated *H. pylori*. Bound antisera was detected with goat anti-rabbit IgG conjugated to alkaline phosphatase. Full details of the methods used may be found in [5].

Restriction Endonuclease Analysis of Genomic DNA. DNA was extracted using the guanidium thiocyanate method, digested and electrophoresed according to previous protocols [3].

Restriction Endonuclease Analysis of Polymerase Chain Reaction Products. PCR was performed according to standard conditions on 100 ng purified *H. pylori* genomic DNA using DNA oligonucleotide primers to specific regions of a number of known genes. After PCR the products were digested without further purification for 2–4 h using a number of restriction endonucleases. Restriction endonucleases were chosen for their known ability to cut the *H. pylori* genome at frequent intervals. The restriction fragments produced were analysed by agarose gel electrophoresis.

Results

SDS-PAGE of Whole Cell Proteins. Figure 1 shows a Coomassie blue stained polyacrylamide gel of a number of *H. pylori* strains isolated from different patients. Major protein bands are evident at 61, 56, 54 and 48 kDa corresponding to the urease B gene product, the flagellin proteins and the HtrA protein. Also present in all strains is a 27-kDa protein. Variation between the strains is evident at 50–200 kDa and at 46–54 kDa.

SDS-PAGE of [^{35}S] Methionine-Labelled Proteins. Figure 2 shows [^{35}S]methionine-labelled protein patterns of a number of single isolates. Again the major protein bands at 61, 56, 54 and 48 kDa are evident. Individual isolates are characterised by variation between 58–200 kDa and 46–55 kDa. Isolates from the same patient have very similar patterns in these regions (results not shown).

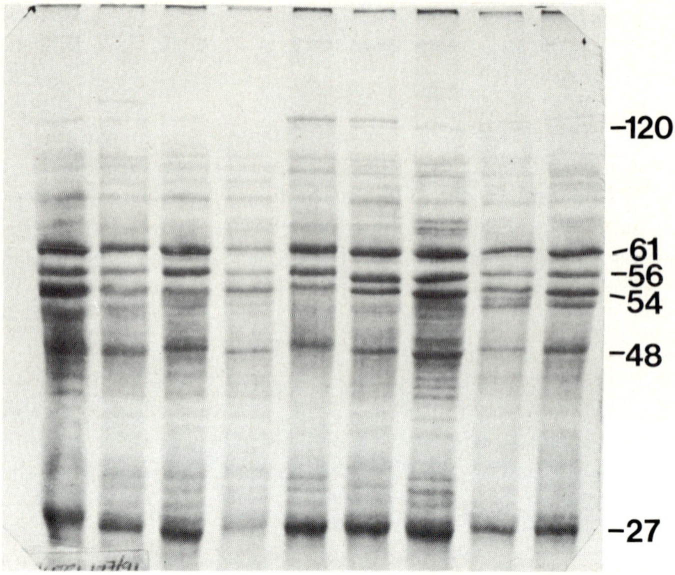

Fig. 1. Coomasie blue stained SDS-PAGE patterns of whole cell proteins of individual isolates of *H. pylori* (molecular weights in kilodaltons as indicated)

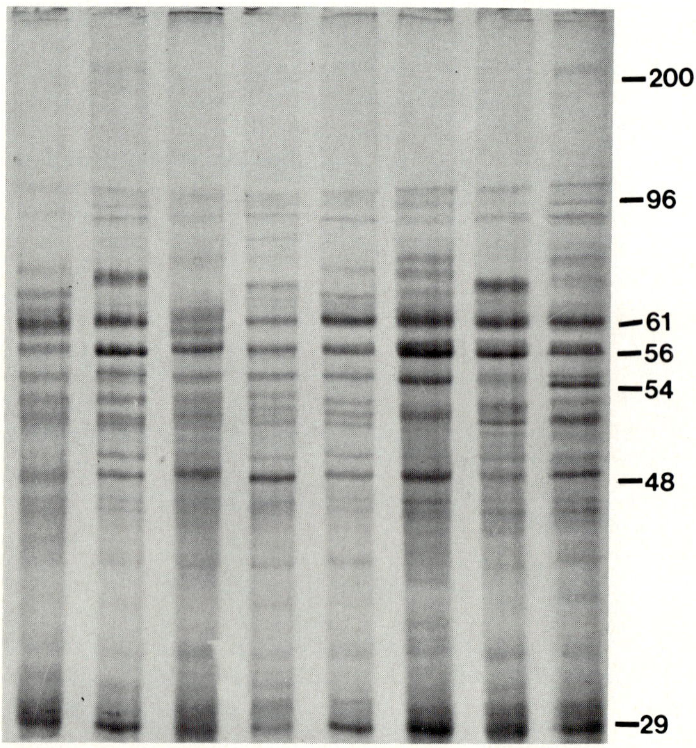

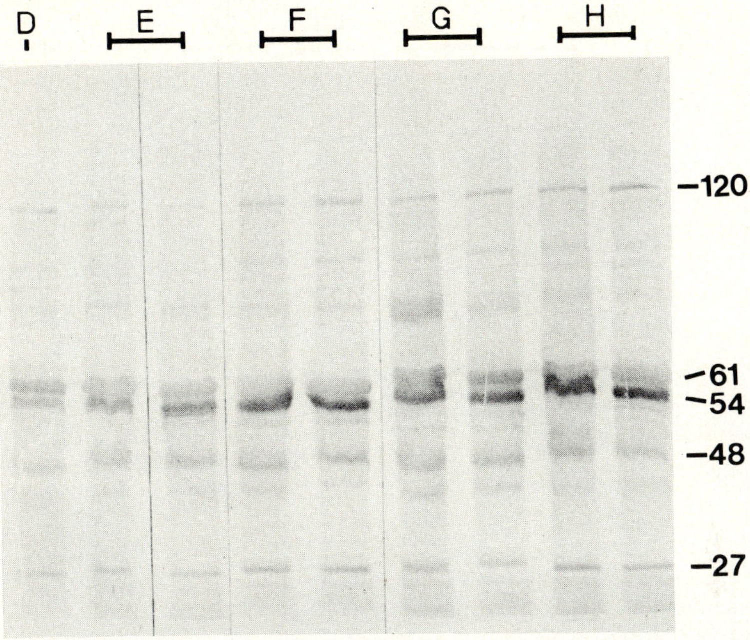

Fig. 3. Immunoblot of whole cell proteins of isolates of *H. pylori* taken from patients before and after treatment (molecular weights in kilodaltons as indicated)

Immunoblot Analysis of Whole Cell Proteins. Figure 3 shows an immunoblot of whole cell proteins detected with rabbit antisera raised against sonicated *H. pylori.* Major protein bands such as the urease (61 kDa) and the flagellin are easily identified as well as a number of other immunogenic proteins in the 48–84 kDa region. Minor differences in the 26–48 and the 58–120 kDa regions allow identification of isolates from the same patient and also differentiate between isolates from different patients.

Restriction Endonuclease Analysis of Genomic DNA. Figure 4 shows DNA fingerprints obtained from pre- and post-treatment isolates of *H. pylori.* As can be seen from the figure restriction fragments from approximately 2 to 23 kb allow accurate fingerprinting of isolates from the same patient and also distinguish between isolates from different patients. This figure also demonstrates the high degree of genomic variation at the sub-species level as has been noted by other workers [6, 7].

Restriction Endonuclease Analysis of Polymerase Chain Reaction Products. Figure 5 shows restriction endonuclease digests of PCR products from the urease gene. As can be seen from the figure PCR of all isolates gives rise to an homogeneous

Fig. 2. SDS-PAGE patterns of [^{35}S]methionine-labelled proteins of individual isolates of *H. pylori* (molecular weights in kilodaltons as indicated)

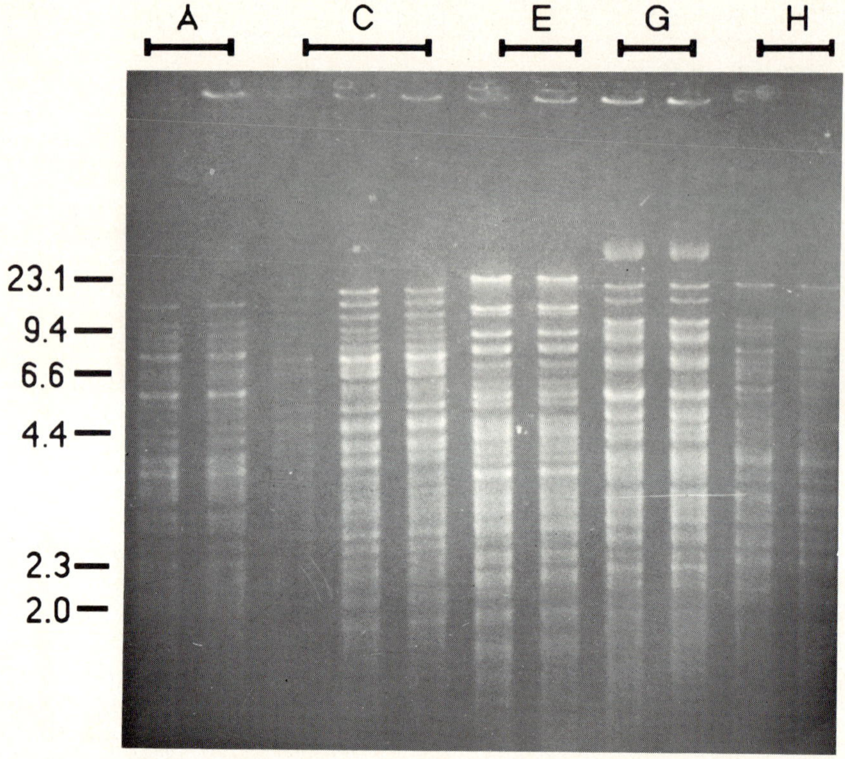

Fig. 4. *Hae*III restriction digest of genomic DNA of isolates of *H. pylori* taken from patients before and after treatment (molecular weights in kilobases as indicated)

917-bp product. However, if the products are digested with a number of restriction endonucleases, as indicated, a number of polymorphisms become apparent allowing fingerprinting of the isolates.

A combination of a number of DNA oligonucleotide pairs and restriction digests are necessary for fingerprinting each *H. pylori* isolate.

Discussion

All molecular fingerprinting methods examined in this study gave good agreement with each other in identifying isolates from the same patient and distinguishing between isolates from different patients.

A number of the isolates examined consistently failed to give clear, resolved SDS-PAGE protein patterns in the 46–54 and 50–200 kDa regions when stained with Coomassie blue (as has been found by other workers [8]). This makes accurate strain identification and fingerprinting difficult. In our hands this problem was overcome by the use of [^{35}S]methionine-labelled proteins which generally gave clearer and more defined band patterns in these regions. We have found that SDS-PAGE of [^{35}S]methionine-labelled proteins is a reprodu-

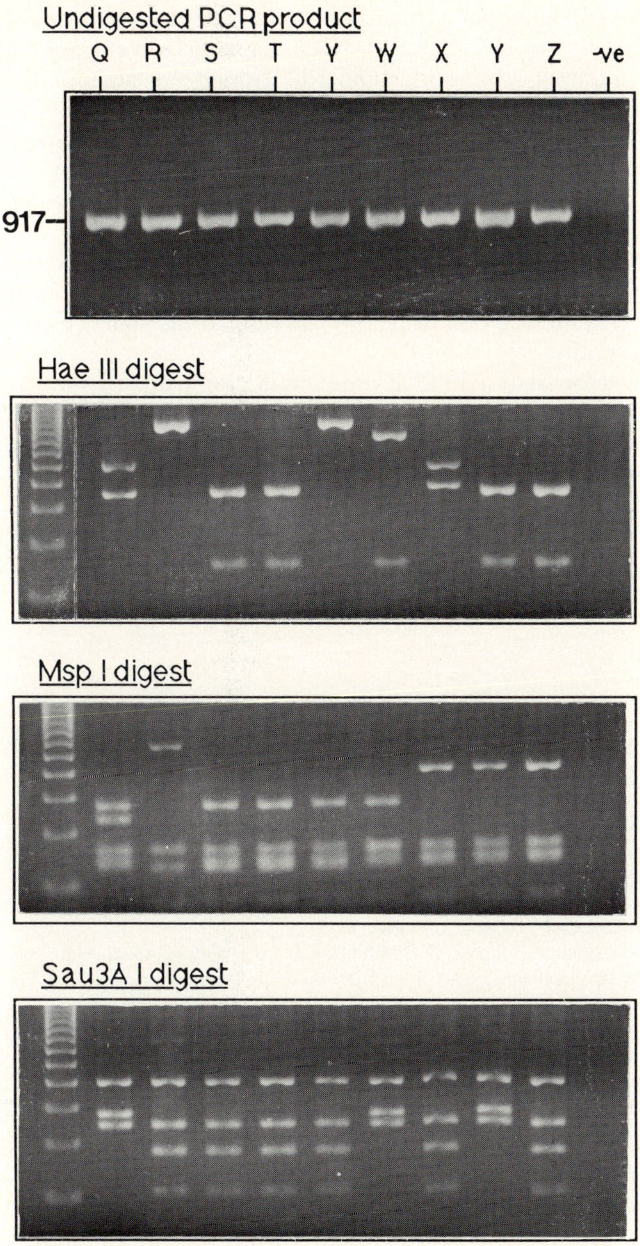

Fig. 5. Restriction endonuclease analysis of polymerase chain reaction fragments of the urease B gene of a number of individual isolates of *H. pylori* (*lane 1* of each digest: 100 basepair ladder)

cible method that is technically simple to perform. Although the method requires some time to produce good autoradiograph images and involves the use of radioactive isotopes, we feel that this method may represent a standardised approach that may be employed in dffferent laboratories.

Immunoblot analysis of whole cell proteins is a technically difficult method to perform requiring lengthy incubation periods. Clear, highly resolved patterns are difficult to obtain, and inter-laboratory standardisation of the method may be difficult due to antigenic variation.

Restriction endonuclease analysis of genomic DNA is a rapid and inexpensive method of fingerprinting *H. pylori*. The DNA fingerprints produced are reproducible and highly discriminatory. However, the fingerprints are complex and in the case of some restriction endonucleases are difficult to interpret. This problem may be overcome by the use of specific gene probes such as ribosomal RNA genes [3]. However, methods such as these are time consuming to perform and have been found by some workers to be less discriminating than the corresponding DNA fingerprints [9].

Restriction endonuclease analysis of PCR products is a rapid and reproducible fingerprinting method that is easy to perform and produces simple and easy to interpret DNA fingerprints. It is possible to perform this technique on boiled extracts of bacterial colonies making the method more applicable to clinical situations. Having by-passed the requirement for a relatively complicated genomic DNA preparation we feel that this method will find wider application in the fingerprinting of *H. pylori* and other bacteria.

References

1. Owen RJ, Desai M (1990) Preformed enzyme profiling of *Helicobacter pylori* and *Helicobacter mustelae* from human and animal sources. Lett Appl Microbiol 11: 103–105
2. Owen RJ, Costas M, Morgan DD et al. (1989) Strain variation in *Campylobacter pylori* detected by numerical analysis of one-dimensional electrophoretic protein patterns Antonie van Leeuwenhoek. J Microbiol 55: 283–287
3. Morgan DD, Owen RJ (1990) Use of DNA restriction endonuclease digest and ribosomal RNA gene probe patterns to fingerprint *Helicobacter pylori* and *Helicobacter mustelae* isolated from human and animal hosts. Mol Cell Probes 4: 321–334
4. Tabaqchali S, O'Farrell S, Holland D, Silman R (1986) Method for typing *Clostridium difficile* based on polyacrylamide gel electrophoresis of [^{35}S]methionine labelled proteins. J Clin Microbiol 23: 197–198
5. Clayton CL, Wren BW, Mullany P, Topping A, Tabaqchali S (1989) Molecular cloning and expression of *Campylobacter pylori* specific antigens in *Escherichia coli* K-12. Infect Immun 57: 623–629
6. Langenberg W, Rauws EAJ, Widjojokusomo A, Tytgat GNJ, Zanen HC (1986) Identification of *Campylobacter pylori* isolates by restriction endonuclease DNA analysis. J Clin Microbiol 24: 414–417
7. Majewski SIH, Goodwin CS (1988) Restriction endonuclease analysis of the genome of *Campylobacter pylori* with a rapid extraction method: evidence for considerable genomic variation. J Infect Dis 157: 465–471
8. Owen RJ, Bickley J, Costas M, Morgan DR (1991) Genomic variation in *Helicobacter pylori*: application to identification of strains. Scand J Gastroenterol 26 [Suppl 181]: 43–50
9. Fraser J, Owen RJ, Morgan DD, Costas M, Morgan DR (1990) Assessment of DNA and protein molecular fingerprinting methods for strain identification of *Helicobacter pylori*. In: Malfertheiner P, Ditschuneit H (eds) *Helicobacter pylori*, gastritis and peptic ulcer. Springer, Berlin Heidelberg New York

Developments in Ribotyping of *Helicobacter pylori*

R.J. Owen

Introduction

In 1986 Langenberg and colleagues [5] showed that chromosomal DNA restriction endonuclease digest analysis provided a sensitive method of discriminating between isolates of *Helicobacter pylori.* Since then such data have been used increasingly to characterize clinical isolates of *H. pylori* in treatment and epidemiological studies (for reviews see [3,9]). The total DNA patterns are generally complex and difficult to apply to large numbers of strains, but in 1990 Morgan and Owen [6] demonstrated that simpler fingerprints can be obtained by highlighting specific DNA sequences, namely ribosomal (r)RNA genes, within total digests. Subsequent studies provided further evidence that rRNA gene probe patterns (ribopatterns) are a simple but highly discriminatory electrophoretic fingerprint for *H. pylori* [9–12, 16]. The aim of the present report is to describe some recent developments and applications of ribopatterns to typing *H. pylori.*

Materials and Methods

Media and Growth Conditions. The *H. pylori* isolates used were from gastric and duodenal sites of patients in the United Kingdom, Canada, South Africa, Nigeria and Italy. Organisms were grown routinely on Oxoid brain-heart infusion agar supplemented with 5% v/v horse blood and 1% Isovitalex for 2 days at 37°C in microaerobic conditions (5% O_2; 5% CO_2; 2% H_2; 88% N_2) in a Variable Atmosphere Incubator (Don Whitley Scientific, Shipley, Yorkshire, UK). Strains were preserved at − 196°C on glass beads in Nutrient Broth 2 (Oxoid, CM67) containing 10% v/v glycerol.

DNA Preparation. Chromosomal DNA was isolated and purified using the guanidium thiocyanate reagent method [14].

DNA Digestion and Electrophoresis. All DNA samples (5 μg) were digested for 4 h at 37°C with *Hae*III and *Hind*III (2–3 U/μg DNA). The digested DNA was

National Collection of Type Cultures, Central Public Health Laboratory, 61 Colindale Avenue, London NW9, 5HT, UK

Gasbarrini/Pretolani (Eds.)
Basic and Clinical Aspects of H. pylori Infection

electrophoresed at 30 V for 16 h in a horizontal 0.7% (w/v) agarose gel in a buffer containing 89 m*M* Tris hydrochloride, 89 m*M* boric acid, and 2 m*M* disodium ethylenediaminetetraacetic acid (EDTA), pH 8.3. After electrophoresis the gels were stained with ethidium bromide and photographed with Polaroid 667 film.

Preparation of Biotinylated Probe cDNA. The biotinylated cDNA probe was prepared from *Escherichia coli* 16-S and 23-S rRNA (BDH, UK), using Moloney mouse leukaemia virus reverse transcriptase (Gibco-BRL). Biotinylation was by the incorporation of biotin-16dUTP [15].

Southern Blotting and Hybridization. After electrophoresis and photography the gels were transferred to nylon membranes (Hybond-N, Amersham International) by means of either the standard capillary transfer or vacuum methods. The membranes were then hybridized by standard procedures for 18 h at 42°C using the biotinylated cDNA probe [15]. The membranes were washed and the hybridized probe detected colorimetrically with the BlueGene (Gibco-BRL) nonradioactive detection kit.

Band Size Estimation. DNA fragment sizes in the blot hybridization patterns were calculated from migration distances either by the DNA SIZE program described previously [8] or by an automated gel reader and analysis system (IBI, New Haven, Conn., USA). Biotinylated lambda phage (GIBCO-BRL) digested with *Hin*dIII was used to provide the size markers on each gel.

Computation of Strain Similarities. To compare ribopatterns from different membranes, the bands were coded according to size to minimize errors when determining similarities by computer-assisted methods of analysis. The blot hybridization patterns were screened for bands within 21 dfff erent size ranges up to 10 kb and positive (presence) and negative (absence) results were recorded. Bands of faint intensity were excluded. Double bands falling within a given range were scored as a single band. Computed similarities among strains were estimated by means of the Dice coefficient (negative matches excluded) and clustering of strains was based on the unweighted pair group method to facilitate the generation and the plotting of a dendrogram [17]. All computations were performed using the DNAGE program, a modification of previously described software [21].

Results and Discussion

Restriction Endonucleases Used. Restriction endonucleases differ widely in the ability to cut chromosomal DNA from *H. pylori* and to yield total digest patterns and ribopatterns suitable for molecular fingerprinting purposes:

- DNA cut completely by: *Hae*III, *Hin*dIII
- DNA cut to some extent by: *Bam*HI, *Bst*EII, *Eco*RI, *Msp*I, *Pvu*II, *Stu*I
- DNA not cut by: *Acc*I, *Alu*I, *Bsc*I, *Cfo*I, *Pst*I, *Rso*I, *Sac*II, *Sal*I, *Sph*I, *Taq*I, *Xho*I

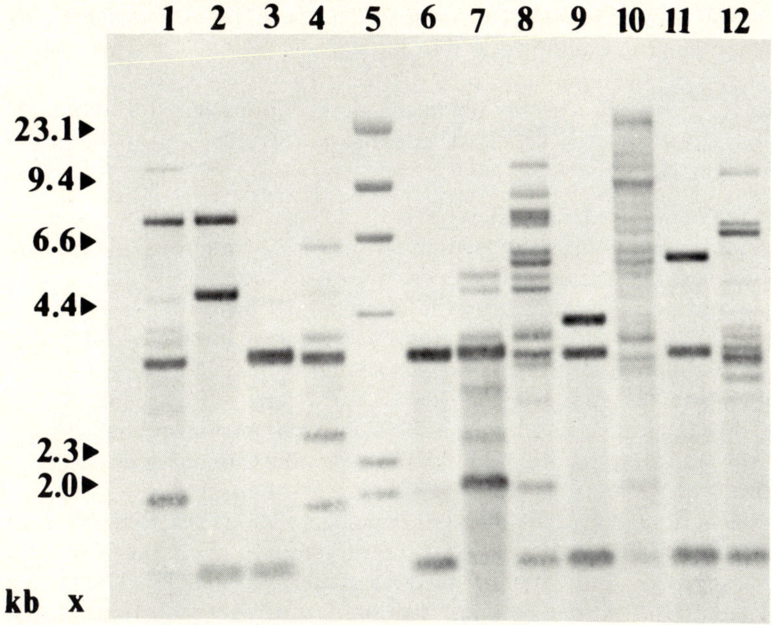

Fig. 1. The rRNA gene patterns (ribopatterns) for *Hin*dIII digests of chromosomal DNA probed with biotinylated cDNA from 16 + 23*S* rRNA from *H. pylori* NCTC 11638. The strains (*lanes 1–4, 6–12*) were provided by Dr N. Figura, University of Siena, Italy [12]. *Lane 5*, *Hin*dIII digest of bacteriophage – DNA.

Studies on over 200 strains of *H. pylori* show that the tetranucleotide recognition sequence cutting enzyme *Hae*III and the hexanucleotide cutter *Hin*dIII yield the most generally usable patterns. *Hae*III ribopatterns commonly comprise five to eight well resolved fragments in the range 1–10 kb [11, 12]. However, *Hae*III does not cut DNA from about 25% of *H. pylori*, which is most likely due to some degree of selective methylation of the *Hae*III sites. In contrast, *Hin*dIII cuts DNA from most strains yielding ribopatterns that differ considerably in complexity from simple two to three fragment patterns to those containing multiple (> 10) fragments (Fig. 1). The latter ribopatterns appear to be characteristic of particular strains and due to partial cutting of the DNA by *Hin*dIII, which may be caused by residual inhibitors such as guanidium thiocyanate, carried over in the DNA extraction procedure.

Ribotyping Probes. The 16*S* rRNA gene sequences of *E. coli* and *H. pylori* are about 80% homologous [13] so ribotyping of *H. pylori* was initially performed using *E. coli* 16 + 23*S* rRNA as the cDNA template for reverse transcription [8, 9]. Sometimes referred to as a "universal probe" [18], *E. coli* rRNA gene sequences have been used to obtain ribopatterns for a variety of bacterial species [4, 7]. Subsequently, we discovered that the hybridization signal intensity, the number of bands detected and the reproducibility of detection with the biotin-labelled cDNA probe were significantly improved if *H. pylori* 16 + 23*S* rRNA was used as the template for cDNA synthesis. The use of the *E. coli* rRNA gene probe was therefore discontinued in this context.

Results on H. pylori. The results obtained on the ribopatterns of about 250 isolates of *H. pylori* from a variety of patients and countries over the past 3 years are summarized below:

- Species are genotypically diverse.
- Most patients are colonized by a single strain with a uniform genotype, but possibly several DNA subtypes.
- Duodenal and antral isolates from the same patient have similar genotypes (no consistent variation between anatomical sites in genotypes or subtypes).
- Strains from different individuals are genotypically distinct, except for some family members.
- Sequential isolates are generally the same before and after treatment so ulcer relapse or treatment failure is most probably due to recrudescence not reinfection.
- Differences in ribopatterns are reflected in polyacrylamide gel electrophoresis protein patterns, but the latter are less discriminatory.
- No consistent associations exist between ribopatterns or individual fragments in ribopatterns and enzyme biotypes, motility, cytotoxin production, patient symptoms, or geographical origin of strains.

The primary result of our studies is that *H. pylori* exhibits a diversity of genotypes when conserved rRNA genes are used as molecular markers. This heterogeneity arises despite the fact that strains within *H. pylori* exhibit a relatively high intra-specific overall DNA homology [1]. *H. pylori* appears to be unusual in this respect because other bacterial species generally show greater intraspecific uniformity in their ribopatterns to the extent that in *Campylobacter* and *Acidovorax* some fragments can be regarded as species-specific markers (R.J. Owen, unpublished results).

A novel aspect of our most recent research has been the application of numerical methods to code and compare ribopatterns from different isolates of *H. pylori*. There was no evidence of correlations between such patterns as particular bands within ribopatterns and phenotypic subsets based on enzymic biotyping, motility, cytotoxin production, site of isolation, patient diagnosis or geographical location. An important development from this work is that it has enabled us to show that each individual has a unique strain type with the possible exceptions of some family members, and to define genomic subtypes *H. pylori* within individuals. Furthermore, comparisons of isolates from different anatomical sites in the same individual have shown intersite heterogeneity in *H. pylori* subtypes as well as the presence of different subtypes on repeat biopsy from the same or adjacent anatomical sites (Fig. 2).

*Conclusions. Hae*III ribopatterns provide an excellent basis for fingerprinting strains in small scale studies such as family groups or treatment studies but are too discriminatory for large-scale purposes with as yet no rational basis for grouping strains. By contrast, *Hin*dIII ribopatterns are generally simpler, and as strains from diverse origins can be sorted into groups with common genotypes

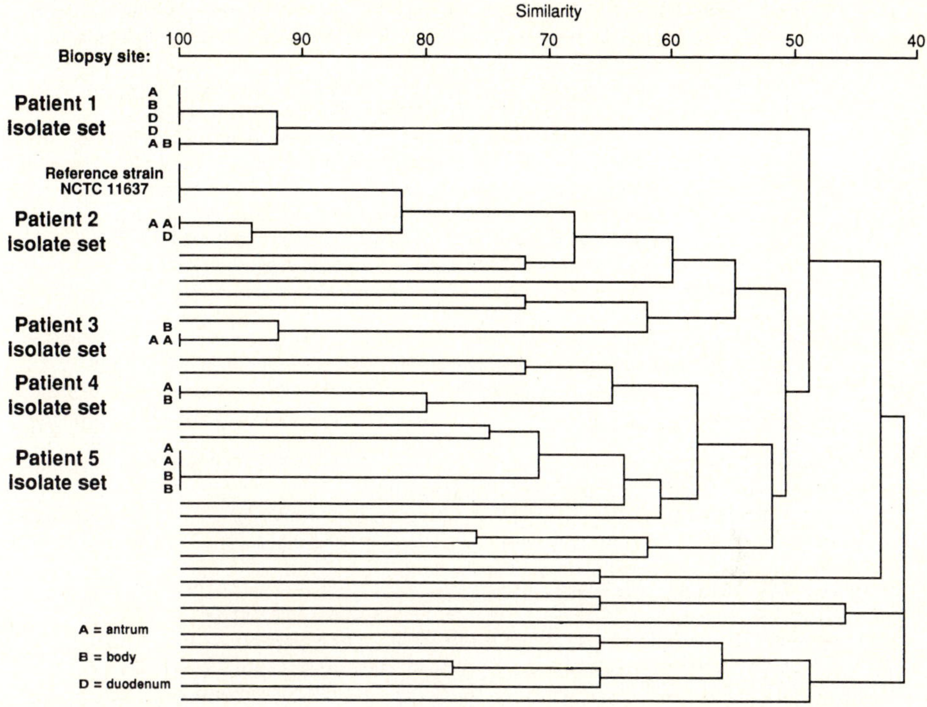

Fig. 2. Dendrogram of a numerical analysis of *H. pylori* ribopatterns (*vertical axis*) from different patients and anatomical sites. *Numbers on horizontal axis*, percentage similarities as determined by the Dice coefficient. The strains were from biopsies provided by Dr E. Prewett, Royal Free Hospital, London, UK [16].

[11], such ribopatterns may provide the basis for future epidemiological typing studies.

Acknowledgements. J. Bickley, M. Moreno and M. Desai are thanked for their excellent technical assistance. The Procter and Gamble Company (Cincinnati) is thanked for financial support.

References

1. Bukholm G, Nedenskov-Sorensen P, Bovre K (1989) DNA-DNA hybridization incompatibility of *Campylobacter pylori* with other *Campylobacter* and *Wolinella* species. APMIS 97: 472–474
2. Costas M (1990) Numerical analysis of sodium dodecyl sulphate – polyacrylamide gel electrophoretic protein patterns for the classification, identification and typing of medically important bacteria. Electrophoresis 11: 382–391
3. Costas M, Owen RJ, Bickley J, Morgan DR (1991) Molecular techniques for studying the epidemiology of infection by *Helicobacter pylori*. Scand J Gastroenterol 26 [Suppl 181]: 20–32
4. Grimont F, Grimont PAD (1986) Ribosomal ribonucleic acid gene restriction patterns as potential taxonomic tools. Ann Inst Pasteur Microbiol 137B: 165–175
5. Langenberg W, Rauws EAJ, Widjojokusomo A et al. (1986) Identification of *Campylobacter pylori* isolates by restriction endonuclease analysis. J Clin Microbiol 24: 414–417

6. Morgan DD, Owen RJ (1990) Use of DNA restriction digest and ribosomal RNA gene probe patterns to fingerprint *Helicobacter pylori* and *Helicobacter mustelae* isolated from human and animal hosts. Molec Cell Prob 4: 321–334
7. Owen RJ (1989) Chromosomal DNA fingerprinting – a novel method of species and strain identification applicable to microbial pathogens. J Med Microbiol 30: 89–99
8. Owen RJ, Beck A (1987) Evaluation of three procedures using a laser densitometer and microcomputer for estimating molecular sizes of restriction endonuclease digest fragments and application to *Campylobacter jejuni* chromosomal DNA. Lett Appl Microbiol 4: 5–8
9. Owen RJ, Bickley J, Costas M, Morgan DR (1991) Genomic variation of *Helicobacter pylori*: application to identification of strains. Scand J Gastroenterol 26 [Suppl 181]: 43–50
10. Owen RJ, Bickley J, Moreno M et al. (1991) Biotype and macromolecular profiles of cytotoxin-producing strains of *Helicobacter pylori* from antral gastric mucosa. FEMS Microbiol Lett 79: 199–204
11. Owen RJ, Bickley J, Lastovica A et al. (1992) Ribosomal RNA gene patterns of *Helicobacter pylori* from surgical patients with healed and recurrent peptic ulcers. Epidemiol Infect 108: 39–50
12. Owen RJ, Figura N, Moreno M (1992) Biotype and DNA fingerprints of cytotoxigenic *Helicobacter pylori* from patients with gastritis and peptic ulceration in Italy. Eur J Epidemiol 8: 15–21
13. Pitcher DG, Saunders NA, Owen RJ (1989) Rapid extraction of bacterial genomic DNA with guanidium thiocyanate. Lett Appl Microbiol 8: 151–156
14. Paster BJ, Dewhirst FE (1988) Phylogeny of campylobacters, wolinellas, *Bacteroides gingivalis*, and *Bacteroides ureolyticus* by 16*S* ribosomal ribonucleic acid sequencing. Int J Syst Bacteriol 38: 56–62
15. Pitcher DG, Owen RJ, Dyal P, Beck A (1987) Synthesis of a biotinylated DNA probe to detect ribosomal RNA cistrons in *Providencia stuartii*. FEMS Microbiol Lett 48: 283–287
16. Prewett EJ, Bickley J, Owen RJ, Pounder RE (1992) DNA patterns of *Helicobacter pylori* isolated from gastric antrum, body, and duodenum. Gastroenterology 102: 829–833
17. Sneath PHA, Sokal RR (1973) Numerical taxonomy. Freeman, San Francisco
18. Stull TL, LiPuma JJ, Edlind TD (1988) A broad spectrum probe for molecular epidemiology of bacteria: ribosomal RNA. J Infect Dis 157: 280–286

The 130-kDa Vacuolating Cytotoxin-Associated Protein Is a Component of Cytotoxic *Helicobacter pylori* Organisms

M. Bugnoli[1], D. Armellini[1], R. Rappuoli[1], A. Rossolini[2], Z.Y. Xiang[3], and N. Figura[2]

Introduction

Helicobacter pylori (HP) is the agent of type B gastritis and a cofactor in the development of peptic ulcer and probably also of gastric cancer. Certain HP strains produce a toxin which induces intracellular vacuolization on mammalian cells in vitro. Proteins associated with vacuolating activity (VA) have molecular weights of 130, 95, and 80 kDa and can be detected in broth and in concentrated broth culture filtrates (CBCF) of cytotoxic strains [1].

Toxigenicity could be involved in the development of ulcerative lesions in dyspeptic patients. In fact, HP strains isolated from patients with peptic ulcer are significantly more often toxigenic than are those isolated from patients without ulcer with chronic gastritis only [3]. In addition, patients with duodenal ulcer have serum antibodies to the major 130-kDa cytotoxin-associated protein (p130), while patients without duodenal ulcer have antibodies to p130 at a significantly lower frequency [2]. Serum samples from patients infected by cytotoxic HP organisms (CTHP) also neutralize VA of CBCF. This suggests that the toxin is also produced in vivo, and that it is immunogenic.

In this study we demonstrate that p130 is a component of CTHP organisms, and that could be the major responsible of vacuolization, since a polyclonal antibody raised in mouse to p130 (MPA) inhibits VA of CBCF and of a whole cell HP suspension on cells in culture.

Material and Methods

Six cytotoxic (including CCUG 17874) and five noncytotoxic HP strains were used in this study. Strains were isolated on Columbia agar with 7% horse blood, 1% Vitox (Oxoid), and the Skirrow selective supplement. Strains were stored in Wilkins-Chalgren broth with 20% glycerol at −85°C. For all tests, ultrasonicates (US), CBCF, and whole cell guanidine extracts (GE) of bacteria were used.

HP extracts were prepared by treating whole bacterial suspension in phosphate-buffered saline (PBS) with guanidine 6 *M* at room temperature in

[1] Sclavo Research Center, Via Fiorentina 1, 53100 Siena, Italy
[2] Istituto di Malattie Infettive, Università di Siena, Italy
[3] Shanghai Hospital, Shanghai, China

Gasbarrini/Pretolani (Eds.)
Basic and Clinical Aspects of H. pylori Infection

agitation for 1 h. The supernatant, obtained by centrifugation in Beckman rotor JA 20 at 7000 rpm at 4°C for 30 min, was dialysed against PBS at 4°C for 16 h. After dialysis the insoluble material was pelletted by centrifugation as described above. The supernatant also contained an enriched fraction of 130-kDa protein as seen by sodium dodecyl sulfate polyacrylamide gel electrophoresis (SDS-PAGE). Electrophoresis was performed according to the method of Laemmli in Mini Protean II (Bio-Rad Laboratories). Proteins were denatured at 100°C for 5 min in sample buffer containing dithiothreitol, were stacked in 3% acrylamide gel, and separated by using 7% acrylamide (200 V). Proteins were stained with Coomassie brillant blue R-250. Separated proteins were also electrophoretically transferred on to nitrocellulose sheets (Schleicher and Schuell) with a constant current of 200 mA for 30 min. Nitrocellulose strips were blocked with PBS containing 3% defatted dry milk and 0.1% Triton X-100 at room temperature for 60 min. Strips were then incubated at room temperature for 16 h with MPA to 130-kDa protein diluted 1:5000 or with sera, diluted 1:200, from 11 patients infected by CTHP strains, from seven patients infected by non-CTHP organisms, and from five patients considered noninfected on the basis of negative results of culture, microscopic examination, and rapid urease activity of gastric biopsies, and of serology. Sera and MPA were diluted in PBS with 3% milk and 0.1% Triton (Blotto). Then strips were washed in Blotto for 30 min, and were incubated with peroxidase conjugated goat anti-mouse total IgG (Cappel) or with alkaline phosphatase conjugated goat anti-human IgG (Cappel) diluted 1:2500 in Blotto at room temperature for 90 min. Finally, the strips were washed in PBS with 0.5% Triton for 20 min and then with PBS alone. The Enhanced Chemiluminescence kit (ECL, Amersham) was used to reveal the reaction with the strips incubated with peroxidase conjugated antibody, and BCIP-MBT system (Bio-Rad) with the strips incubated with alkaline phosphatase conjugated antibody.

The GE of HP strains induced vacuolization on HeLa cells in vitro. Thus 130-kDa protein band of GE of HP CCUG 17874 was electroeluted from polyacrylamide gel and used to immunize mice. Animals were each given 30 μg protein intraperitoneally, emulsionated with Freund complete adjuvant. Injections were repeated weekly three times. The second dose was given after injection of 0.8 ml pristane per mouse. The antibodies were recovered in ascit fluid taken from the abdominal cavity.

The test of inhibition of VA was carried out in the following manner: HeLa cells were grown in Dulbecco's modified Eagle's medium (MEM) supplemented with 10% fetal calf serum (Hyclone), 100 U penicillin G, and 50 μg streptomycin per milliliter, in normal air with 5% CO_2 at 37°C. Confluent cells were trypsinized and 2×10^5 cells/ml were seeded into six-well polystyrene tissue culture plates (Costar). Cells were incubated over night, then were washed three times with MEM without antibiotics, and CBCF or whole HP suspension were added. For VA inhibition test, HP CCUG 17874 from a 48-h culture was washed three times in MEM without antibiotics, suspended in MEM up to a concentration of 5×10^7 organisms/ml, and mixed with MPA diluted 1:100 to 1:400. CBCF was diluted 1:8, which represented eightfold the vacuolization titer (the highest dilution at which 50% of cells were vacuolated), and then mixed with MPA diluted 1:4–1:256. Mixtures were incubated at 37°C for 60 min and at 4°C for a further 60 min; they were then added to HeLa cells which had been previously washed three times with MEM without antibiotics. After o.n. incubation at 37°C, cells were inspected for vacuolization and HP adhesion by optic microscope. Cells were also fixed with methanol and acetone (3:1) for 10 min, stained with acridine orange, and observed with epifluorescent microscope at X1000.

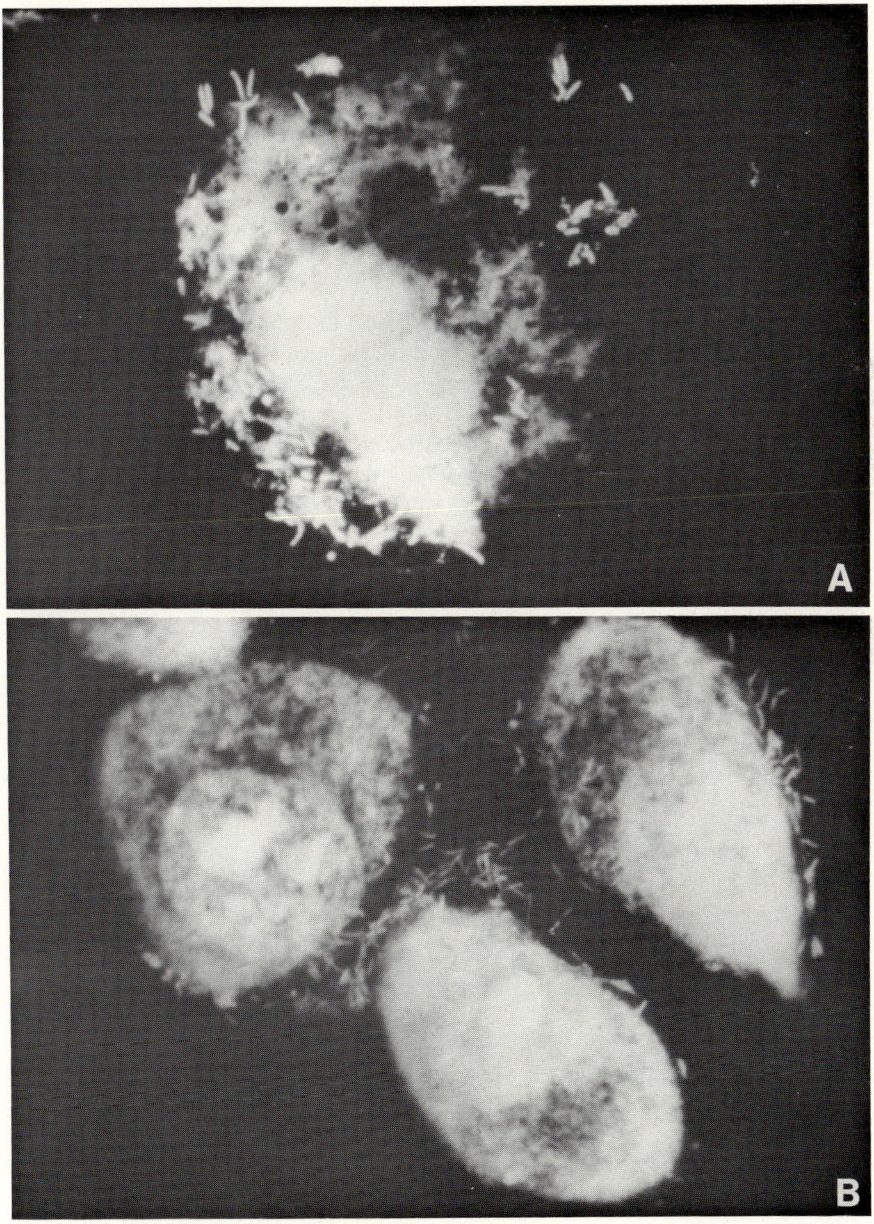

Fig. 1. Inhibition of vacuolization exerted by HP whole cell suspension of HeLa cells by mouse polyclonal antibody diluted 1:400 (**B**). **A** Control cells without mouse antibody. Acridine orange stain

Results and Discussion

A protein of 130 kDa mass (p130) was stained only in US and GE of the six CTHP strains; p130 was not present in the five non CTHP organisms. By western blotting, p130 was only recognized in US, GE, and CBCF of CTHP strains, and only by the sera collected from the 11 patients infected by CTHP bacteria. Sera from patients infected by non-CTHP strains did not react with any 130-kDa protein, but generally recognized 61-, 54-, and 29-kDa proteins (as well as sera from the 11 patients) present in CTHP and non-CTHP strains. Sera from noninfected patients did not react at all with any protein.

PMA reacted only with 130-kDa protein in US, GE, and CBCF of CTHP strains alone. In addition, it neutralized VA of GE and CBCF of the type strain up to a dilution of 1:64. It also prevented vacuolization induced by a whole cell suspension of HP CCUG 17874 at a dilution ⩾1:400 (Fig. 1A). The adhesion was not inhibited at all by MPA.

We started this study from the observation that p130 was a component of the type HP strain CCUG 17874 which induces vacuolization on cells in vitro. As a result, we saw that all CTHP organisms share this polypeptide, that it is generally retained by the bacteria, and that it is present in minimal amount in broth cultures. In fact, Coomassie blue does not stain any p130 in CBCF run in SDS-PAGE. In addition, when we grew a CTHP strain in *Brucella* broth with 0.1% β-cyclodextrin without fetal calf serum, blood or blood products, no VA was observed, and no p130 was detected in concentrated broth cultures. We also suspended a CTHP organism in MEM with and without fetal calf serum, centrifuged it after 2 h of incubation, and filtered the suspension. VA was observed only in filtrates which contained serum. Finally, the treatment of HP CCUG 17874 with tripsin (which degrades bacterial superficial proteins) completely destroyed p130.

In conclusion, p130 is the marker of vacuolating cytotoxin. It is most probably exposed at the surface of the bacteria and is not secreted, but it is simply splitted in the broth probably by proteases present in the serum added to media for culture.

References

1. Figura N, Bugnoli M, Cusi MG, Pucci AM, Lusini P, Quaranta S, Barberi A, Rossolini A, Di Tommaso AL, De Magistris T, Rappuoli R, Marri L, Musmanno RA, Russi M, Guarna M, Losi M (1990) Pathogenic mechanisms of *Helicobacter pylori*: production of cytotoxin. In: Malfertheiner P, Ditschuneit H (eds) *Helicobacter pylori*, gastritis and peptic ulcer. Springer, Berlin Heidelberg New York, p 86
2. Figura N, Bugnoli M, Guglielmetti P, Musmanno RA, Russi M, Quaranta S (1990) Antibodies to vacuolating toxin of *Helicobacter pylori* in dyspeptic patients. Rev Esp Enferm Dig 78 (S I): 7
3. Figura N, Guglielmetti P, Rossolini A, Barberi A, Cusi G, Musmanno RA, Russi M, Quaranta S (1989) Cytotoxin production by *Campylobacter pylori* strains isolated from patients with peptic ulcers and from patients with chronic gastritis only. J Clin Microbiol 27: 225–226

The Cloning and Partial Sequence Analysis of the Catalase Gene of *Helicobacter pylori*

D.G. Newell[1,3], P.J.M. Nuijten[2], A.R. Stacey[3], and S.L. Hazell

Introduction

Helicobacter pylori expresses significant quantities of a catalase, which may be an important virulence factor, modifying the effectiveness of the host polymorphonuclear cell responses to the organism at the gastric mucosal surface. Little is known about the structure of this enzyme. Hazell et al. [2] have shown that the native catalase is a tetramer with polypeptide subunits of 50 kDa. In addition, from other catalases it must also be assumed that is a metalloprotein containing a variable number of iron atoms.

The aim of this study was therefore to define at the molecular level the structure of this enzyme and thus provide the opportunity to define its role as a virulence factor in the same way as has been achieved for *H. pylori* urease.

Production of Monoclonal Antibodies Against Catalase

Monoclonal antibodies were produced from mice immunised with the catalase containing fraction (fraction 17) of sonicated organisms fractionated on a Superose 6 FPLC column as previously described [6]. This fraction contains a variety of polypeptides, but the major polypeptide was approximately 51–54 kDa. It is also known that the flagellin of *H. pylori* is present in this fraction 17 [6]. All the monoclonal antibodies produced and tested reacted with fraction 17 and the acid extract antigen of *H. pylori* [4], but only CP30, 30/2C6 and CP2J appeared to be specific for catalase purified according to the chromatographic techniques previously described [2]. By western blotting both CP30 and CP2J immunolabelled a single 54-kDa polypeptide in fraction 17 and in the purified catalase. This is also the approximate molecular weight of *H. pylori* flagellin [1], but the anti-*H. pylori* flagellin antibody 30.3B11 (Newell, unpublished data) did not react with purified catalase.

[1] Central Veterinary Laboratory, Weybridge, UK
[2] Institute for Infectious Diseases and Immunology University of Utrecht, The Netherlands
[3] PHLS, Centre for Applied Microbiology and Research Porton Down, Salisbury SP4 OJG UK
[4] School of Microbiology, University of New South Wales, Australia

Gasbarrini/Pretolani (Eds.)
Basic and Clinical Aspects of H. pylori Infection

Construction of a Genomic Library of *H. pylori*

An expression library of *H. pylori* chromosomal DNA was constructed in pEX plasmid vectors [3, 7]. Briefly, the *H. pylori* chromosomal DNA was isolated and partly digested with Sau 3AI giving DNA fragments with an average length of 2kb. These fragments were ligated in the pEX vectors linearized with *Bam*H1 and dephosphorylated with calf intestinal phosphatase. Ligation mixtures were electrophorated in *Escherichia coli* pop 2136. This resulted in a library of 130 000 clones, of which 80% were recombinant. Any recombinant containing an open reading frame from *H. pylori* should then lead to protein fusions with β-galactosidase.

Characterisation of Two pEX Clones that React with the Monoclonal Antibody CP30

More than 100 000 colonies of the pEX *H. pylori* library were screened with monoclonal antibody CP30. Two positive clones, Hp7 and Hp2, were isolated and characterised. The expression product of clone Hp7 was fusion protein with β-galactosidase, having a molecular weight of about 130 kDa. However, clone Hp2 produced a 30 kDa non-fusion protein which reacted only with CP30 but not with any other monoclonal antibody tested and not anti-β-galactosidase antibodies.

Nucleotide Sequencing of the 5′ End of the Catalase Gene

Initially the nucleotide sequence of clone Hp2 was determined. From this the open reading frame was deduced, and it was realised, on the basis of the expected size of the protein, that not all the gene was present in this clone. Clone Hp7, which overlapped with Hp2 by 300 bp, was then sequenced. Obviously the epitope recognised by monoclonal antibody CP30 was enclosed in this overlapping region. Although the overlapping region was identical in sequence, the downstream region showed an interruption of the reading frame. This open reading frame encodes a protein of 30 kDa, smaller that the expected 50–54 kDa for the catalase subunits. We therefore concluded that due to a possible cloning artefact the C-terminal end of the gene had not been obtained.

Comparison of the N-Terminal Sequences of Various Catalases

The sequence obtained, from clone Hp2, of the *H. pylori* catalase was compared with various catalases using the Sequence Databank in Nijmegen, the Netherlands. The open reading frame deduced from this sequence had a striking resemblance to the catalases of human and *E. coli* with 58% and 47% homology, respectively.

Antigenicity of *H. pylori* Catalase

One of the aims of previous studies has been to identify surface antigens of *H. pylori* for serodiagnostic purposes and for studying the specificity of immune responses. The immunogenicity of the native and recombinant catalases was therefore investigated using ELISA or western blotting techniques. Initially the catalase looked a promising antigen reacting with rabbit polyclonal antibodies directed against *H. pylori* but not those directed against *C. jejuni*, suggesting species specificity. The sensitivity and specificity of this antigen were assessed in 45 patients of known *H. pylori* status, established by culture and histology of endoscopy biopsies, serology using a standard technique and [^{14}C] urea breath test [5]. None of the sera from *H. pylori* negative patients reacted with the purified native catalase by ELISA. Only 5 of the sera from the 22 *H. pylori* positive patients (23%) had antibodies directed against this antigen. None of these seropositive patients had antibodies which reacted with the recombinant catalase (clone Hp2) as shown by western blotting, indicating that anti-catalase antibodies are either directed against the C-terminus end of the protein or, more likely, are directed against discontinuous epitopes.

Conclusion

In conclusion, part of the catalase gene of *H. pylori* has been cloned and expressed in *E. coli*, but the 3′ end has yet to be cloned. The *H. pylori* catalase gene promotor seems to be active in *E. coli* because clone Hp2 is a non-fusion protein. The catalases are evolutionary conserved enzymes as indicated by the homology between the *E. coli*, *H. pylori* and human genes. Finally, although the catalase is antigenic in some *H. pylori* positive patients the recombinant polypeptides are not suitable as diagnostic antigens. Work is in progress to complete the sequencing of this gene so that defined mutants can be produced for virulence investigations at a latter date.

References

1. Geis G, Leying H, Suerbaum S, Mai U, Offerkuch W (1990) Ultrastructure and chemical analysis of *Campylobacter pylori* flagella. J Clin Microbiol 27:436–441
2. Hazell SL, Evans DJ, Graham DY (1991) *Helicobacter pylori* catalase. J Gen Microbiol 137:57–61
3. Kusters JG, Jager EJ, van der Zeijst BAM (1990) Improvement of the cloning linker of the bacterial expression vector pEX. Nucleic Acid Res 17:8007

4. Newell DG (1987) Identification of the outer membrane proteins of *Campylobacter pyloridis* and antigenic cross reactivity between *C. pyloridis* and *C. jejuni*. J Gen Microbiol 133: 163–170
5. Newell DG, Hawtin PR, Stacey AR, MacDougall MH, Ruddle AC (1991) Estimation of prevalence of *Helicobacter pylori* infection in an asymptomatic elderly population comparing [^{14}C] urea breath test and serology. J Clin Pathol 44: 385–7
6. Stacey AR, Hawtin PR, Newell DG (1990) Antigenicity of fractions of *Helicobacter pylori* prepared by fast protein liquid chromatography and urease capture by monoclonal antibodies. Eur J Clin Microbiol Infect Dis 9: 732–737
7. Stanley KK, Luzio JP (1984) Construction of a new family of high efficiency bacterial expression vectors; identification of cDNA clones coding for human liver proteins. EMBO J 3: 1429–1434

Binding of *Helicobacter pylori* to Extracellular Matrix Proteins

A.P. Moran[1], P. Kuusela[2], and T.U. Kosunen[2]

Introduction

The extracellular matrix is composed of molecules and molecular complexes secreted by eukaryotic cells, whose components have adhesive properties, linking cells to one another or to the matrix. Extracellular matrices are typically composed of various types of collagens, the non-collagenous glycoproteins fibronectin and laminin, and different proteoglycans [17]. Since the first report of an interaction between a bacterium and a matrix protein [7], increased interest has arisen in the possibility that extracellular matrix proteins could act as receptors for bacterial adherence. In fact, a diverse range of bacteria, including staphylococci, streptococci, enterobacteria, *Bacillus subtilis*, *Mycobacterium tuberculosis*, *Treponema pallidum*, *Vibrio cholerae*, and *Campylobacter jejuni* have been shown to bind various extracellular matrix proteins [15].

It is well established that adherence is an important event in the pathogenesis of *Helicobacter pylori* [6]. The precise molecular mechanisms involved in recognition have not, to date, been fully elucidated. Although haemagglutinin activity [2, 4] and gastric glycolipid-binding [9, 11, 12] by *H. pylori* have been reported, the interaction of the bacterium with extracellular matrix proteins has received only limited attention [1]. We therefore investigated the interaction of *H. pylori* with soluble and immobilized extracellular matrix proteins.

Materials and Methods

Bacteria and Cultivation Conditions. H. pylori strains used in this investigation and their sources are shown in Table 1. Bacteria were grown on blood agar (Trypticase Soy agar, 6% horse blood) supplemented with 10% IsoVitaleX (BBL, Cockeysville, MD, USA) which was incubated in an atmosphere of 5% O_2, 10% CO_2, and 85% N_2 at 37°C for 42 h. Bacteria were harvested in 0.1 *M* phosphate-buffered saline (PBS), pH 7.3.

Proteins. Laminin (PBL, Gaithersburg, MD, USA), fibronectin, isolated from human plasma [3], and collagens, types I, III, IV, and V (Sigma, St. Louis, MO,

[1] Department of Microbiology, University College Galway, Galway, Ireland
[2] Department of Bacteriology and Immunology, University of Helsinki, 00290 Helsinki, Finland

Gasbarrini/Pretolani (Eds.)
Basic and Clinical Aspects of H. pylori Infection

Table 1. Strains used in this investigation

Strain	Source	Country of isolation
NCTC 11637	A	Australia
NCTC 11638	A	
C-5430	B	Canada
C-5437	B	
C-5790	B	
C-7058	B	
C-7066	B	
S-7	C	Sweden
S-23	C	
S-25	C	
S-27	C	

A, National Collection of Type Cultures, London, UK, B, H. Lior, Laboratory Centre for Disease Control, Ottawa, Canada, C, D. Danielsson, Medical Centre Hospital, Örebro, Sweden.

USA) were used in binding assays. Bovine serum albumin (BSA; Sigma) served as a negative control in binding assays. For use in adherence assays with soluble proteins, the selected proteins were labelled with ^{125}I by the iodogen procedure [10]. Alternatively, areas of 38 mm^2 on glass slides were coated with the extracellular matrix components under conditions which produced equal surface concentrations for each protein [8, 16].

Assay for Binding to Soluble Proteins. Bacteria (2×10^9) were incubated with 10 ng ^{125}I-labelled proteins in 1.0 ml PBS containing 1% (wt./vol.) BSA (PBS-BSA) at 20°C for 1.5 h. Subsequently, suspensions were centrifuged (15 000*g*, 5 min), the bacterial pellet saved and finally washed once with PBS-BSA. The amount of ^{125}I in the pellet, and hence the amount of protein bound to the bacteria, was measured by liquid scintillation counting.

Assay for Binding to Immobilized Proteins. Bacterial suspensions (100 μl) were applied to the immobilized proteins on glass slides, and incubated under aerobic (ambient atmosphere) or microaerobic (see above) conditions, at 20°C for 1.5 h. After incubation, glass slides were washed with PBS-BSA and bound bacteria stained with 1% (wt./vol.) crystal violet in ethanol. Attached bacteria were quantified by photomicroscopy; the mean bacterial count was calculated in six randomly chosen microscopic fields, and thus by relating the size of each microscopic field ($4.8 \times 10^3\,\mu m^2$) to that of the total coated area (38 mm^2) the total number of bound bacteria could be determined.

Estimation of the Percentage of Coccoid and Other Aberrant Forms in Suspensions. A sample (100 μl) of each bacterial suspension was examined by light microscopy before their use in adherence testing. Another sample of equal volume was incubated on an uncoated slide under aerobic conditions as in binding assays. Duplicate heat-fixed smears of these suspensions were stained with 0.1% (wt./vol.) aqueous carbol fuchsin for 5 min. The percentage of coccoid forms and other aberrant forms (e.g. rods without spiral morphology or short, squat rods) were estimated in three fields of vision per smear and the average of these estimations recorded for each sample. Approximately 600 bacteria were counted per sample.

Results

We evaluated the ability of 11 strains from three widely separated geographical regions (Australia, Canada, and Sweden) to bind to soluble and immobilized laminin, fibronectin and various collagens (I, III, IV and V). None of the strains tested bound these soluble proteins. On the other hand, some strains (NCTC 11637, C-5430, C-5437) adhered to immobilized fibronectin and laminin. When the assay for binding to immobilized proteins was performed under aerobic conditions, repeated experiments showed binding which was variable and irreproducible (Table 2), or failed to demonstrate bacterial adherence. In contrast, when testing was performed under microaerobic conditions, binding of *H. pylori* strains to fiibronectin and laminin was reproducible (Table 3). In addition,

Table 2. Attachment of *H. pylori* strains to extracellular matrix components at 2.0 pmol concentration under aerobic conditions: number of bacteria ($\times 10^5$) attached[a] (means ± ranges)

	Experiment 1			Experiment 2		
Immobilized protein	NCTC 11637	C-5430	C-5437	NCTC 11637	C-5430	C-5437
Laminin	73.9 ± 8.6	15.9 ± 1.9	—	14.9 ± 0.4	3.0 ± 0.6	—
Fibronectin	5.1 ± 0.6	10.2 ± 2.9	5.1 ± 2.0	—	1.7 ± 0.1	2.5 ± 0.1
Collagen I	—	—	—	—	—	—
Collagen III	—	—	—	—	—	—
Collagen IV	—	—	—	—	—	—
Collagen V	—	—	—	—	—	—
BSA	—	—	—	—	—	—

[a] 8×10^7 bacteria were added to each protein-coated area.

Table 3. Attachement of *H. pylori* strains to extracellular components at 2.0 pmol concentration under microaerobic conditions: number of bacteria ($\times 10^5$) attached[a] (means ± ranges)

	Experiment 1			Experiment 2		
Immobilized protein	NCTC 11637	C-5430	C-5437	NCTC 11637	C-5430	C-5437
Laminin	99.0 ± 17.6	35.2 ± 11.3	—	98.7 ± 15.3	34.0 ± 9.5	—
Fibronectin	8.9 ± 4.7	30.9 ± 11.1	15.7 ± 3.6	9.3 ± 2.6	29.3 ± 6.1	14.9 ± 5.2
Collagen I	—	3.2 ± 1.3	—	—	3.1 ± 0.5	—
Collagen III	—	—	—	—	—	—
Collagen IV	—	—	—	—	—	—
Collagen V	—	—	7.8 ± 1.0	—	—	7.8 ± 1.0
BSA	—	—	—	—	—	—

[a] 8×10^7 bacteria were added to each protein-coated area.

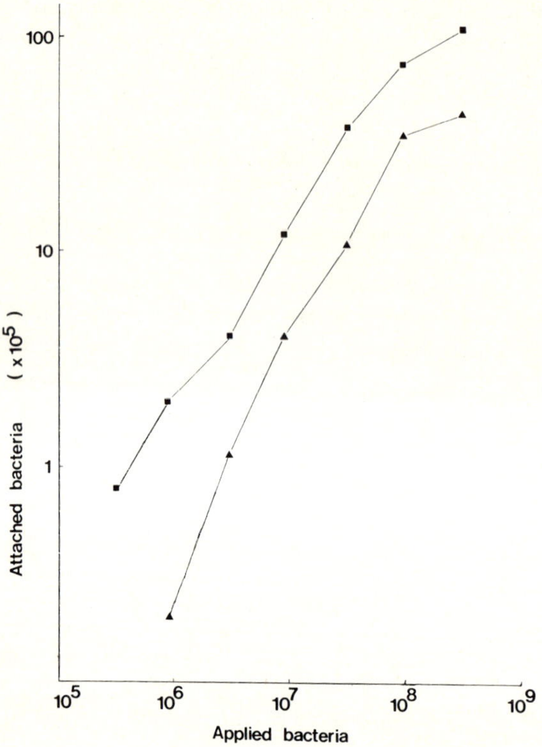

Fig. 1. Titration of the binding of *H. pylori* NCTC 11637 to laminin (▲, 0.5 pmol; ■, 2 pmol)

adherence to other proteins was observed, i.e. C-5430 to collagen I and C-5437 to collagen V. Furthermore, under microaerobic conditions an identical spectrum of bacterial binding to surfaces coated with 0.5 pmol protein was obtained.

Under microaerobic conditions, titration showed that the number of adhering bacteria increased with bacterial concentration until a saturation point was reached, as shown in Fig. 1 for the binding of *H. pylori* NCTC 11637 to laminin. Such a saturation phenomenon reflects the presence of a limited number of sites available on the protein for bacterial binding and also demonstrates the specificity of this adhesion.

Differences in the protein-binding abilities of *H. pylori* strains under aerobic and microaerobic conditions correlated with higher production of coccoid and other aberrant forms of these bacteria under aerobic conditions (Fig. 2).

Discussion

The data presented favour the possibility that laminin, fibronectin and certain collagens may mediate attachment of some *H. pylori* strains in vivo. We were unable to demonstrate binding to soluble ^{125}I-labelled laminin, fibronectin or

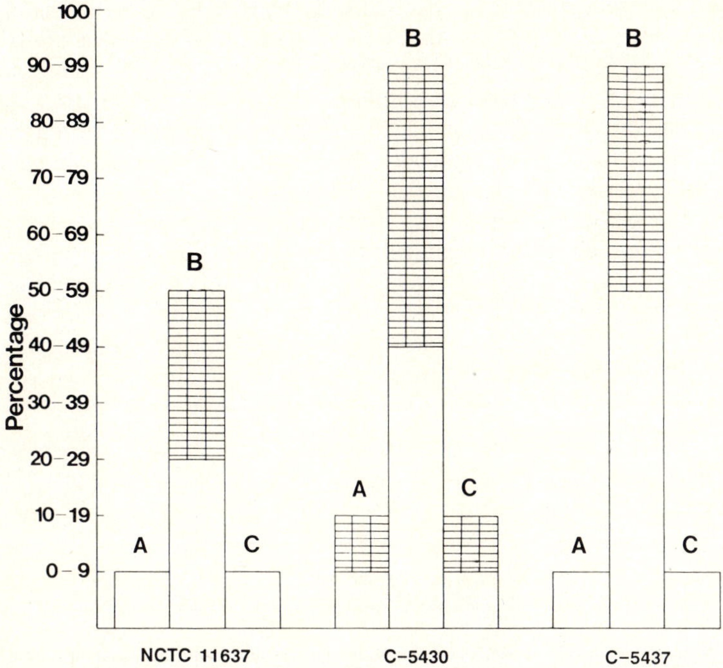

Fig. 2. Production of aberrant and degenerate coccoid forms by *H. pylori* strains during adherence tests. *A*, Before adherence test; *B*, after adherence testing with aerobic conditions; *C*, after adherence testing with microaerobic conditions. *Unshaded area*, coccoid forms; *shaded areas*, other aberrant forms

various collagens, in agreement with a previous study [1], but were able to demonstrate attachment to immobilized laminin, fibronectin and some collagens. Varying the procedure for iodination of the proteins did not influence the lack of binding, suggesting that another factor is involved. It may be that, although open and extended when immobilized, the conformations of the proteins are different in the soluble phase, thus not revealing the binding site for these bacteria. Such a phenomenon has been observed with other bacteria, for example, binding of *C. jejuni* to fibronectin [8].

As these bacteria are microaerophilic, the requirement of microaerobic conditions by *H. pylori* to demonstrate reproducible binding in vitro suggests that an active process is involved, i.e. certain metabolic activity is required. The latter conclusion is supported by the fact that decreased binding was correlated with production of aberrant forms by these oxygen sensitive microorganisms. Alternatively, the receptor/adhesin on the bacterial surface may be modified or even absent from aberrant forms.

The extracellular matrix may form sheets, called basement membranes, which influence the polarization of eukaryotic cells, including the three-dimensional organization of tissues, serve as barriers to cell movement, and participate is filtration of macromolecules [5, 13, 14]. Basement matrices are assemblies of networks of type IV collagen and laminin, linked together by interactions of these components with each other, with entactin/nidogen, and with heparan sulphate proteoglycans [14, 18]. The ability of *H. pylori* to attached to immobilized laminin, and binding to heparan sulphate as previously reported [1], suggest that the bacterium could adhere to basement membranes. The latter is worthy of further investigation, especially the relationship of such binding with altered pathophysiology of the mucosa during infection.

The ability of *H. pylori* to interact with more than one extracellular matrix protein, and previously reported haemagglutinin activity [2, 4] and gastric glycolipid-binding [9, 11, 12] suggests that these bacteria may use several adherence mechanisms. Finally, it will be of interest to attempt to correlate varied binding properties of clinical isolates with pathophysiological manifestations to ascertain which are associated with virulence.

Acknowledgements. This work was supported financially by the Sigrid Jusélius Foundation, Yrjö Jahnsson Foundation, and University of Helsinki.

References

1. Ascencio F, Wei S, Fransson LÅ, Wadström T (1990) Heparan sulfate binding to *Helicobacter pylori*: a possible tissue colonization mechanism. Rev Esp Enferm Dig 78 [Suppl 1]: 54
2. Emödy L, Carlsson Å, Ljungh A, Wadström T (1988) Mannose-resistant hemagglutination by *Campylobacter pylori*. Scand J Infect Dis 20: 353–354
3. Engvall E, Ruoslahti E (1977) Binding of soluble form of fibroblast surface protein, fibronectin, to collagen. Int J Cancer 20: 1–5
4. Evans DG, Evans DJ, Moulds JJ, Graham DY (1988) *N*-Acetylneuraminyllactose-binding fibrillar hemagglutinin of *Campylobacter pylori*: a putative colonization factor antigen. Infect Immun 56: 2896–2906
5. Farquhar MG (1983) The glomerular basement membrane. A selective macromolecular filter. In: Hay ED (ed) Cell biology of extracellular matrix. Plenum, New York, pp 335–378
6. Fauchère JL, Rosenau A, Bonneville F (1989) Virulence factors of *Campylobacter pylori*. Gastroenterol Clin Biol 13: 59B–64B
7. Kuusela P (1978) Fibronectin binds to *Staphylococcus aureus*. Nature 276: 718–720
8. Kuusela P, Moran AP, Vartio T, Kosunen TU (1989) Interaction of *Campylobacter jejuni* with extracellular matrix components. Biochim Biophys Acta 993: 297–300
9. Lingwood CA, Law H, Pellizarri A, Sherman P, Drumm B (1989) Gastric glycerolipid as a receptor for *Campylobacter pylori*. Lancet II: 238–241
10. Markwell MAK, Fox CF (1978) Surface-specific iodination of membrane proteins of viruses and eucaryotic cells using 1,3,4,6-tetrachloro-3α,6α-diphenylglycouril. Biochemistry 17: 4807–4817
11. Saitoh T, Natomi H, Zhao W, Okuzumi K, Sugano K, Iwamori M, Nagai Y (1991) Identification of glycolipid receptors for *Helicobacter pylori* by TLC-immunostaining. FEBS Lett 282: 385–387
12. Slomiany BL, Piotrowski J, Samanta A, VanHorn K, Murty VLN, Slomiany A (1989) *Campylobacter pylori* colonization factor shows specificity for lactosylceramide sulfate and GM3 ganglioside. Biochem Int 19: 929–936
13. Timpl R (1986) Recent advances in the biochemistry of glomerular basement membranes. Kidney Int 30: 293–298
14. Timpl R (1989) Structure and biological activity of basement membrane proteins. Eur J Biochem 180: 487–502

15. Westerlund B (1991) Interaction of *Escherichia coli* with mammalian extracellular matrix. Thesis, University of Helsinki, Finland
16. Westerlund B, Kuusela P, Risteli J, Risteli L, Vartio T, Rauvala H, Virkola R, Korhonen TK (1989) The O75X adhesin of uropathogenic *Escherichia coli* is a type IV collagen-binding protein. Mol Microbiol 3: 329–337
17. Yamada KM, Akiyama SK, Hasegawa T, Hasegawa E, Humphries MJ, Kennedy DW, Nagata K, Urushihara H, Olden K, Chen W-T (1985) Recent advances in research on fibronectin and other cell attachment proteins. J Cell Biochem 28: 79–97
18. Yurchenco PD, Schittny JC (1990) Molecular architecture of basement membranes. FASEB J 4: 1577–1590

Therapeutic Approaches

Helicobacter pylori: Clinical Aspects

J.J. Misiewicz

Introduction

Helicobacter pylori (Hp) is now recognised as one of the most common chronic bacterial infections affecting humans worldwide. There is very strong evidence connecting Hp infection with the presence of gastritis [17]. Depending on the distribution of the organism in the stomach and the duodenum (it can colonise in the duodenal cap in the presence of gastric metaplasia), Hp can give rise to antritis, corpusitis, pangastritis, or duodenitis. Most of these inflammatory states affecting the gastric mucosa in the stomach or in the duodenum have clinical equivalents, but the guidelines for the clinical and therapeutic management of the associated conditions have not yet been worked out fully. Moreover, there is as yet no final agreement concerning the most effective and safest way of treating Hp infection in the clinic. The incidence of Hp infection in the community varies according to geographical location and seems dependent on the socio-economic status of the community in question. This Hp point prevalence rates are higher in the emergent countries and are associated with low income, poor housing conditions and polluted water supply [7–9].

From the clinical point of view, the aim of treatment is eradication of the organism, rather than its temporary suppression with subsequent early recolonisation. It is now generally agreed that eradication should be defined as the absence of Hp 4 weeks after the end of therapy, although the test, or tests, to be used for this purpose have not been universally agreed.

At the time of writing, most workers have used some sort of triple regime, comprising bismuth, metronidazole or tinidazole, and an antibiotic (usually tetracycline or a penicillin) to achieve eradication. The main difficulty at present in practical therapeutics of Hp is metronidazole resistance, and this will govern the success rate in the rate of healing of duodenal ulcer (DU), attainable with anti-Hp treatment. For example, in 15/17 patients with metronidazole sensitive Hp the organism was eradicated and the ulcer healed, while a similar outcome was recorded in only 1/9 DU patients colonised by a metronidazole resistant strain [10]. However, using regimens comprising, for example, omeprazole 40 mg daily with amoxycillin 500 mg q.i.d. on days 1–14, DeNol 1 q.i.d. on days 1–7 and ciprofloxacin 750 mg b.d. on days 8–14, it is possible to produce clearance in 84% and eradication in 74% of subjects harbouring metronidazole resistant strains of Hp (median follow up 3.5 months, range 2.4–6 months) [11].

Department of Gastroenterology and Nutrition Central Middlesex Hospital, London, UK

Gasbarrini/Pretolani (Eds.)
Basic and Clinical Aspects of H. pylori Infection

The optimal length of treatment remains to be worked out in large-scale, head-to-head controlled trials. It is possible to achieve impressive eradication rates after only 1 week of therapy; regimens shorter than 7 days are probably not viable. For example, of 106 patients treated with a 1-week regimen comprising tripotassium dicitratobismuthate 120 mg q.d.s. and amoxycillin 500 mg q.d.s. on days 1–7, with metronidazole 400 mg five times daily on days 5–7, an overall eradication rate of 72% was recorded (median follow up 9.3 months, range 2–12 months). The failed treatments were due to the presence of metronidazole resistant organisms [12].

For the clinician therefore, the presence of resistance constitutes a major problem especially as Hp acquires metronidazole resistance very easily [5]. The prevalence of metronidazole resistance varies with geographical location and with the gender of the patient; metronidazole resistance is more common in women, presumably because of previous exposure to antibiotics for pelvic and urinary tract infections, and in emergent countries, where antibiotics are used freely for enteric infections and are available without prescription. Recent evidence suggests that regimens administered for 2 weeks, comprising either dual, or triple therapy, may yet provide the most effective duration of treatment for the eradication of Hp.

Bismuth therapy raises interesting questions concerning DU healing and relapse, which merit further investigation. Eradication rates after bismuth monotherapy are very low, and even suppression rates consistently underrun healing rates of DU. Moreover, the incidence of relapse of DU after a healing course of bismuth is lower than after H_2 receptor antagonists [14]. On the other hand, investigations using the [C^{13}] urea breath test indicate that the recurrence of Hp after bismuth is very prompt, and that recurrence is not prevented by varying the length of treatment with bismuth from 1 to 4 weeks [13]. The reasons for this are not clear. It is possible that absorption of bismuth is followed by retention of this compound in the body, with the formations of a depot of bismuth and prolonged pharmacological effect; this is possible, although it does not seem very likely, because absorption of bismuth is low in most subjects. Pharmacological effects of bismuth unrelated to its anti-Hp effects may play a part. Another possibility is that the suppression of Hp by a course of bismuth, with consequent decrease in mucosal inflammation may lead to more complete healing and epithelialisation of the ulcer, so that the ulcer scar is better able to withstand ulcerogenic factors, including the recolonisation by Hp.

One practical spinoff of recognition of Hp as an important aetiological factor in DU is the possibility of using screening for Hp as a means of decreasing the work load of endoscopy units. Such procedures would be applicable to patient aged 45 years or under and not taking nonsteroidal anti-inflammatory drugs (NSAIDs) – if serologically negative to Hp, endoscopy might be omitted in the investigation of their abdominal symptoms. In one such prospective study, the saving of endoscopic procedures would have amounted to 25%, no gastric cancers or peptic ulcers would have been missed, but 11 instances of oesophagitis, 7 of erosions and 1 of duodenitis would not have been diagnosed ($n = 293$; five gastric cancers in this series were all over 45 years old) [18]. As demand for endoscopy services is increasing, the cost effectiveness of such approach to the management of dyspepsia merits further study, although it must be remembered that patients demand for endoscopic investigation can be quite strong.

The ideal situation from the clinical point of view therefore, would be to first determine whether the patient needs eradication therapy. Clinicians differ in their attitude to Hp eradication at first presentation of DU. The impression is that, rightly or wrongly, at present only a minority of gastroenterologists use Hp eradication at first presentation of DU and that most reserve this treatment for the management of recurrent, or H_2 blocker resistant ulcers – the latter indication seems non-controversial. Indications for Hp eradication in non-ulcer dyspepsia, duodenitis, or gastric ulcer have not yet been established. Indeed, because of the ease with which metronidazole resistance can be produced, the treatment of these conditions should, at present, be restricted to research settings, so that properly worked guidelines can be established.

If the patient merits anti-Hp treatment and has a DU, the simplest approach is to assume that for all practical purposes it is highly likely that Hp colonisation is present. Thus anti-Hp therapy can be administered without prior Hp diagnosis, and the result of treatment checked 4 or more weeks after the end of the therapy by the breath test, examination of endoscopic biopsy for urease activity and/or histopathology and bacterial culture, or perhaps by serology, if initial anti-Hp antibody concentrations were established initially. This approach will probably eradicate Hp in some 70% of patients thus treated, but in those harbouring metronidazole-resistant Hp the treatment is likely to fail.

There seem to be two strategies available to deal with this difficulty. Firstly, all patients could be endoscoped and biopsied before the treatment and the sensitivity of Hp to metronidazole determined. This strategy increases the endoscopic workload and the number of invasive procedures for the patient, but enables the clinician to choose a drug schedule suitable for metronidazole resistant organisms. However, it must be borne in mind that even under ideal circumstances a number of bacterial cultures will fail, and so time and effort will have been wasted. The second option is to use a drug regimen that deals effectively with both metronidazole resistant and sensitive Hp. There are some indications from recent work that is may be possible to design such a regime, which would then be the main treatment choice. Whichever strategy is adopted, it seems essential to check for Hp eradication, otherwise subsequent management of the patient cannot be properly effected.

There is increasing evidence from various studies linking the presence of Hp corpusitis with the increased risk of gastric cancer [1–4, 15–17, 19]. Whether Hp acts simply as a marker for other factors, all seemingly associated with disadvantaged populations, or whether it acts together with other carcinogens by producing chronic atrophic gastritis, is not clear. Nor is it clear whether, at least in the West, such associations should lead to prospective eradication therapy in individuals found to be Hp positive; unfortunately, at present this policy would be impracticable in the Third World, where in fact it is needed most. Perhaps eradication treatment should be offered to first-degree relatives of propositi with existing gastric cancer, to those with a strong family history of malignant disease, and to those in whom precancerous histological changes are found at endoscopic gastric biopsy. The testing of these propositions in properly controlled prospective investigations is a daunting prospect.

References

1. Barker DJP, Coggon D, Osmond C, Wickham C (1990) Poor housing in childhood and high rates of stomach cancer in England and Wales. Br J Cancer 61: 575–578
2. Burstein M, Monge E, Leon Barua R et al. (1991) Low peptic ulcer and high gastric cancer prevalence in a developing country with a high prevalence of infection by *Helicobacter pylori*. J Clin Gastroenterol 13: 154–156
3. Forman D (1991) The etiology of gastric cancer. IARC Sci Publ (1991): 22–32
4. Forman D, Sitas F, Newell DG et al. (1990) Geographic association of *Helicobacter pylori* antibody prevalence and gastric cancer mortality in rural China. Int J Cancer 46: 608–611
5. Glupczynski Y, Burette A (1990) Drug therapy for *Helicobacter pylori* infection: problems and pitfalls. Am J Gastroenterol 85: 1545–1551
6. Glupczynski Y, Burette A (1992) Letter. Lancet 339: 54–55
7. Graham DY, Malaty HM, Evans DG, Evans DJJ, Klein PD, Adam E (1991) Epidemiology of *Helicobacter pylori* infection in intestinal- and diffuse-type gastric adenocarcinomas. J Natl Cancer Inst 83: 640–643
8. Klein PD, Graham DY, Gaillour A, Opekun AR, Smith EO (1991) Water source as risk factor for *Helicobacter pylori* infection in Peruvian children. Gastrointestinal Physiology Working Group. Lancet 337: 1503–1506
9. Li YY, Hu PJ, Du GG, Hazell SL (1991) The prevalence of *Helicobacter pylori* infection in the Peoples Republic of China. Am J Gastroenterol 86: 446–449
10. Logan RPH, Polson RJ, Baron JH, Misiewicz JJ (1991) Follow up after anti-*Helicobacter pylori* treatment. Lancet 337: 562–563
11. Logan RPH, Gummett PA, Karim QN, Walker MM, Baron JH, Misiewicz JJ (1991) A treatment regimen for metronidazole resistant *Helicobacter pylori*. Ital J Gastroenterol 23: 110
12. Logan RPH, Gummett PA, Misiewicz JJ, Walker MM, Polson RJ, Karim NQ, Baron JH (1991) One week's treatment for duodenal ulcer. Gut 32: A1207
13. Logan RPH, Gummett PA, Polson RJ, Baron JH, Misiewicz JJ (1990) What length of treatment with tripotassium dicitrato-bismuthate (TDB) for *Helicobacter pylori*? Gut 31: A1178
14. Martin DF, Hollanders D, May SJ, Ravenscroft MM, Tweedle DEF, Miller JP (1981) Difference in relapse rates of duodenal ulcer after healing with cimetidine or tripotassium dicitrato bismuthate. Lancet i: 7–10
15. Nomura A, Stemmermann GN, Chyon PH, Kato I, Perez-Perez GI, Blaser MJ (1991) *Helicobacter pylori* infection and gastric carcinoma among Japanese Americans in Hawaii. N Engl J Med 325: 1132–1136
16. Parsonnet J, Friedmann DG, Vandersteen DP et al. (1991) *Helicobacter pylori* infection and the risk of gastric carcinoma. N Engl J Med 325: 1127–1131
17. Rauws EAJ, Langenberg W, Honthoff HJ, Zanen HC, Tytgat GNJ (1988) *Campylobacter pyloridis*-associated chronic active antral gastritis. A prospective study of its prevalence and the effects of antibacterial and anti-ulcer treatment. Gastroenterology 94: 33–40
18. Sobala GM, Crabtree JE, Pentith JA, Rathbone JB, Shallcross TM, Wyatt JI, Dixon MF, Heatley RV, Axon ATR (1991) Screening dyspepsia by serology to *Helicobacter pylori*. Lancet 338: 94–96
19. Wotherspoon AC, Ortiz-Hidalgo C, Falzon MR, Isaacson PG (1991) *Helicobacter pylori*-associated gastritis and primary B-cell gastric lymphoma. Lancet 338: 1175–1176

H_2 Receptor Antagonists: Is There a Place in the Treatment of *Helicobacter pylori* Infection?

C. Scarpignato[1], M. Felder[2], and G. Dobrilla[2]

Introduction

Helicobacter pylori (H.p.) is an important human pathogen causing type B gastritis [25], and it is in some way implicated in the pathogenesis of peptic disease [7, 9]. It is now clear that healing of a duodenal ulcer without persistent H.p. eradication is unequivocally followed by early relapse [5, 26, 33]. As a consequence, H.p. clearance and eradication is one of the goals of the medical therapy, and in this connection it is certainly of interest to examine the effect of antiulcer drugs on H.p. clearance and eradication.

Several diverse drugs are now available to accelerate peptic ulcer healing [3]. Acid lowering compounds have been for years the most popular medications, in keeping with Schwartz's dictum "no acid – no ulcer". Among these, H_2 receptor antagonists are the most widely employed compounds because of their proven efficacy and safety. These drugs inhibit acid secretion by blocking competitively H_2 receptors located on the parietal cells [32]. From a theoretical viewpoint, H_2 blockers might affect H.p. status by a direct action or through indirect mechanisms, connected with the inhibition of acid secretion or with the healing effect. We present evidence for and against each of these possible mechanisms.

Is There Any Direct Effect of H_2 Receptor Antagonists on *Helicobacter pylori* Organisms?

A wide range of antimicrobial agents are active against *H. pylori* when tested in vitro at a neutral pH. These include tetracyclines, beta-lactams, most quinolones, macrolides, nitroimidazoles as well as other agents [12, 23, 24]. Unfortunately, the bismuth salts are the only antiulcer agents which display antibacterial activity against H.p. [19, 23, 24]. H_2 blockers, such as cimetidine and ranitidine, are *practically* devoid of such effect [19, 23] (Table 1). In an electron microscopic

[1] Institute of Pharmacology, School of Medicine and Dentistry, University of Parma, Parma, Italy
[2] Division of Gastroenterology and Digestive Endoscopy, Regional General Hospital, Bolzano, Italy

Gasbarrini/Pretolani (Eds.)
Basic and Clinical Aspects of H. pylori Infection

Table 1. In vitro susceptibility of *H. pylori* to antiulcer drugs (from [19])

Agent	Minimum inhibitory concentration (MIC), mg/l	
	MIC_{90}	MIC range
Acid-suppressing agents		
Mg/Al-containing antacid (Maalox)	> 1000	> 1000
Ranitidine	1280	320–1280
Cimetidine	3200	400–3200
Famotidine	> 1024	128 → 1024
Omeprazole	> 1000	> 1000
Misoprostol	> 1000	> 1000
Topically Active Agents		
Colloidal tripotassium dicitrato bismuthate[a]	32	8–64
Bismuth subnitrate[a]	64	8–128
Bismuth salicylate[a]	32	8–128
Sofalcone	50	25–50
Carbenoxolone	> 1000	> 1000
Sucralfate	320	400 → 320
Metronidazole[a,b]	32	0.06–128
Furazolidone[a]	0.25	≤ 0.03–0.5

[a] Activity against *H. pylori*
[b] About 25% of strains less sensitive.

study performed on bacterial cultures, Armstrong et al. [1] – while showing significant alterations in bacterial morphology and ultrastructure caused by the different antimicrobials – were unable to fiind any morphological change after incubation of the H.p. cells with cimetidine at the concentration of up to 2000 mg/l.

In 1988 Humphreys and colleagues [16] found that seven patients who were initially H.p. positive became negative after 6 weeks on therapy with cimetidine 400 mg twice daily. However, they also found that five patients who were initially negative became positive using this regimen. These findings can be explained by the weak antibacterial effect of cimetidine or better by sampling error, while the occurrence of colonization in patients on cimetidine could be explained by the more favorable conditions of a less acid environment. One year later Graham and coworkers [11] evaluated several antiulcer compounds in vivo through the use of the urea breath test (UBT; table 2) and confirmed that cimetidine as well as ranitidine are ineffective against H.p. because patients remained positive after drug treatment. In agreement with these data, the majority of studies showed no change in H.p. status of patients treated with H_2 receptor blockers [4, 6, 13–15, 20, 21]. Despite healing, almost all the patients treated with cimetidine, ranitidine or famotidine [4, 14, 15] remained H.p. positive, and there was so significant change in the inflammatory status of their gastric mucosa. One can therefore conclude that these compounds have no *intrinsic* activity against H.p. either in vitro or in vivo.

Table 2. Effect of various drugs on *H. pylori* assessed by the urea breath test (from [11])

Drug	Dosage (mg/day)	Duration (days)	Urease results after therapy[a]
Ferrous sulfate	1300	7	Positive
Ferrous sulfate	1300	7	Positive
Ferrous sulfate	1300	7	Positive
Ferrous sulfate	1300	4	Negative
Ferrous sulfate	1300	7	Positive
Ferrous sulfate	700	3	Positive
Ferrous sulfate	700	3	Positive
Ferrous gluconate	1200	3	Positive
Zinc sulfate	700	3	Positive
Bismuth subsalicylate	2096	10	Negative
Bismuth subsalicylate	2096	10	Negative
Bismuth subsalicylate	2096	10	Negative
Bismuth subnitrate	600	3	Negative
Misoprostol	0.80	4	Positive
Misoprostol	0.80	4	Positive
Misoprostol	0.80	4	Positive
Misoprostol	0.80	4	Positive
Misoprostol	0.80	4	Positive
Misoprostol	0.80	4	Positive
Sucralfate	4000	1	Positive
Maalox	120 ml	1	Positive
Ranitidine	300	1	Positive
Cimetidine	1200	1	Positive
Furazolidone	49	4	Negaive
Furazolidone	49	4	Borderline
Furazolidone	49	4	Negative
Gold	6	2	Positive
Gold	6	2	Positive
Ursodeoxycholic acid	4000	2	Positive
Ursodeoxycholic acid	4000	2	Positive

[a] Urea breath test was positive in all before therapy

Indirect Effects of H_2 Receptor Antagonists on *Helicobacter pylori* Organisms

It has been suggested that gastric metaplasia develops in the duodenum as a result of exposure to high levels of acid entering the lumen. Patrick et al. [29] were able to relate the frequency (but not the extent) of gastric metaplasia to maximal acid output. The extensive gastric metaplasia in patients with Zollinger-Ellison syndrome [28] and its reversion by highly selective vagotomy [38] further support a response to acid injury. The metaplastic gastric epithelium allows H.p. to colonize the duodenal mucosa, where it produces an acute inflammatory response. Acid-induced gastric metaplasia in the duodenum and H.p. associated gastritis seem therefore to be synergistic in the pathogenesis of duodenitis [38].

With these data at hand, one might speculate that a prolonged reduction in the duodenal acid load (obtained through the use of an antisecretory regimen) may indirectly reduce H.p. colonization of the duodenum. However, despite ulcer healing, short-term treatment with H_2 antagonists proved to be ineffective in reversing the gastric metaplasia in the duodenal bulb [22]. Conversely, from other therapeutic regimens, indeed, H_2 blockers are unable to obtain both clearance and eradication of H.p. organisms [31]. It is likely that only a long-term eradication could be followed by improvement of metaplasia.

By inhibiting acid secretion, H_2 receptor antagonists increase intragastric pH in a time- and dose-dependent fashion [32]. The question thus arises as to whether these compounds can modify H.p. status by affecting the activity of coadministered antimicrobial agents.

H.p. leaves usually within the gastric mucus between tight junctions and attached to epithelial cell [35]. Its localization is very deep in the gastric pits, where the access of antimicrobials is very poor. The reasons why antibiotics can be ineffective are as follows [10]:

- Low compliance
- Altered drug distribution and insufficient tissue concentration with pure penetration within the mucus layer
- Bacterial resistance
- Drug interactions
- Stationary state (no multiplications)
- Presence of binding proteins
- Presence of inactivating enzymes
- Acidic pH
- Anaerobic environment

The altered drug distribution and insufficient tissue concentration with poor penetration within the mucus layer and the reduced activity in the acid environs of the gastric mucosa are those that can be influenced by the administration of H_2 receptor antagonists.

Effect on the Activity of Antimicrobial Agents. McNulty [25] recently studied the activity of various antimicrobial agents over the range of pH 5–8 at which H.p. survives (Table 3). Penicillin was ten fold less active at the most acidic pH than at neutral pH, with a MIC_{90} of 0.5 mg/l at pH 5–6 and 0.33 mg/l at pH 7.5. There was a ten fold change in the activity of ampicillin and a 16-fold change in the activity of cephalexin between pH 5.5 and 7.5. Similar results were obtained with ciprofloxacin and erythromycin base. There was little change in the activity of tetracycline and nitrofurantoin; metronidazole and bismuth were unaffected by pH. By raising luminal pH, H_2 blockers – coadministered with antimicrobials – should be able to increase their bactericidal activity against H.p. in vivo.

Effect on Tissue Concentration of Antimicrobial Agents. Besides increasing the activity of antimicrobials, H_2 antagonists could also enhance their concentration within the gastric mucosa. In a guinea pig model, Westblom and Duriex [37] showed cimetidine to be capable of enhancing antibiotic concentrations in gastric mucosa. Indeed, 2 h after cimetidine administration, the pH of gastric

Table 3. Effect of pH on the activity of antimicrobial agents against *H. pylori* (from [25])

Agent	Isolates (*n*)	MIC_{90}(mg/l) pH 7.5	pH 6.0	pH 5.5
Penicillin	20	0.03	0.5	0.5
Ampicillin	20	0.06	0.25	0.5
Cephalexin	17	2	16	32
Erythromycin	20	0.06	2	8
Ciprofloxacin	20	0.12	0.5	2
Tetracycline	17	0.12	0.25	0.5
Nitrofurantoin	17	1	2	2
Metronidazole[a]	15	2	2	2
Bismuth subcitrate	17	16	8	—

[a] Sensitive isolates.

mucosa was increased from 1.7 to about 6, and mucosal concentrations of clindamycin were more than five times higher in comparison with those observed in basal conditions, despite serum levels were virtually identical (Fig. 1). By looking at the tissue concentration–time curves in basal conditions and after cimetidine administration (Fig. 2), a marked increase in tissue availability of clindamycin in cimetidine-treated animals is clearly evident. Plotting clindamycin concentrations at various time intervals against mucosal pH revealed a significant nonlinear correlation between these two parameters: the higher the mucosal pH the higher was tissue concentration of the antibiotic.

Why can an H_2 antagonist enhance mucosal concentration of clindamycin? This molecule is a weak base with a pK_a of 7.7 and is known to concentrate

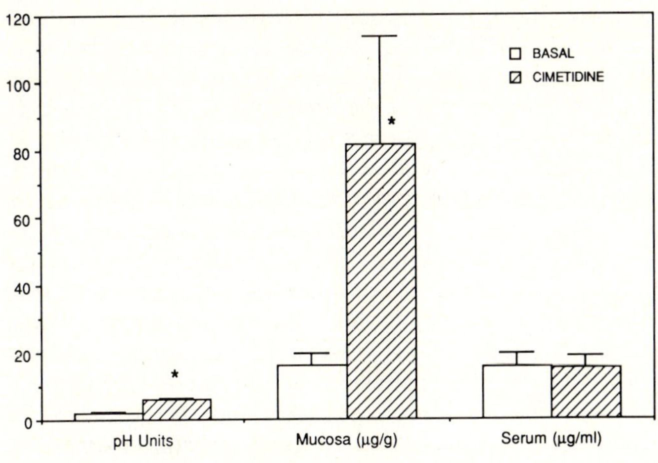

Fig. 1. Mucosal pH and clindamycin concentrations in basal conditions 2 h after cimetidine (4 mg/kg i.m.) administration (and 1 h after clindamycin injection, 100 mg/kg i.m.) in guinea pigs. (From data in [37])

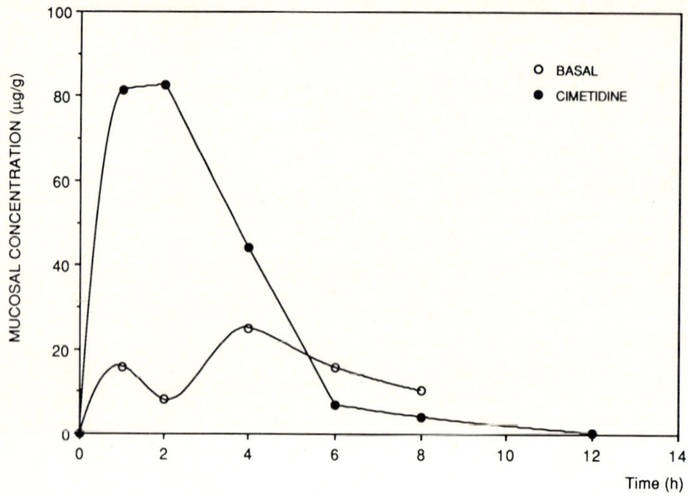

Fig. 2. Clindamycin concentration in guinea pig gastric mucosa in basal conditions and after cimetidine administration. (From [37])

in acidic compartments [18]. All weak bases are accumulated within the gastric mucosa, thus providing evidence for the existence of an acidic storage pool [8]. Under basal conditions (i.e., normally secreting cells), the acidic storage pool is almost full and dilutes the V_d of antibiotics accumulated within the pool, thus delaying their release into the lumen. When acid secretion is blocked or strongly reduced by an antisecretory compound, the acid storage pool is empty, and there is no acid to trap antibiotics. The net result is that more antibiotic is free to travel across the luminal side, thus establishing higher concentrations.

H_2 Antagonists plus Antimicrobials in the Treatment of Helicobacter pylori *Infection: Clinical Relevance.* Based on the above in vitro and in vivo data, one could predict that addition of an H_2 antagonist to an antimicrobial compound should enhance its activity against H.p. There are some trials with combined therapies in the literature, but unfortunately the antimicrobial alone was rarely tested. Therefore confirmation of synergistic action is not yet available.

Bayerdorffer and colleagues [2] first showed that addition of ofloxacin to a standard ranitidine regimen markedly improves the clearance rate of H.p. and also significantly increases healing of resistant duodenal ulcers (Fig. 3). In this trial a group with ofloxacin alone was not included, so one can merely say that ofloxacin increased the clearing capacity of ranitidine but cannot state that ranitidine *potentiated* the effect of the antimicrobial. A recent paper from Russian investigators [17] showed that addition of oxacillin to ranitidine was very effective not only in clearing the micro-organisms but also in eradicating them. There was, however, no significant difference in healing rate between the two treatments. Similar results were obtained when a cephalosporin (cefixime) was added to cimetidine [34]. In this and in the previous study the clearance rate approached 80%, which is indeed a very high figure, certainly superior to that one can expect with the antimicrobial alone. Here again, however, the lack of

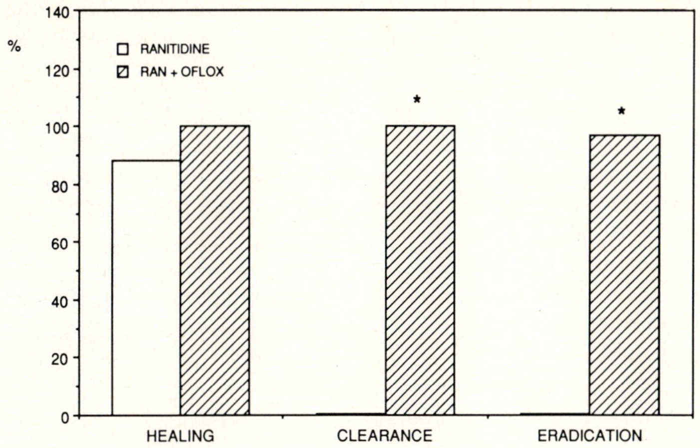

Fig. 3. Effect of a 10-day addition of oxacillin (500 mg q.i.d.) to ranitidine (300 mg nocte for 4 weeks) on healing and H.p. status in H.p. positive duodenal ulcer patients. (From data in [17])

a group treated with oxacillin or cefixime alone does not allow any definite conclusion about synergism between H_2 blockers and antimicrobials.

The only trial well done in this respect is that of Wagner and colleagues [36], who studied bismuth subsalicylate (BSS) and ranitidine alone or in combination in patients with antral gastritis or peptic ulcer. As expected, ranitidine did not show any effect on H.p. status whereas BSS alone was more active in clearing rather than eradicating the micro-organisms. Ranitidine, however, failed to potentiate the action of the bismuth salt (Fig. 4). It is worthwhile to remember that

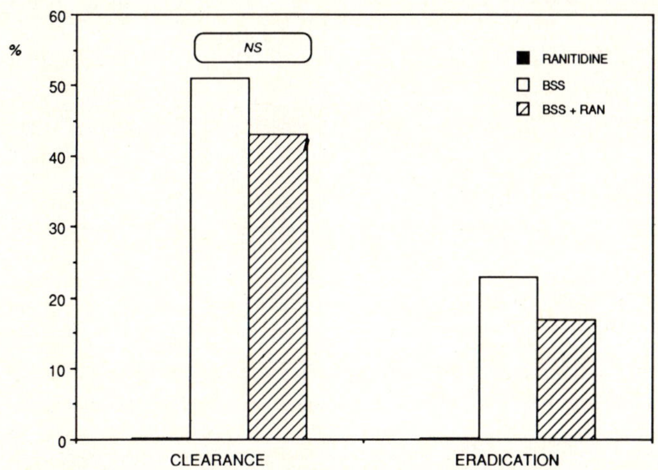

Fig. 4. Effect of a 4 week treatment with ranitidine (300 mg daily), BSS (1800 mg daily) or ranitidine + BSS on H.p. status in patients with antral gastritis or peptic ulcer. There was no statistical significance between results obtained with BSS alone and with BSS + ranitidine. (From data in [36])

the mechanism of the bactericidal action of bismuth is different from that of the other antimicrobials and that its activity is independent from environmental pH.

Does Ulcer Healing Per se Influence Helicobacter pylori *Status?* The ulcer lesion per se is not colonized by H.p., thus healing per se cannot influence the H.p. status. However, the ulcer lesion may be associated with motility disorders which might favor gastric metaplasia (and thus H.p. colonization) through an increased duodenal acid load due to enhanced gastric emptying and a reduced acid clearance of the duodenal bulb [30]. Healing is often associated with reversal of impaired gastroduodenal motility [27], thus reducing the likelihood of gastric metaplasia which represents indeed the link for colonization of duodenal mucosa by H.p.

Conclusions

Available data unequivocally show that H_2 receptor antagonists are devoid of antibacterial activity against H.p. However, in spite of lacking in vitro activity against the organisms these compounds may have a role in H.p. infections as adjunct therapeutic agents since they might increase antibacterial activity and gastric mucosal concentrations of antibiotics with basic characteristics (e.g., clindamycin, erythromycin). Nevertheless, there is a urgent need for well-designed clinical trials to prove or disprove this hypothesis.

References

1. Armstrong JA, Wee SH, Goodwin CS et al. (1987) Response of *Campylobacter pyloridis* to antibiotics, bismuth and an acid-reducing agent in vitro – an ultrastructural study. J Med Microbiol 24: 343–350
2. Bayerdorffer E, Pirlet T, Sommer A et al. (1988) Ofloxacin therapy of resistant duodenal ulcer. Z Gastroenterol 26: 155–159
3. Bianchi Porro G, Lazzaroni M (1992) Peptic ulcer disease: medical treatment. In: Gustavsson S, Kumar D, Graham DY (eds) The stomach. Churchill Livingstone, Edinburgh, pp 246–265
4. Blanco M, Pajares JM, Jimenez ML et al. (1988) Effect of acid inhibition on *Campylobacter pylori*. Scand J Gastroenterol 23 [Suppl 142]: 107–109
5. Coghlan JG, Tobin A, O'Morain C (1989) *Campylobacter pylori* and ulcer treatment. In: Rathbone BJ, Heatley RV (eds) *Campylobacter pylori* and gastroduodenal disease. Blackwell Scientific, Oxford, pp 232–245
6. Coppola FV, Boero MG, Recchia S et al. (1989) *Campylobacter pylori* in antral gastritis: therapeutic response to colloidal bismuth subcitrate versus ranitidine. A six month follow-up. In: Mégraud F, Lamouliatte H (eds) Gastroduodenal pathology and *Campylobacter pylori*. Elsevier, Amsterdam, pp 587–590
7. Doley CP (1991) *Helicobacter pylori* and duodenal ulcer. In: Marshall B, McCallum RW, Guerrant RL (eds) *Helicobacter pylori* in peptic ulceration and gastritis. Blackwell Scientific, Oxford, pp 129–138
8. Ekblad EBM, Warnock DG, Licko V (1989) Accumulation of weak base in gastric mucosa provides evidence for an acidic storage compartment. Am J Physiol 257: G359–G368
9. Graham DY (1989) *Campylobacter pylori* as a pathogenetic factor in duodenal ulcer: the case for Scand J Gastroenterol 24 [Suppl 160]: 46–52

10. Graham DY, Börsch GMA (1990) The who's and when's of therapy for *Helicobacter pylori.* Am J Gastroenterol 85: 1552–1555
11. Graham DY, Klein PD, Opekun AR et al. (1989) In vivo susceptibility of *Campylobacter pylori.* Am J Gastroenterol 84: 233–238
12. Hui WM, Ho J, Lam SK (1988) Persistence of *Campylobacter pylori* during remission and subsequent relapse in duodenal ulcer. Gastroenterology 94: A196
13. Hirschl AM, Pletschette M (1989) Antibiotic treatment of *Campylobacter pylori* infection. In: Rathbone BJ, Heatley RV (eds) *Campylobacter pylori* and gastroduodenal disease. Blackwell Scientific, Oxford, pp 217–224
14. Hui WM, Lam SK, Ho J et al. (1989) Effect of sucralfate and cimetidine on duodenal ulcer-associated antral gastritis and *Campylobacter pylori.* Am J Med 86 [Suppl A]: 60–65
15. Hui WM, Lam SK, Ho J et al. (1991) Effect of omeprazole on duodenal ulcer-associated antral gastritis and *Helicobacter pylori.* Dig Dis Sci 36: 577–582
16. Humphreys H, Bourke S, Dooley C et al. (1988) Effect of *Campylobacter pylori* in peptic disease: a randomised prospective trial. Gut 29: 279–283
17. Isakov VA, Grigoriev PYa, Yakovenko EP (1990) Treatment of *Helicobacter pylori* positive duodenal ulcers. Lancet 2: 755–756
18. Klempner MS, Styrt B (1983) Alkalinization of the intralysosomal pH by clindamycin and its effect on neutrophil function. J Antimicrob Chemother 12 [Suppl C]: 39–50
19. Lambert JR (1990) Effect of antiulcer drugs on *Helicobacter pylori.* Drug Investigation 2 [Suppl 1]: 52–55
20. Madsen JE, Vetvik K, Aase S (1991) *Helicobacter pylori* and chronic active inflammation of the duodenum and stomach in duodenal ulcer patients treated with ranitidine, misoprostol, or an acid-neutralizing agent. Scand J Gastroenterol 26: 465–470
21. Malfertheiner P, Bode G, Vanek E et al. (1987) *Campylobacter pylori* – besteht ein Zusammenhang mit der peptischen Ulcuskrankheit? Dtsch Med Wochenschr 112: 493–497
22. Malfertheiner P, Bode G, Stanescu A et al. (1989) Gastric metaplasia in the duodenum – a persistent condition following ulcer healing. Abstract book of the symposium on gastroduodenal disease and *Campylobacter pylori.* Charlottesville, Virginia, A21
23. Malfertheiner P, Pieramico O (1992) *Helicobacter pylori.* In: Gustavsson S, Kumar D, Graham DY (eds) The stomach, Churchill Livingstone, Edinburgh, pp 297–311
24. Marshall B (1991) Treatment of *Helicobacter pylori.* In: Marshall B, McCallum RW, Guerrant RL (eds) *Helicobacter pylori* in peptic ulceration and gastritis, Blackwell, Oxford, pp 160–186
25. McNulty CAM (1989) Pathogenicity of *Campylobacter pylori* – a causative factor in gastritis? Scand J Gastroenterol 24 [Suppl 160]: 3–6
26. Miller JP, Faragher EB (1989) The potential impact of *Campylobacter pylori* in the treatment of duodenal ulcer disease. Scand J Gastroenterol 24 [Suppl 160]: 39–45
27. Moore JG, McIntyre B, Alazraki N (1985) Gastric emptying of combined liquid-solid meals in healed duodenal ulcer. Dig Dis Sci 30: 1134–1138
28. Parrish JA, Rawlins DC (1965) Intestinal mucosa in the Zollinger-Ellison syndrome. Gut 6: 286–289
29. Patrick WJA, Denham D, Forrest PM (1974) Mucous changes in the human duodenum: a light and electron microscopic study and correlation with disease and gastric acid secretion. Gut 15: 767–776
30. Pieramico O, Malfertheiner P (1990) Gastroduodenal motility in relation to peptic ulcer pathogenesis and *Helicobacter pylori* infection. In: Malfertheiner P, Ditschuneit H (eds) *Helicobacter pylori,* gastritis and peptic ulcer. Springer, Berlin Heidelberg New York, pp 306–311
31. Rauws EAJ, Tytgat GNJ (1990) Natural history and long-term monitoring of therapeutic attempts to eradicate *Helicobacter pylori.* In: Malfertheiner P, Ditschuneit H (eds) *Helicobacter pylori,* gastritis and peptic ulcer. Springer, Berlin Heidelberg New York, pp 448–451
32. Scarpignato C (1991) Pharmacological basis of therapeutics. In: Galmiche JP, Jian R, Mignon M, Ruszniewski P (eds) Non-ulcer dyspepsia: pathophysiological and therapeutic approaches. Libbey Eurotext, Paris, pp 201–225
33. Scarpignato C, Galmiche JP (1988) Mucosal coating agents: pharmacology and clinical use. In: Bianchi Porro G (ed) Topics in digestive disease, vol 1. Cortina International/Raven, Verona/New York, pp 73–133

34. Tatsuta M, Ishikawa H, Iishi H et al. (1990) Reduction of gastric ulcer recurrence after suppression of *Helicobacter pylori* by cefixime. Gut 31:973–976
35. Tytgat GNJ, Rauws EAJ, Langenberg W et al. (1988) Significance of *Campylobacter pyloridis*. In: Bianchi Porro G (ed) Topics in digestive disease, vol 1. Cortina International/Raven, Verona/New York, pp 59–71
36. Wagner S, Freise J, Bar W et al. (1989) Epidemiologie und therapie der *Campylobacter pylori* infection. Dtsch Med Wochenschr 114:407–413
37. Westblom TU, Duriex DE (1991) Enhancement of antibiotic concentrations in gastric mucosa by H_2-receptor antagonist. Implications for treatment of *Helicobacter pylori* infections. Dig Dis Sci 36:25–28
38. Wyatt JI, Rathbone BJ, Dixon ME et al. (1987) *Campylobacter pyloridis* and acid-induced gastric metaplasia in the pathogenesis of duodenitis. J Clin Pathol 40:841–848

Proton Pump Inhibitors in the Management of *Helicobacter pylori*-Related Diseases

M. Deltenre, E. De Koster, and J.F. Nyst

Proton pump inhibitors (PPIs) might soon become the most prescribed drugs in reflux esophagitis and peptic ulcer disease (PUD). In many comparative clinical trials, they were shown to heal ulcerous lesions more rapidly than H_2-receptor antagonists. They are so far the most potent non-surgical means to suppress gastric acidity, long recognized as a key factor in PUD. Their possible role in the treatment of the other key factor in PUD, *Helicobacter pylori* (HP) infection, is a very attractive field in clinical research. So far, few papers have been published about this topic, and this review deals mainly with personal experience, letters to editors and abstracts (out of 32 references, only 5 are full papers). We summarize our current knowledge about the potential role of PPIs in the treatment of HP infection. So far, this crucial (and sometimes very emotional) question has no definite answer. There is a mixing of facts, hopes, and wishes, and while reading this chapter one must remember that what is true today will often be wrong tomorrow.

In Vitro Antibacterial Activity of Proton Pump Inhibitors

Several in vitro experiments [2, 8, 10, 18, 19, 24] revealed that omeprazole, lansoprazole, and pantoprazole have some antibacterial activity against HP (Table 1). The minimal inhibitory concentration (MIC) ranges between 8 and 64 μg/ml for omeprazole and between 8 and 128 μg/ml for pantoprazole. According to the data of Iwahi et al. [10], lansoprazole might be twice as potent as omeprazole. These MIC values are close to those previously described for colloidal bismuth subcitrate (CBS). Nevertheless, the regimen with CBS treatment is usually 120 mg q.i.d. versus 20, 30 or 40 mg once daily for PPI. Moreover, no one knows exactly what amount of pure PPI (if any) reaches the gastric mucosa and mucus layer. Finally, there is a high variability in the experimental conditions for testing antimicrobial activity. Glupczynski et al. [8] found no synergy between omeprazole and antibiotics, but Vogt et al. [29] did: the MIC of omeprazole decreased from 32–128 mg/l to 4–32 mg/l when combined with various antibiotics (trimethoprim, metronidazole, ampicillin). Again, the clinical relevance of such an observation remains questionable. A remarkable study by Bode [2] reported

Gastroenterology Unit, University Hospital Brugmann, ULB/VUB Brussels, Place Van Gehuchten 4, 1020 Brussels, Belgium

Gasbarrini/Pretolani (Eds.)
Basic and Clinical Aspects of H. pylori Infection

Table 1. In vitro activity of PPI (in μg/ml) against HP

Reference	Omeprazole	Lansoprazole	Pantoprazole
Iwahi [10]	—	3.13–12.50 (MIC)	—
Paradis [19]	25 (MIC_{50})	—	—
Megraud [18]	64 (MIC_{50})	32 (MIC_{50})	—
Glupczynski [8]	8–32 (MIC)	—	—
Suerbaum [24]	8–32 (MIC)	—	8–128 (MIC)

morphological changes of HP under increasing concentration of omeprazole (from 0.2 to 256 μg/ml). A viable, nongrowing, coccoid form of HP is induced by omeprazole which acts in vitro as a bacteriostatic. Once more, is there pure omeprazole in the gastric mucus layer after a single daily intake of 20 or 40 mg per os?

In Vivo Omeprazole Reduces the Bacterial Load of Antral Mucosa

So far, in the field of PPI and HP, only omeprazole has been studied in vivo. This fact, observed by Veldhuyzen van Zanten et al. in a short series of human antral biopsies [27], was also reported by Catalano et al. [3]. It has been beautifully confirmed by Logan and coworkers. In a first study of 36 patients [15], these authors reported the results of the [^{13}C] urea breath test before treatment, after a 2-week course of omeprazole 40 mg daily and 2 weeks after treatment. In the group of HP positive patients ($n = 28$), mean pretreatment value of excess $^{13}CO_2$/ml was 25.3. It was significantly ($p < 0.05$) reduced at the end of the omeprazole course (19.2) but rose again to 25.7 2 weeks after the treatment. In HP negative patients ($n = 8$), the mean excess $^{13}CO_2$/ml was 1.9 before treatment and remained unchanged 2 weeks after treatment. No false-positive breath test has been induced by the omeprazole course. In a second study [16], these authors confirmed that the transient reduction of bacterial load by omeprazole was observed mainly in the antrum. They wisely advised performing biopsies both in the antrum and the fundus in eradication studies. The same observation has been published by Stolte and Bethke [23] in a retrospective histological study of 134 HP carriers treated by omeprazole for peptic ulcers or reflux esophagitis.

In Vivo Clearance of *Helicobacter pylori* with Omeprazole

The clearance (or transient elimination) of HP in patients treated by PPI has been widely reported [1, 4, 7, 9, 17, 20, 26, 28, 30]. In some early studies [17], the term "eradication" was even misused. The cumulative results of these small series that include patients with nonulcer dyspepsia and patients with active duodenal ulcer show a 50% mean clearance rate with a 20 mg omeprazole 4-week regimen in a total of 114 cases (Table 2). There is a striking variability between the

Table 2. HP clearance rates after 4 weeks of omeprazole 20 mg once daily

Reference	*n* HP + patients	Clearance
Biasco [1]	18	55%
Collins [4]	22	50%
Ferrini [7]	10	60%
Rokkas [22]	20	60%
Vandelli [26]	20	0%
Vigneri [28]	24	75%

Table 3. HP clearance rates after 4 weeks of omeprazole 40 mg once daily

Reference	*n* HP + patients	Clearance
Goh [9]	15	100%
Mainguet [17]	9	77%
Pretolani [21]	15	13%
Wagner [30]	13	15%

different series (range 0–75%). The same results were observed in a total of 52 patients treated by a 40 mg omeprazole 4-week course (Table 3): the mean clearance rate was 50% (13%–100%). Our group observed 16% clearance in 31 patients with either 20 or 40 mg daily for weeks. Such discrepancies could be explained only by differences in the methodology. The sensitivity of culture greatly varies between research centers. Moreover, the delay between the cessation of omeprazole therapy and HP reassessment is crucial and could be a question of days. As previously underlined, biopsies must be taken both from the antrum and the fundus.

Finally, the mechanisms of the decreasing of the bacterial load in patients treated by omeprazole remain unclear: Does HP need an acid environment to survive? Is in vitro antibacterial activity of omeprazole reproduced in vivo? The hypothesis of overgrowth of contaminants [23] could explain false-negative cultures, but why should histology be negative?

Omeprazole along is unable to eradicate HP, except perhaps in some sporadic cases, but the kinetics of HP reappearance after an omeprazole course is not known. Rokkas and coworkers [22] reported a case of false-negative culture up to 2 months after the end of omeprazole treatment.

Can Omeprazole Help Antibiotics in Eradicating *Helicobacter pylori*?

The antimicrobial activity of many drugs is pH dependent. The combination of an antibacterial agent with a potent inhibitor of acid secretion could, by including a significant increase in pH, potentiate the activity of the antibiotic. The minimal inhibitory concentration of amoxycillin, erythromycin, and ciprofloxacin in vitro decreases by a factor of 10 when pH increases from 3.5 to 5.5. Moreover, a lower volume of gastric secretion might increase the antibacterial agent's local concentration. The association of omeprazole and CBS has been disappointing in our hands (no eradication in 9/9 patients [6]. Labenz et al. [11] found that *omeprazole* 40 mg once daily *plus ciprofloxacin* 500 mg b.i.d was inefficient (3 eradications out of 20 patients). To date, macrolides have been little investigated. The association *omeprazole plus clarithromycin* might be promising, and the study of Petrino et al. [20] revealed a 100% clearance rate in a group of 12 HP-positive duodenal ulcer patients, but no data were given about possible eradication. Our group, eager to find a solution to the problem of tinidazole-resistant HP carriers, obtained 50% eradication in 18 patients treated by *omeprazole* 40 mg once daily plus *erythromycin ethylsuccinate solute* 500 mg q.i.d. and CBS 120 mg q.i.d. for week [5]. No posttreatment resistance to erythromycin was observed. Eradication rate with "maxitherapy" (*omeprazole* 40 mg once daily, CBS 120 mg q.i.d., *amoxicillin solute* 500 mg q.i.d., and *minocyclin* 100 mg b.i.d. for 1 week) was not better, and we observed 50% eradication in 12 patients [5].

So far, the bitherapy with *amoxicillin-omeprazole* has been the more frequently investigated association. A preliminary pilot study was done by Unge et al. and published in 1989 [25]. In this double-blind study, a subgroup of nine HP-positive patients with nonulcer dyspepsia received omeprazole 40 mg once daily plus 750 mg amoxicillin tables b.i.d. for 2 weeks. Four weeks after the cessation of therapy, five out of eight evaluable patients in that subgroup were still HP negative. In the same study, the eradication rate was 1/7 in a group of patients treated by amoxicillin alone (750 mg b.i.d.) and 0/8 in patients receiving omeprazole along (40 mg once daily). These encouraging results were later confirmed by Lamouliatte et al. [13], who reported a 53% eradication with a different regimen: omeprazole 20 mg once daily and amoxicillin suspension 500 mg q.i.d. for 4 weeks. It must be stressed that in this study 27 patients were included and 20 were evaluable at the end of therapy (17 of whom were cleared). Of the 17 cleared patients 14 were reassessed 4 weeks after the end of the treatment and nine were still negative.

Much higher eradication rates have recently been described. Bayerdorffer and colleagues (1991, personal communication) reported, in a group of duodenal ulcer patients treated with high doses of omeprazole (40 mg b.i.d.) plus amoxicillin, an 82% eradication rate. The subsequent 9-month remission rate of the ulcer disease is reportedly as high as 90%. No data are currently given about the evolution of antral gastritis in these cases. Labenz et al. [12] reported a tremendous eradication rate (83%), using omeprazole 20 mg b.i.d. and amoxicillin suspension (500 mg q.i.d.). Eradication was assessed by culture, urease test, and histology on biopsies both from the antrum and the body. The same authors did not observe further benefit by using higher dosages of omeprazole.

We observed quite opposite results. In 1989 a pilot study was abandoned after 13 HP-positive patients with nonulcer dyspepsia had been included. They received omeprazole 40 mg once daily plus amoxicillin suspension 500 mg q.i.d. for a 1-week course. [^{14}C] urea Breath test results were positive in all 13 cases before the treatment and remained positive in all 13 patients at least 4 weeks after the end of the treatment. In another pilot study, five consecutive patients with duodenal ulcer were treated by omeprazole 40 mg once daily and amoxicillin suspension 500 mg q.i.d. for 2 weeks. At the end of the treatment, biopsies (Sydney system) showed negative results both on histology and on culture in all cases (clearance rate 100%). All ulcers were healed. Follow-up endoscopy and biopsies at least 5 weeks after the end of the treatment revealed that all five patients were again HP positive.

How can one explain such differences in results? Compliance problems could be evoked in our studies but a 100% clearance rate at the end of therapy shows that the drugs were taken by the patients. Moreover, the specificity of culture is 100%, and false-positive results of culture are quite impossible. As far as the urea breath test is concerned, Logan et al. [15] showed that omeprazole does not induce false-positive results at least 2 weeks after the end of therapy, as discussed above.

One explanation could be that methodology problems, obvious in clearance studies, could have been exported to eradication trials. A washout period of 4 weeks after therapy (both for amoxicillin *and* omeprazole) is mandatory before assuming eradication since, as previously discussed, omeprazole alone may induce bacterial clearance. Biopsies must be taken from the antrum *and* fundus as shown by isotopic studies, and follow-up biopsies after 6 or 9 months should show a significant regression of antral gastritis if eradication is maintained. Since clearance temporarily reduces ulcer relapse rate (for instance after CBS monotherapy), reduced early relapse rates do not confirm eradication. Discrepancies among the different studies do not seem related to omeprazole dosage, but there could be a problem of timing for amoxicillin intake. We observed that clearance rate by omeprazole alone depends neither of the daily dose nor cumulative dose of omeprazole but increases with a longer duration of treatment. It could be more efficient to give antibiotics at the end of an omeprazole therapy when the bacterial load might be the lowest. The preliminary results of an interesting Swedish multicenter, study has recently been reported by Unge (1991, personal communication). So far, 233 consecutive patients with duodenal ulcer have been included. All the patients receive omeprazole 40 mg for 4 weeks. For the last 2 weeks, they are randomized in two groups: either amoxicillin 1.5 g/day or placebo. The first results show an eradication rate of 54% in the amoxicillin group versus 4% in the placebo group, and the 6-month remission rate of duodenal ulcer disease is, respectively, 70% and 36%. Finally, Lamouliatte et al. [14], comparing long-term results of omeprazole-amoxicillin-tinidazole and ranitidine-amoxicillin-tinidazole in 49 randomized duodenal ulcer patients, found no significant difference in healing rate of the ulcer nor in HP eradication rate. Six months after the end of treatment, eradication persisted in 93% of the patients, equally in each group. These excellent results are probably related to the low proportion of tinidazole-resistant strains (3 out of 49 cases included), but acid suppression by omeprazole or ranitidine might, at least theoretically, play a role. If eradication with Omeprazole-Amoxicillin is as high as reported by Bayerdorffer (1991, personal communication) or Labenz et al. [12], one can ask the question: why should we need tinidazolc? A provocative study, comparing the bitherapy (omeprazole-amoxicillin) with tritherapy (ranitidine-amoxicillin-tinidazole) should be very interesting.

Conclusion

PPIs are no doubt a very efficient treatment of upper gastrointestinal tract ulcerations. If they could bring a definite help for HP eradication, they should have, besides their role in the treatment of lesions, a key role in the treatment of ulcer disease and perhaps, in the prevention of gastric cancer. Very interesting and attractive data strongly suggest that PPIs (mainly omeprazole) can help antibiotics (mainly amoxicillin) to eradicate HP, but some investigators have not found any benefit of this association. Moreover, among studies that showed favorable results reported eradication rates from 50% to 83%, Posology differences might interfere as well as differences between HP strains. To date, the most prominent contribution of PPIs in HP-related research has been to reveal important methodological pitfalls, obvious in the studies of HP clearance with omeprazole alone. If these methodology problems can be ruled out in eradication studies, PPIs could be called *the* solution in the treatment of gastroduodenal ulcer disease.

References

1. Biasco G, Miglioli M, Barbara L, Corinaldesi R, DiFebo G (1989) Omeprazole, *Helicobacter pylori*, gastritis and duodenal ulcer. Lancet 2(8676): 1403
2. Bode G, Malfertheinert P, Lettner I, Nilius M, Ditschuneit H (1991) The influence of omeprazole on growth, morphology and viability of *Helicobacter pylori* in vitro (abstract). Ital J Gastroenterol 23 [Suppl 2]: 35
3. Catalano F, Rizzo G, Ayoubi Khajekini MT, Branciforte G, Liberti A, Ricci A (1991) Chronic antral *Helicobacter pylori* positive gastritis: effect of omeprazole therapy (abstract). Ital J Gastroenterol 23 [Suppl 2]: 101
4. Collins R, Keane C, O'Morain C (1991) Omeprazole and colloidal bismuth subcitrate +/− adjuvant antibiotics in the treatment of *Helicobacter pylori* associated duodenal ulcer disease (abstract). Gastroenterology 100 (512): A48
5. De Koster E, Burette A, Nyst JF, Glupczynski Y, Deprez C, Deltenre M (1990) H. Pylori treatment. The macrolide trail: one week erythromycin + CBS + omeprazole. (Abs) Rev Esp Enferm Dig 78 [Suppl I]: 118–119
6. De Koster E, Burette A, Nyst JF, Glupczynski Y, Deprez C, Jonas C, Otero J, De Reuck M, Deltenre M (1991) HP treatment: bismuth, omeprazole, antibiotics (abstract). Gastroenterology 100 (512): A52
7. Ferrini G, Larcinese G, Costantini N (1990) Efficiency of treatment with ranitidine, CBS, sucralfate and omeprazole in patients with *Helicobacter pylori* (abstract). Rev Esp Enferm Dig 78 [Suppl I]: 106
8. Glupczynski Y, Goutier S, Labbé M (1991) In vitro interaction between bismuth subcitrate, omeprazole, urease inhibitors and various antimicrobial agents against *Helicobacter pylori* (abstract). Gastroenterology 100, (5/2): A583
9. Goh KL, Parasakthi N, Peh SC, Tan KK, Anderson PE, Wong NW, Puthucheary SD (1991) Healing of duodenal ulcers with omeprazole is associated with clearance of *Helicobacter pylori* (abstract). Gastroenterology 100 (5/2): A71
10. Iwahi T, Satoh H, Nakao M et al. (1991) Lansoprazole, a novel benzimidazole proton pump inhibitor and its related compounds have selective activity against *Helicobacter pylori*. Antimicrob Agents Chemother 35: 490–496
11. Labenz J, Gyenes E, Peitz U, Borsch G (1991) Ciprofloxacin-omeprazole treatment for eradication of *Helicobacter pylori*. Z Gastroenterol 29: 143–145

12. Labenz J, Gyenes E, Ruhl GH, Borsch G (1991) Combined amoxicillin/omeprazole treatment (two weeks) for eradication of *Helicobacter pylori* (abstract). Ital J Gastroenterol 23 [Suppl 2]: 108–109
13. Lamouliatte H, de Mascarel A, Mégraud F, Barberis C, Bernard PH, Cayla R, Quinton A (1990) Omeprazole improves amoxicillin therapy directed towards *Helicobacter pylori* associated chronic gastritis (abstract). Proceedings of 1990 AGA, San Antonio, abstract nr 907
14. Lamouliatte H, Bernard PH, Boulard A, Mégraud F, de Mascarel A, Quinton A (1991) Controlled study of omeprazole-amoxicillin-tinidazole vs ranitidine-amoxicillin-tinidazole in *Helicobacter pylori* associated duodenal ulcers. Final and long term results (abstract). Ital J Gastroenterol 23 [Suppl 2]: 9
15. Logan RPH, Gummett PA, Misiewicz JJ, Walker MM, Karim NQ, Baron JH (1991) The urease activity of *H. pylori* before, during & after treatment with omeprazole (abstract). Gastroenterology 100 (5/2): A112
16. Logan RPH, Gummett PA, Walker MM, Karim NQ, Baron JH, Misiewicz JJ (1991) The effect of omeprazole on the dynamics of *H. pylori* infection (abstract). Ital J Gastroenterol 23 [Suppl 2]: 110
17. Mainguet P, Delmée M, Debongnie JC (1989) Omeprazole, *Campylobacter pylori* and duodenal ulcer. Lancet 2 (8659): 389–390
18. Mégraud F, Bouchard F, Lamouliatte H (1991) Proton pump inhibitors have an antimicrobial activity against *Helicobacter pylori* (abstract). Gastroenterology 100 (5/2): A123
19. Paradis A, Goldie J, Veldhuyzen van Zante SJO et al. (1990) The in vitro inhibitory effect of omeprazole on *Helicobacter pylori*: a bimodal distribution? (Abstract). Rev Esp Enferm Dig 78 [Suppl I]: 97
20. Petrino R, Di Napoli A, Boero M, Gazzera C, Chiandussi L (1991) Omeprazole + claritromicin treatment of *Helicobacter pylori* associated duodenal ulcer (abstract). Gastroenterology 100 (5/2): A140
21. Pretolani S, Bonvicini F, Careddu N, Cilla D, Acampora P, Gasbarrini A, Gasbarrini G (1990) Resistant ulcers and *Helicobacter pylori* gastritis: effect of treatment with omeprazole (abstract). Rev Esp Enferm Dig 78 [Suppl I]: 105
22. Rokkas T, Karameris A, Archavlis E, Tamvakopulos D, Giannikos N (1991) Omeprazole effectiveness on *Helicobacter pylori* in duodenal ulcer patients (abstract). Gastroenterology 100 (5/2): A148
23. Stolte M, Bethke B (1990) Elimination of *Helicobacter pylori* under treatment with omeprazole. Z Gastroenterol 28: 271–274
24. Suerbaum S, Leying H, Klemm K, Opferkuch W (1991) Antibacterial activity of pantoprazole and omeprazole against *Helicobacter pylori*. Eur J Clin Microbiol Infect Dis 10: 93–94
25. Unge P, Gad A, Gnarpe H, Olsson J (1989) Does Omeprazole improve antimicrobial therapy directed towards gastric *Campylobacter pylori* in patients with antral gastritis? Scand J Gastroenterol 24 [Suppl 167]: 49–54
26. Vandelli A, Cariani G, Santini D, Fontana G (1991) Omeprazole and *helicobacter*-like organisms in duodenal ulcer (abstract). Gastroenterology 100 (5/2): A179
27. Veldhuyzen van Zanten SJO, Miarczynski D, Hunt RH, Riddell RH (1991) Omeprazole decreases the nuumber of *Helicobacter pylori* and concomitant inflammation in patients with *Helicobacter*-associated gastritis (abstract). Gastroenterology 100 (5/2): A847
28. Vigneri S, Scialabba A, Termini R, Pisciotta G, Scarpignato E, Tessaro P, DiMario F, Naccarato R (1990) Efficacy of omeprazole in healing duodenal ulcer and eradicating *Helicobacter pylori*. (Abs) Rev Esp Enferm Dig 78 [Suppl I]: 115
29. Vogt K, Wiedersatz P, Hahn H (1991) In vitro interaction of omeprazole with antibiotics against *Helicobacter pylori* (abstract). Ital J Gastroenterol 23 [Suppl 2]: 48
30. Wagner S, Varrentrapp M, Gebel M, Bar W, Schmidt F W (1990) New aspects in the treatment of *Helicobacter pylori* Infection? (Abstract). Rev Esp Enferm Dig 78 [Suppl I]: 116–117

Pharmacology of Bismuth-Containing Medicines Used to Treat *Helicobacter pylori* Infections

D.W.R. Hall

Introduction

Although bismuth-containing compounds have been used for centuries, it is only in recent years that a systematic investigation into their clinical efficacy and mechanisms of action has been carried out. This was stimulated by scientific advances in the fields of diarrhoea and peptic ulcer. Both the recognition of the importance of *Helicobacter pylori* in the aetiology of peptic ulcer disease [3, 9, 10, 16, 20] and the finding that bismuth-containing medicines (BCMs) have a profound effect on the organism [17, 23, 32] have been a great spur to research into the actions of BCMs. The best known BCMs used to treat *H. pylori* infections are colloidal bismuth subcitrate (CBS: DE-NOL, Telen) and bismuth subsalicylate (BSS; Pepto-Bismol, Iatrox), and to a lesser extent bismuth subnitrate (BSN; Roter). A comparison of the actions of these compounds on *H. pylori* is hampered by the shortage of published information on BSS and BSN. In this review I discuss briefly the chief physical chemical properties of the bismuth compounds, followed by a discussion of their anti-microbial action and their effects on the postulated pathogenic mechanisms of *H. pylori.*

Physicochemical Properties

BSS is composed of microscopic prisms which are almost insoluble in water [7]. In the acid environment of the stomach BSS can react with HCl to form insoluble bismuth oxychloride and salicylic acid [2]. Colloidal bismuth subcitrate is an amorphous powder which forms colloidal solutions in water [7]. In the stomach it can be transformed to bismuth oxychloride and various other compounds containing free carboxyl groups and positively charged bismuth ions [55]. BSN is a micro-crystalline powder that is practically insoluble in water [7].

Anti-Microbial Activity

Minimum Inhibitory Activity. Bismuth salts, in common with other heavy metals, have anti-microbial activity. Various laboratories [18, 27, 34] discovered that *H. pylori* was sensitive to CBS and BSS. Recently comparisons of the sensitivity

Research and Development, Brocades Pharma B.V., Elisabethhof 19, 2350AC Leiderdorp, The Netherlands

Gasbarrini/Pretolani (Eds.)
Basic and Clinical Aspects of H. pylori Infection

Table 1. MICs of bismuth-containing medicines against *H. pylori*

	MIC_{90} (range; μg/ml)[a]		
Substance	Lambert [27]	Vogt [53]	Malfertheiner [31]
Metronidazole	2.0	—	—
Ampicillin	< 0.06	—	—
CBS	4.0	16(4–32)	16(16–32)
BSN	—	> 128(8– > 128)	16(8–32)
BSS	—	64(8–128)	64(16–64)

[a] Mean values as determined by the agar dilution method.

of *H. pylori* to various bismuth salts were made using the agar dilution technique [31, 53]. In Table 1 the MICs are shown for CBS, BSN and BSS, and to show the order of sensitivity they are compared with the MICs of metronidazole and ampicillin [34]. There is good agreement between the studies on the results with CBS and BSS, with CBS apparently showing a numerically lower MIC than BSS. In the case of BSN, Vogt [53] found a substantially higher MIC than Malfertheiner [31]. Differences in methods of suspension of BSN might explain these findings.

Ultrastructural Investigations. A number of ultrastructural studies have been carried out on *H. pylori* that were treated with CBS in vitro and in vivo. *H. pylori* in the presence of CBS showed focal accumulation of particulate bismuth under the cell wall, affecting nearly all organisms by 24 h [1]. In patients treated by single oral doses of CBS or BSS [33] and CBS [50] transmission electron microscopy of antral biopsies after 0.5–2 h showed a loosening of *H. pylori* from the antral epithelium (*H. pylori* apparently losing its adherence properties) and structural distortion by condensation, with fine and gross vacuolization. Furthermore, deposits of electron-dense material (bismuth) on the external surface and beneath the cell wall were seen. Recently van der Voort [54] using liquid culture and ultrastructural analysis of *H. pylori* exposed to CBS, established that the most bactericidal effects were seen in the stationary phase. This suggested that the mechanism of action does not involve replication or protein synthesis, but rather that CBS interfares with reactions involved in maintenance and/or integrity of the cytoplasmic membrane. CBS is bactericidal towards *H. pylori* [51, 54].

Synergy with Other Antibiotics. Synergy between CBS and β-lactam antibiotics and rifampin [51] and clindamycin [52] has been found. It is possible that CBS enhances the penetration of these antibiotics into *H. pylori* since there is evidence that the bismuth from CBS accumulates beneath the cell wall [1, 33, 50], and the mechanism of action of CBS involves effects on the cytoplasmic membrane [54].

Resistance of H. pylori *to Anti-microbials.* Goodwin [19] was unable to train *H. pylori* to become resistant to CBS in vitro. Using an in vitro serial passage technique to select resistant strains of *H. pylori*, it was shown that ciprofloxacin and erythromycin selected resistant strains [21], whereas it was not possible to select organisms resistant to BSS. The MICs of 15 *H. pylori* isolates from duodenal ulcer patients were shown to be unchanged before and after unsuccessful treatment with CBS [19]. This indicates that there was also no development of strains resistant to CBS in vivo.

Virulence Factors

H. pylori possesses a number of potential virulence factors, which could have concomitant pathological consequences for the host. Table 2 summarizes these virulence factors and their pathogenic and pathologic consequences.

Inflammatory Reaction. H. pylori appears to secrete a chemotactic substance (possible N-formyl-methionyl-leucyl-phenylalanine), which could account for the persistent accumulation of polymorphonuclear leukocytes in the gastric mucosa that accompanies *H. pylori* infection [35]. In a recent study peptic ulceration was found to be specifically associated with the mucosal recognition of a 120-kDa *H. pylori* protein [8]. Infection with strains of *H. pylori* that do not express this antigen may partly explain the absence of peptic ulceration in a proportion of infected patients. It has been speculated [4] that the substances produced by *H. pylori* that mediate inflammation are beneficial to the organism by allowing the release of nutrients. The degree of suppression of the inflammatory response by the host would determine the pathological and clinical outcome. BCMs might influence the course of the inflammatory response by interacting directly with the organism or with the released bacterial inflammatory mediators.

Motility. The spiral shape and active flagella of *H. pylori* enables the bacteria to move easily in the viscous mucus environment of gastric mucosa [5, 11], which would enhance the chances of colonization. There is no information available on the effects of drugs on motility.

Adhesion. Adhesion of *H. pylori* to the apical cell membranes of surface gastric epithelium is an important step in the colonization process. Adherence of

Table 2. Pathogenic/pathological consequences of potential *H. pylori* virulence factors

Virulence factor	Pathogenic/pathological consequences
Inflammatory mediators	Inflammation (nutrients?)
Motility	Increases chance of colonization
Cytotoxins	Damages epithelium
Urease	Acid survival; damages epithelium
Mucolytic activity	Degrades mucus
Lipolytic activity	Lysolecithin damages epithelium Decreases hydrophobicity
Adhesion	Contact with epithelium

See text for references.

Table 3. The effect of bismuth-containing medicines on the adhesion of *H. pylori* to various epithelial cell lines

BCM	IC_{50} μg/ml[a] HeLa cells	Hep-2 cells	Int-407 cells
CBS	0.04	0.02	0.01
BSS	> 100	> 100	> 100
BSN	> 100	100	> 100
BST	> 100	> 100	> 100

CBS, Colloidal bismuth subcitrate; BSS, bismuth subsalicylate; BSN, bismuth subnitrate; BST bismuth sodium tartrate.
[a] IC_{50} is the concentration to give 50% inhibition. The BCMs (equivalent amounts of bismuth tested) were incubated directly with L-[^{35}S]-methionine-prelabelled *H. pylori* and [^{3}H] thymidine-prelabelled cell lines for 1 h. After washing and trypsin treatment, the cells were harvested and radioactivity determined. Modified with permission from Kamsteeg et al. [26].

H. pylori to human gastric mucosa has been found in vivo [17] and in cultured epithelial cell lines [37]. It has been suggested that the mechanism of adhesion is via non-specific factors, such as hydrophobic interactions [40] and specific factors, such as adhesins and agglutinins [32] and glycolipid receptors [30, 37, 45]. The precise mechanism and the factors influencing adhesion still need to be established. In the latter respect a recent study points to gastric sulfomucins as one of the host's protective mechanisms against infection, by interferring with attachment of *H. pylori* with the epithelial mucosa [39], and CBS appears to enhance the activity of the sulfomucins [44]. Kamsteeg [26] studied the effect of various bismuth compounds on the adhesion of various strains of *H. pylori* to HeLa and Hep-2 cell lines. CBS was extremely potent with an IC_{50} (concentration to produce 50% inhibition) in the order of 10–40 ng/ml against a number of cell lines (Table 3). On the other hand, BSS and the soluble non-colloidal bismuth sodium tartrate were inactive, while BSN was 5000–10 000 times less potent than CBS. The colloidal properties of CBS seem to be decisive determinants of anti-adhesive activity.

Cytotoxins. H. pylori have been shown to produce materials that exhibit cytotoxic properties. Morphological and ultrastructural abberations were found in cell cultures in vitro [13, 14, 25, 28] and a reduction in the glycocalyx thickness of superficial mucous cells in vivo [6]. Although the role of cytotoxins in the pathogenicity of *H. pylori* is not fully resolved, it is thought that cytotoxin-producing strains are more associated with duodenal ulcer [13]. There is no published information on potential interactions with or inactivation of these cytotoxic materials by BCMs.

Urease. Survival of *H. pylori* in the acidic environment of the stomach is attributed to the ability of *H. pylori* to hydrolyse urea present in gastric juice, to ammonia, thus increasing the local pH [49]. The ammonia produced by *H. pylori* has been suggested to cause functional and morphological alterations in gastric epithelium. A reduction of transmucosal potential difference [36, 49], an enhanced back diffusion of H^+ ions to epithelial cells [22], damage to a mucus-producing gastric cell line [47] and damage to Int 407 and Vero tissue culture cells [56] can be cited as evidence of the toxic effects of ammonia. There appears to be conflicting evidence regarding the actions of BCMs on urease activity. Using a spectrophotometric determination of urease activity Sarosiek [41] found that BSS between approximately 0.4–4 mg/ml produced complete, dose-dependent inhibition of urease. On the other hand, Hughes [24] using an ammonia electrode could find only 25% inhibition at 50 mg/ml BSS. In my own laboratory we found no inhibition of urease activity after 10 min incubation (no pre-incubation) with 10 mg/ml CBS (unpublished). The type of experimental set up could have explained the differences in results with BSS, since it was reported [41] that incubation after pre-incubation of urease and BSS decreased the urease inhibition by 25–40%.

Proteolysis. An extracellular endopeptidase type enzyme from *H. pylori* has been described to degrade gastric mucus [46]. The enzyme is apparently also of significance in vivo, since destruction of the three-dimensional threadlike gastric mucus structure was observed by electron microscopy in patients with *H. pylori* infection [6, 20]. These results were suggested to demonstrate a breakdown of the stable and protective mucus by *H. pylori.* The rapid recovery of the netlike structure was seen after eradication of *H. pylori.* CBS partially inhibited the protease at concentrations between 0.1 and 1 mg/ml [42].

Lipolysis. The superficial epithelium of the stomach is covered by a layer of surface active phospholipids which are considered to constitute the hydrophobic barrier to acid damage [29]. Recently it has been discovered that human stomach mucosa hydrophobicity is greatly reduced in the presence of *H. pylori* infection [48]. *H. pylori* produces lipases and, more importantly, phospholipases [38, 43]. Phospholipases would be capable of degrading the hydrophobic lining, and lysolecithin formed from the action of phospholipase could be cytotoxic to epithelial cells. CBS has been shown to have a relatively weak effect on *H. pylori* lipase activity, but produced potent dose-dependent inhibition of phospholipase activity [38, 43]. It has also been found that clearance of *H. pylori* in patients results in a recovery of the hydrophobicity of the stomach lining to normal levels [15]. On return of the *H. pylori* infection the hydrophobicity decreases.

Conclusions

In the past 5 years there has been an explosive growth of information on *H. pylori,* and a concomitant interest in the actions of BCMs on this bacterium. Table 4 presents an overview of the main actions of CBS and, where the information is available, on BSS and BSN. It can be seen that there is approximately similar anti-microbial activity between the bismuth medicines; however, only CBS displays very potent inhibition of *H. pylori* adhesion. This property of CBS may translate to clinical efficacy; for example, CBS may produce an increased speed of clearance of *H. pylori* in comparison to other BCMs. Whether

Table 4. Summary of the actions of bismuth-containing medicines on *H. pylori*

Activity	BSS	BSN	CBS
MIC (16–64 μg/ml)	√	√	√
No resistance	√	?	√
Synergy in vitro (antibiotics)	?	?	√
Urease inhibition	+/−	?	—
Protease inhibition	?	?	√
Phospholipase inhibition	?	?	√
Anti-adhesion activity	—	—	√

√, Activity present; —, no activity present; ?, no information; +/−, controversial.

the differences in BCM pharmacology on *H. pylori* will result in meaningful differences in clinical efficacy needs to be ascertained by comparative clinical trials.

References

1. Armstrong JA, Wee SH, Goodwin CS, Wilson DH (1977) Response of *Campylobacter pyloridis* to antibiotics, bismuth and an acid-reducing agent in vitro – an ultrastructural study. J Med Microbiol 24: 343–350
2. Bierer DW (1988) Bismuth subsalicylate its history, chemistry and safety. Rev Infect Dis 12: S3–8
3. Blaser MJ (1988) Type B gastritis, aging, and *Campylobacter pylori*. Arch Intern Med 148: 1021–1022
4. Blaser MJ (1991) Pathogenic mechanisms involved in *Helicobacter pylori* infections. Abstract European digestive disease week, 21 Oct 1991
5. Bode G, Malfertheiner P, Ditschuneit H (1988) Pathogenetic implications of ultrastructural findings in *Campylobacter pylori* related gastroduodenal disease. Scand J Gastroenterol 23 [Suppl 142]: 25–39
6. Bode G, Malfertheiner P, Lehnhardt G, Ditschuneit H (1990) Virulence factors of *Helicobacter pylori* – ultrastructural features. In: Malfertheiner P, Ditschuneit H (eds) *Helicobacter pylori*, gastritis and peptic ulcer. Springer, Berlin Heidelberg New York, pp 63–73
7. Budavari S (ed) (1989) The Merck Index, 11th edn. Merck, Rahway
8. Crabtree JE, Taylor JD, Wyatt JI, Heatley RV, Shallcross TM, Tompkins DS, Rathbone BJ (1991) Mucosal IgA recognition of *Helicobacter pylori* 120 kDa protein, peptic ulceration and gastric pathology. Lancet 338: 332–335
9. Dooley CP, Cohen H (1988) The clinical significance of *Campylobacter pylori*. Ann Intern Med 108: 70–79
10. Dooley CP, McKenna D, Humphreys H, Bourke S, Keane CT, Sweeney E, O'Morain C (1988) Histological gastritis in duodenal ulcer: relationship to *Helicobacter pylori* and effect of ulcer therapy. Am J Gastroenterol 83: 278–282
11. Eaton KA, Morgan DR, Kakowka S (1989) *Campylobacter pylori* virulence factors in gnotobiotic piglets. Infect Immun 57: 1119–1125
12. Evans DG, Evans DJ Jr, Moulds JJ, Graham DY (1988) *N*-acetyl-neuraminyllactose-binding fibrillar hemagglutinin of *Campylobacter pylori*: a putative colonization factor antigen. Infect Immun 56: 2896–2906
13. Figura N, Guglielmetti P, Rossolini A, Berberi A, Cusi G, Musmanno RA, Russi M, Quaranta S (1989) Cytotoxin production by *Campylobacter pylori* strains isolated from patients with peptic ulcers and from patients with chronic gastrits only. J Clin Microbiol 27: 225–226
14. Fumarola D, Miragliotta G (1988) Possible pathogenic mechanisms of *Campylobacter pylori*. Eur J Clin Microbiol Infect Dis 7: 579–580

15. Goggin PM, Marrero JM, Jazrawi RP, Corbishley CM, Yu CW, Northfield TD (1990) Effect of *Helicobacter pylori* infection on gastric mucosal hydrophobicity in man. Gastroenterology 98: A49
16. Goodwin CS (1988) Duodenal ulcer, *Campylobacter pylori*, and the "leaking roof" concept. Lancet 2: 1467–1469
17. Goodwin CS, Armstrong JA, Marshall BJ (1986) *Campylobacter pyloridis*, gastritis and peptic ulceration. J Clin Pathol 39: 353–365
18. Goodwin CS, Blake P, Blincow E (1986) The minimum inhibitory and bactericidal concentrations of antibiotics and anti-ulcer agents against *Campylobacter pyloridis*. J Antimicrob Chemother 17: 309–314
19. Goodwin CS, Bell B, McCullough C, Turner M (1989) Sensitivity of *Campylobacter pylori* to colloidal bismuth subcitrate. J Clin Pathol 42: 216–219
20. Graham DY (1989) *Campylobacter pylori* and peptic ulcer disease. Gastroenterology 96: 615–625
21. Haas CE, Nix DE, Schentag JJ (1990) In vitro selection of resistant *Helicobacter pylori*. Antimicrob Agents Chemother 34: 1637–1641
22. Hazell SL, Borody TJ, Lee A (1987) *Campylobacter pyloridis* gastritis. I. Detection of urease as a marker of bacterial colonization and gastritis. Am J Gastroenterol 82: 292–296
23. Hislop I, Glancy R, Armstrong J, Marshall BJ (1984) Histological improvement of active chronic gastritis in patients treated with DE-NOL. Aust NZ Med 14 [Suppl 4]: 907
24. Hughes S, Stewart M, Rhodes JM (1988) Use of an ammonia electrode for rapid quantification of *C. pylori* urease – lack of inhibition by bismuth subsalicylate. Gut 29: A710
25. Hupertz V, Czinn S (1988) Demonstration of a cytotoxin from *Campylobacter pylori*. Eur J Clin Microbiol Infect Dis 7: 576–578
26. Kamsteeg H, Poot LJ, Van Den Berg TP (1990) Activity of colloidal bismuth subcitrate and other bismuth salts against the adhesive properties of *Helicobacter pylori*. Rev Esp Enferm Apar Dig 78 [Suppl 1]: 119–120
27. Lambert JR, Hansky J, Davidson A, Pinkard K, Stockman K (1985) *Campylobacter* like organisms (CLO) – in vivo and in vitro susceptibility to antimicrobial and anti-ulcer therapy. Gastroenterology 88: 1462
28. Leunk RD, Johnson PT, David BC, Kraft WG, Morgan DR (1988) Cytotoxic activity in broth-culture filtrates of *Campylobacter pylori*. J Med Microbiol 26: 93–99
29. Lichtenberger LM, Graziani LA, Dian EJ, Buttler BD, Hills BA (1983) Role of surface-active phospholipids in gastric cytoprotection. Science 219: 1327–1329
30. Lingwood CA, Law H, Pellizzari A, Sherman P, Drumm B (1989) Gastric glycerolipid as a receptor for *Campylobacter pylori*. Lancet I: 238–241
31. Malfertheiner P, Stanescu A, Lehnhard G, Bode G, Kemmer TP, Ditschuneit H (1990) In vivo and in vitro susceptibility of *Helicobacter pylori* to different bismuth formulations, Gastroenterology 98: A82
32. Marshall BJ, McGechie DB, Rogers PA, Glancy RJ (1985) Pyloric *Campylobacter* infection and gastroduodenal disease. Med J Aust 142: 439–444
33. Marshall BJ, Armstrong JA, Francis GJ, Nokes NT, Wee SH (1987) Antibacterial action of bismuth in relation to *Campylobacter pyloridis* colonization and gastritis. Digestion 37 [Suppl 2]: 16–30
34. McNulty CAM, Dent J, Wise R (1985) Susceptibility of clinical isolates of *Campylobacter pyloridis* to 11 antimicrobial agents. Antimicrob Agents Chemother 28: 837–838
35. Mooney C, Keenan J, Munster D, Wilson I, Allardyce R, Bagshaw P, Chapman B, Chadwick V (1991) Neutrophil activation by *Helicobacter pylori*. Gut 32: 853–857
36. Murakami M, Yoo JK, Inada M, Miyake T (1988) Effect of ammonia on the gastric mucosa in rats: pathophysiological importance of urease in gastric ulcer disease. Jpn J Pharmacol 47: 330–332
37. Neman-Simha V, Megraud F (1988) In vitro model for *Campylobacter pylori* adherence properties. Infect Immun 56: 3329–3333
38. Ottlecz A, Romero JJ, Graham DY, Lichtenberger LM (1991) Inhibitory effect of bismuth (Bi^{3+}) salts on *Helicobacter pylori* phospholipase activity. Gastroenterology 100: A136
39. Piotrowski J, Slomiany A, Murty VLN, Fekete Z, Slomiany BL (1991) Inhibition of *Helicobacter pylori* colonization by sulfated gastric mucin. Biochem Int 24: 749–756
40. Pruul H, Goodwin CS, McDonald PJ, Lewis G, Pankhurst D (1990) Hydrophobic characterisation of *Helicobacter* (*Campylobacter*) *pylori*. J Med Microbiol 32: 93–100

41. Sarosiek J, Roche JK, Marshall BJ, McCallum RW (1990) Urease enzyme inhibition by bismuth subsalicylate: a putative antibacterial mechanism. Gastroenterology 98: A119
42. Sarosiek J, Bilski J, Murty VLN, Slomiany A, Slomiany BL (1989) Colloidal bismuth subcitrate (DE-NOL) inhibits degradation of gastric mucus by *Campylobacter pylori* protease. Am J Gastroenterol 84: 506–510
43. Slomiany BL, Kasinathan C, Slomiany A (1989) Lipolytic activity of *Campylobacter pylori*: effect of colloidal bismuth subcitrate (DE-NOL). Am J Gastroenterol 84: 1273–1277
44. Slomiany BL, Piotrowski J, Murty VLN, Ehrlich J, Slomiany A (1991) CBS enhances gastric mucin capacity to interfere with *H. pylori* colonization factor. Gastroenterology 100: A165
45. Slomiany BL, Piotrowski J, Semanta A, Van Horn K, Murty VLN, Slomiany A (1989) *Campylobacter pylori* colonization factor shows specificity for lactosylceramide sulfate and GM3 ganglioside. Biochem Int 19: 929–936
46. Slomiany BL, Bilski J, Sarosiek J, Murty VLN, Dworkin B, Van Horn K, Zielenski J, Slomiany A (1987) *Campylobacter pyloridis* degrades mucin and undermines gastric mucosal integrity. Biochem Biophys Res Commun 144: 307–314
47. Smoot DT, Mobley HLT, Chippendale GR, Lewison JF, Resau JH (1990) *Helicobacter pylori* urease activity is toxic to human gastric epithelial cells. Infect Immun 58: 1992–1994.
48. Spychal RT, Goggin PM, Marrero JM, Saverymuttu SH, Yu CW, Corbishley CM, Maxwell JD, Northfield TD (1990) Surface hydrophobicity of gastric mucus in peptic ulcer disease. Gastroenterology 98: 1250–1254
49. Thomson L, Tasman-Jones C, Morris A, Wiggins P, Lee S, Forlong C (1989) Ammonia produced by *Campylobactoer pylori* neutralizes H^+ moving through gastric mucus. Scand J Gastroenterol 24: 761–768
50. Tijtgat GNJ, Rauws EAJ, De Koster E (1988) *Campylobacter pylori*. Scand J Gastroenterol 23 [Suppl 155]: 68–81
51. Van Caekenberghe DL, Breyssens J (1987) In vitro synergistc activity between bismuth subcitrate and various antimicrobial agents against *Campylobacter pyloridis* (*C. pylori*). Antimicrob Agents Chemother 31: 1429–1430
52. Vogt K, Hahn H (1990) Synergism between clindamycin and colloidal bismuth subcitrate against *Helicobacter* (*Campylobacter*) *pylori* in vitro. Zentralbl Bakteriol 274: 246–249
53. Vogt K, Warrelmann M, Hahn H (1989) The minimum inhibitory concentrations of various bismuth salts against *Campylobacter pylori*. Zentralbl Bakteriol 271: 304–310
54. Voort vd LHM, Bos vd AP, Kamsteeg H (1990) In vitro bactericidal effects of colloidal bismuth subcitrate on *Helicobacter pylori*. Rev Esp Enferm Apar Dig 78 [Suppl 1]: 103
55. Wagstaff AJ, Benfield P, Monk JP (1988) Colloidal bismuth subcitrate. A review of its pharmacodynamic and pharmacokinetic properties, and its therapeutic use in peptic ulcer disease. Drugs 36: 11–16
56. Xu JK, Goodwin CS, Cooper M, Robinson J (1990) Intracellular vacuolization caused by the urease of *Helicobacter pylori*. J Infect Dis 161: 1302–1304

Bismuth and *Helicobacter pylori*

P. Malfertheiner[1], M. Nilius[1], and U. Kreusel[2]

Historical Background

The first preparative method in making bismuth salts accessible for therapeutic purposes goes back to Georg Agricola, in the 16th century [1]. In 1786 Odier first administered "magisterium bismuti" (bismuth subnitrate) as a "safe, infallible remedy against gastric spasm", in a dose of 24 g per day [2]. The nineteenth century brought the wide use of bismuth compounds for the treatment of syphilis. In the 1850s, treatment of dispeptic symptoms with bismuth compounds was made popular by Chambers in England and Kussmaul in Germany, administering bismuth subnitrate in doses up to 400 g [2].

The enthusiasm for bismuth compounds waned as cases with bismuth intoxication were reported. The first cases of intoxication seen in ileostomy and colostomy patients under treatment with bismuth subgallate were reported in Australia in 1973 [3, 4]. A large number of cases with bismuth encephalopathy were observed in France [5]. Despite many questions concerning other factors perhaps interferring with bismuth toxicity, bismuth salts were taken off the market in these countries. After a period of apprehension bismuth salts enjoyed a revival as reliable antiulcer drugs in the 1980s. With the discovery of *Helicobacter pylori* and the documented antibacterial activity of bismuth salts these began a new carrier.

Chemical Properties

Bismuth is the heaviest nonradioactive element and is located in the fifth main group of the periodic system together with nitrogen, phosphorus, arsenic, and antimony. It exists in the oxidation states -3, $+3$ and $+5$, but in biological systems it exhibits only the oxidation state $Bi\ 3+$ [7, 8]. The tendency to electropositivity and the basic character of the elements increases from nitrogen to bismuth. For this reasons bismuth halides (general formula BiX_3) in aqueous solution hydrolyse to insoluble compounds of the general formula BiOX. The various bismuth salts are derived from bismuth subnitrate, which in solution

[1] Department of Internal Medicine I, University of Ulm, 89081 Ulm, Germany
[2] Department of Inorganic Chemistry, Technical University of Munich, Germany

Gasbarrini/Pretolani (Eds.)
Basic and Clinical Aspects of H. pylori Infection

Table 1. Properties of different bismuth compounds

Compound	Solubility	Bismuth content %
Bi subcarbonate	Water insoluble	80–82.5
Bi subnitrate	Water insoluble	72–79
Bi aluminate	Water insoluble	53.4
Bi subsalicylate	Water insoluble	56.5–60
Bi subcitrate	Water soluble	52.5
Bi subgallate	Lipid soluble	46–53

reacts with soluble basic salts to form bismuth subcarbonate, subgallate, subsalicylate, or subcitrate.

Table 1 presents the chemical properties of some bismuth compounds suitable for therapy. The two most important bismuth compounds for therapy are colloidal bismuth subcitrate (CBS) and bismuth subsalicylate (BSS). CBS is the only bismuth salt with high solubility in water. The ionic architecture of bismuth citrate complexes, with a three-dimensional network in the crystal lattice, explains the high water solubility of CBS [9] (Fig. 1). Moreover, the hydroxy group also coordinates strongly to the metal centre. These strong covalent Bi–O bonds cause a high chemical resistance of CBS in gastric juice. Basic BSS is more sensitive to hydrolysis and decomposes in hydrochloric acid into insoluble BiOCl and free salicylic acid [9]. According to Pearson [10], the Bi^{3+} cation belongs to the group of "soft acids,". Therefore, bismuth reacts preferably with soft polarizable ligands such as sulphur. The most likely Bi^{3+} binding sites in biological systems are therefore sulphur atoms. Bismuth thiolate

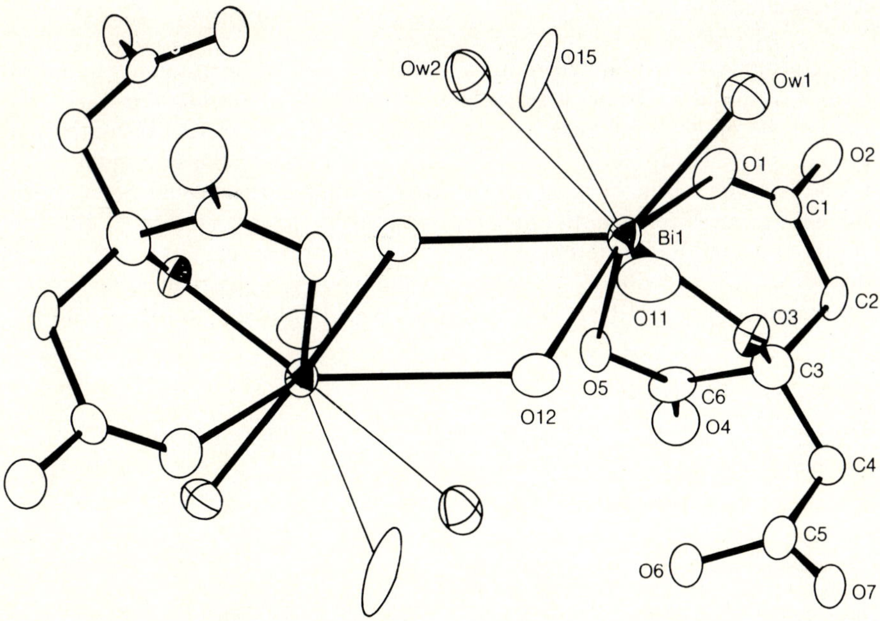

Fig. 1. Three-dimensional network in the crystal structure of potassium bismuth citrate. (From [9])

complexes are stable in acid solutions (pH < 2), in contrast to bismuth carboxylates which decompose (unpublished observations).

Mechanisms of Action of Bismuth Salts

The pharmacological actions of bismuth have been investigated in a limited way. Bismuth reacts readily with sulfhydryl groups, which may explain the interaction of bismuth with proteins; this may account for the cytoprotective effect. CBS has been shown to bind epidermal growth factor in a pH-dependent manner and to accumulate in the ulcerated area of gastric and duodenal mucosa [11]. In an electron microscopic study electron-dense precipitates formed by CBS in the presence of hydrochloric acid were found in contact with the gastric mucus and on the epithelial surface of the duodenum and proximal jejunum [12, 13]. In addition, CBS protects gastric mucus and epidermal growth factor from peptic luminal degradation and stimulates bicarbonate secretion from both gastric and duodenal mucosa as well as prostaglandin E_2-synthesis [11, 14, 15]. We have demonstrated a dose-dependent decrease in *H. pylori* adhesion to human surface mucus cells in vitro with CBS [16]. The suggestion that bismuth compounds other than CBS inhibit the proteolytic activity of gastric juice lacks confirmation. Different studies have in fact shown that the antipeptic activity of bismuth aluminate and bismuth carbonate is scarce [17–19].

Antibacterial Effects

H. pylori growth is inhibited more potently by bismuth compounds than that of any of the other bacteria studied so far. However, considerable variations exist in the minimal inhibitory concentration (MIC) of different bismuth compounds [20–22] (Table 2). Ultrastructural studies show the accumulation of bismuth complexes in the bacterial wall and within the periplasmatic membrane. Bacteria exposed to bismuth appear structurally disintegrated (Fig. 2). Bismuth compounds inhibit bacterial enzymes such as urease, catalase and alcohol dehydrogenase as well as *H. pylori* associated lypolytic activity in a dose-dependent manner [23–26]. Bacterial synthesis of ATP is inhibited in *Escherichia coli*,

Table 2. MIC of bismuth salts for *H. pylori*

Compound	MIC 90 (mg/l)	Reference
Bi subcitrate	16–32	[22]
	32	[21]
	8	[29]
	12	[20]
Bi subsalicylate	64	[21]
	25	[20]
Bi subgallate	32	[21]
Bi subnitrate	> 128	[21]

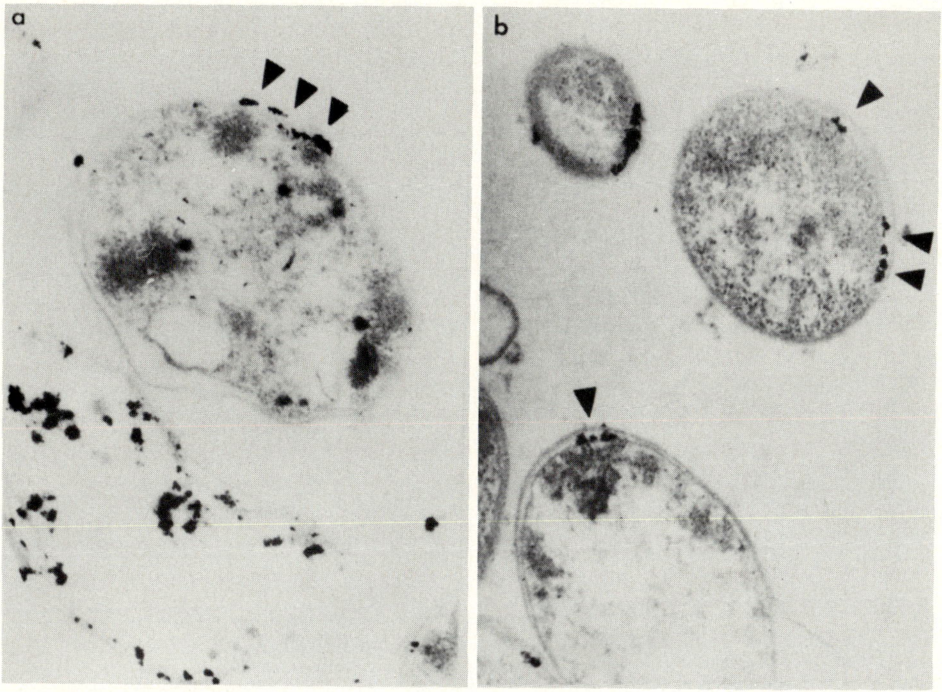

Fig. 2a, b. Bismuth incorporation into *Helicobacter pylori* bacteria

and preincubation of *H. pylori* with CBS decreases adhesion to HeLa cells in vitro [27, 28]. These inhibitory effects of CBS are likely due to its binding to sulfhydryl groups of the proteins, with a consequent alteration of their function.

In Vitro Experiments

The antibacterial effect of bismuth compounds on *H. pylori* has been studied in several in vitro experiments [21, 22, 35] to define the MIC of the various bismuth compounds. Such studies are commonly performed either with the agar dilution test or by broth dilution methods. To determine the effect of bismuth salt against *H. pylori* we performed in vitro studies with two different methods: the agar dilution method and kill-kinetic studies, so-called time-dependent killing curves.

Agar Dilution Method

We performed in vitro experiments with 10 different *H. pylori* strains and 12 different bismuth compounds. Data for the MIC are shown in Table 3.

The strains showed varing susceptibility to the various bismuth compounds. A similar effect was seen in only three of the 12 compounds; the MIC of bismuth

Table 3. MIC of different bismuth compounds tested with ten *H. pylori* strains (μg/ml)

Salts	1[a]	2	3	4	5[a]	6[b]	7	8	9[b]	10
Bismuth subcitrate	16	16	16	16	16	16	16	16	16	16
Bismuth aluminate 1	64	64	64	63	32	64	64	64	32	128
Bismuth aluminate 2	32	64	256	256	32	256	64	64	64	128
Bismuth aluminate 3	64	128	256	256	64	> 512	256	256	512	256
Bismuth aluminate 4	> 512	> 512	> 512	> 512	> 512	> 512	> 512	> 512	> 512	> 512
Bismuth subnitrate 1	32	64	128	64	16	64	16	64	64	64
Bismuth subnitrate 2	8	8	16	16	8	16	8	16	32	16
Bismuth subsalicylate	16	32	64	64	32	16	64	16	64	32
Bismuth subgallate	> 512	> 512	> 512	> 512	> 512	> 512	> 512	> 512	> 512	> 512
Bismuth subcarbonate	> 512	> 512	> 512	> 512	> 512	> 512	> 512	> 512	> 512	> 512
Bismuth subnitrate 3 + bismuth aluminate 2	32	128	128	128	32	64	64	64	256	218
Bismuth nitrate 1 + bismuth subgallate	128	256	256	128	128	512	256	512	> 512	256

[a] Bi-sensitive strain.
[b] Bi-insensitive strain.

aluminate 4, bismuth subgallate and bismuth subcarbonate was higher than 512 μg/ml. Two strains were more sensible to bismuth than all others, whereas two strains were resistant to most of the tested bismuth compounds. The combination of bismuth subnitrate with bismuth aluminate showed a similar MIC as bismuth aluminate but was less effective than bismuth subnitrate alone.

Table 4. MIC of *H. pylori* strains tested with different bismuth compounds

	MIC range	MIC_{50}	MIC_{90}
Bismuth subcitrate	16–32	16	16
Bismuth aluminate 1	32–64	64	64
Bismuth aluminate 2	32–256	64	256
Bismuth aluminate 3	64–512	256	512
Bismuth aluminate 4	> 512		
Bismuth subnitrate 1	16–128	32	64
Bismuth subnitrate 2	8–32	8	16
Bismuth subsalicylate	16–64	32	64
Bismuth subgallate	> 512		
Bismuth subcarbonate	> 512		
Bismuth subnitrate 3 + Bismuth aluminate 2	32–256	64	128
Bismuth subnitrate 1 + Bismuth subgallate	128–> 512	256	512

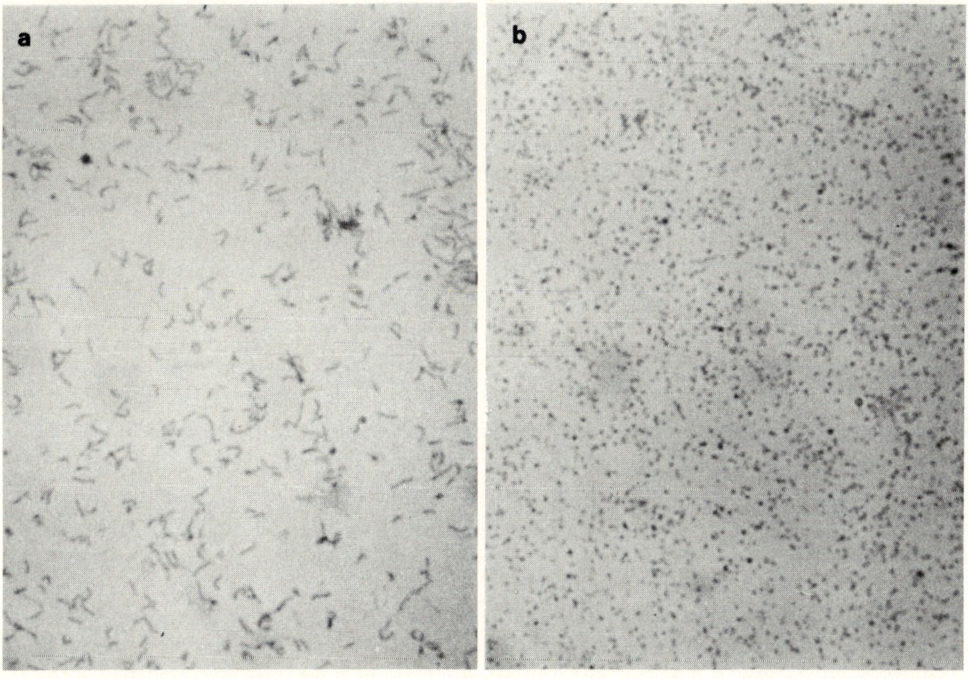

Fig. 3. Helical form of *Helicobacter pylori* (**a**) and CLF (b)

The second combination of bismuth subnitrate with bismuth subgallate was also less effective than bismuth subnitrate alone but more effective than bismuth gallate. This finding does not favour of a synergistic effect of bismuth salt combinations (Table 4).

The MIC above 512 μg/l for bismuth subgallate and bismuth subcarbonate observed in our experiments contrasts with better results by others who have reported an MIC of 4–64 μg/l for bismuth-subgallate and one of 12–50 μg/ml for bismuth subcarbonate [21, 36]. The reason for this discrepancy may lie in the different solubility of these bismuth compounds in acids or organic solubilizers by the other investigators, altering the original compound.

Despite its general acceptance, the MIC may not sufficiently reflect the antibacterial efficacy of bismuth compounds. Using morphological methods one can observe the formation of coccoid-like forms (CLF) even at doses of bismuth compounds with an MIC of 90 (Fig. 3). The CLF are thought to have the potential for survival. The formation of CLF and the insufficient penetration of bismuth compounds through the mucus layer may account for the frequent failure of *H. pylori* eradication with bismuth salts in vivo.

Time-Dependent Killing Curves

A more appropriate method for testing the bactericidal effect of bismuth compounds is the time-dependent killing curve. Kill-kinetic studies were made with CBS and three different *H. pylori* strains. CBS concentrations between 0.2 and 256 μg/ml were tested. The MIC of CBS varied from 2 μg/ml (strain KI) to 16 μg/ml (strains FA and TSI; Fig. 4). These results are in agreement with other studies using with the agar dilution method [21, 29, 36].

Using time-dependent killing curves we observed another interesting detail of *H. pylori* bacteria treated with CBS. Whereas a CBS dose of 16 μg/ml in two *H. pylori* strains was bacteriostatic during the whole incubation period, in strain KI a slight recovery was seen after an incubation period of 16 h and a CBS concentration of 2 μg/ml. This demonstrates that the growth-inhibitory effect of CBS is time and strain dependent.

Solubility of Different Bismuth Salts in Gastric Juice

An essential question concerning the bioavailability of bismuth compounds is their solubility in the gastric juice. To answer this question we performed experiments using atomic absorption spectrometry to test the solubility of different bismuth salts in pooled gastric juice samples obtained from patients during endoscopic examination (Fig. 5). With CBS which is water soluble the highest concentrations of solubilized bismuth were obtained in gastric juice with a wide range of pH (Fig. 5). All bismuth compounds insoluble in water were also scarcely dissolved in gastric juice. With the pH adjusted to 7, most of these salts showed a better solubility, which continued, however, to be much lower compared to CBS.

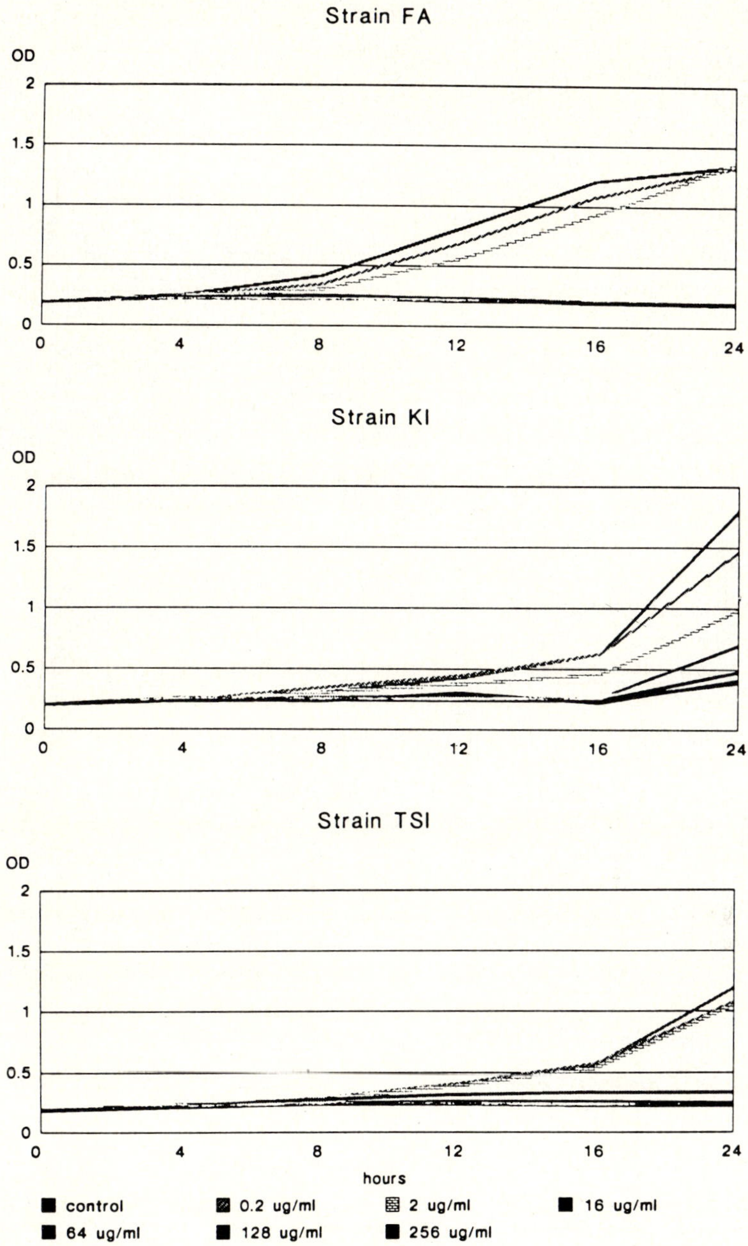

Fig. 4. Time-dependent killing curves of three *Helicobacter pylori* strains, treated with CBS

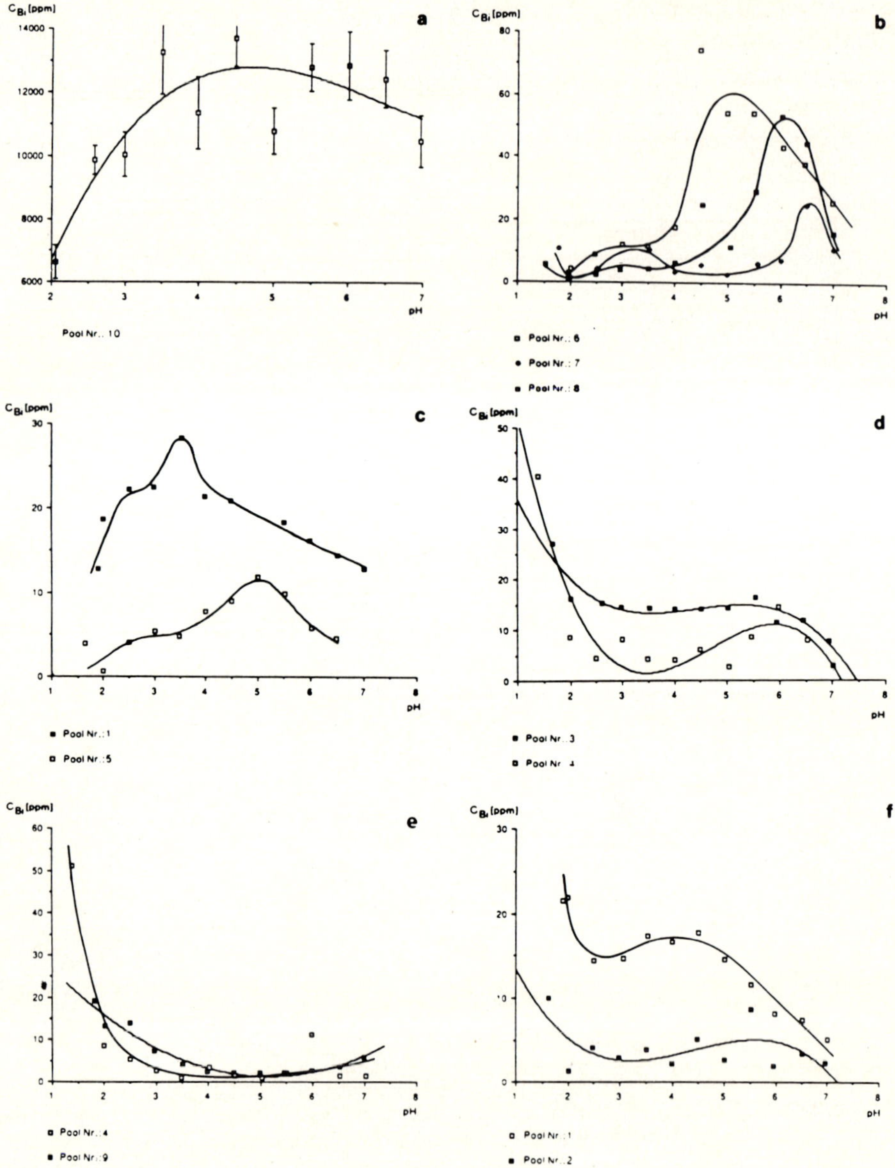

Fig. 5a–e. Solubility curves of different bismuth compounds in gastric juice. **a** CBS. **b** BSS. **c** Bi aluminate. **d** Bi subcarbonate. **e** Bi subgallate. **f** Bi subnitrate

Therapeutic Effects

Bismuth compounds are currently employed for the treatment of peptic ulcer and non-ulcer dyspepsia.

Peptic Ulcer Treatment

Several studies have confirmed the high efficacy of CBS for healing peptic ulcerations in the stomach and duodenum, with a success rate comparable to that of H_2 receptor antagonists [37,38]. A definite advantage with bismuth therapy is the significant reduction in the frequency of duodenal ulcer relapses compared to H_2 receptor antagonists [38–40]. After numerous attempts to explain this, *H. pylori* was identified as the key factor. In fact, following *H. pylori* eradication duodenal ulcer relapses declined significantly in some patients with CBS [41]. Since *H. pylori* in the majority of patients is eliminated only after bismuth monotherapy (*H. pylori* elimination occurs in up to 80%), but not permanently eradicated (eradication rate 15%), the relapse rate of duodenal ulcers is reduced but not abolished with bismuth compounds alone. The concept of *H. pylori* infection as a determinant for duodenal ulcer relapse has been confirmed definitely by studies using combined bismuth antibiotic therapy [42–44]. In fact, eradication of *H. pylori* by this treatment has reduced duodenal ulcer relapses to almost zero [42,43,45]. Because of this significant therapeutic effect with *H. pylori* eradication in duodenal ulcer disease bismuth monotherapy is no longer the primary option, but it is a key drug in combination with antibiotics. While studies continue to seek optimal combination treatments for curing *H. pylori* infection, triple therapy with CBS or BSS, amoxicillin/tetracyclin and metronidazole is still the most effective [44].

Gastritis and Non-ulcer Dyspepsia

Initial reports of an effective elimination of *H. pylori* by CBS and BSS, followed by the regression of inflammatory changes in the gastric mucosa [7,46,47], have prompted the use of a number of bismuth salts for anti-*H. pylori* treatment. Besides the variation in chemical properties, dosages and duration of treatment the different bismuth salts induce *H. pylori* elimination in 50%–83% [48,49]. While the elimination of *H. pylori* is achieved in up to 80% of cases, the few studies reporting eradication rates have been disappointing, showing results of 10%–30% [48]. The efficacy of bismuth salts for the relief of symptoms in patients with non-ulcer dyspepsia (NUD) and chronic gastritis has been studied by several investigators, but the results are still equivocal. Future studies aimed at eradicating *H. pylori* infection in patients with NUD may use either bismuth-antibiotic combinations or other drug combinations (e.g. proton pump inhibitors and antibiotics). Such studies are awaited to confirm a role for *H. pylori* infection as a potential cause of NUD.

Table 5. Side effects of bismuth compounds

Compound	Side effect	Reference
Bi subcarbonate	Bismuth encephalopathy	[52]
Bi subgallate	„	[50]
Bi subnitrate	„	[51]
Bi subsalicylate	„	[51]
Bi-thioglycollate	Nephrotoxicity	[55]
Bi subcitrate	„	[57]
Bi-thioglycollate	Liver toxicity	[58]
Bi subsalicylate	Stomatitis	[59, 60]
Bi subsalicylate	Erythema	[61, 62]
Bi subsalicylate	Local pigmentation	[63]
Bi subnitrate	Osteoarthropathy	[64]
Bi subcarbonate	„	[56]

Side Effects

Major concerns regarding bismuth toxicity arose due to reports on bismuth encephalopathy and nephrotoxicity reported in France and Australia [50, 51]. An epidemic-like outbreak of bismuth-associated encephalopathy occurred in France between 1962 and 1978 following the intake of bismuth salts, including bismuth subgallate, subcarbonate and subnitrate, but the incriminated doses were extremely high, up to 20 g elemental bismuth per day [50, 52]. In spite of the suggestive role of bismuth in the cases of encephalopathy in France the exact etiology of these intoxications has never been clarified, and other factors may be taken in consideration besides bismuth [52].

Nephrotoxicity has been reported after the use of bismuth trithioglycollamate and dialylacetate, but renal failure was reversible [53]. Several reports on nephrotoxicity, osteoarthropathy and neuropathy were ascribed to overdosage of different bismuth salts, generally with recovery after discontinuation of drug intake [54]. Table 5 presents the main toxic effects of bismuth salts.

Bismuth salts currently on the market are usually taken in doses of 400–1200 mg/day and can be regarded as safe. Bismuth plasma concentrations below 50 mg/l are considered as safe [65]. The peak bismuth plasma concentrations immediately following exposure to CBS may reach values above 100 mg/l, but these decrease rapidly [13]. There is no evidence that these peaks are associated with side effects.

A variety of minor side effects have been reported following bismuth intake, including obstipation, abdominal cramps, cutaneous rush and cephalgia. Darkening of the tongue, gingiva and faeces due to bacterial degradation of bismuth salts to bismuth sulfide are purely cosmetic and reversible.

Conclusion

Bismuth salts, despite a long history, have undergone a revival with the discovery of *H. pylori*. The current use of bismuth salts as monotherapy may be recommended for dyspeptic syndromes associated with *H. pylori* infection. For ulcer disease, where eradication is crucial, bismuth compounds need to be combined with antibiotics.

Acknowledgements. We thank Dr. G. Bode for performing the electron microscopy and Mrs. Christine Attenberger for preparing the manuscript.

References

1. Von Lippmann EO (1930) Die Geschichte des Wismuts zwischen 1400 und 1800. Springer, Berlin Heidelberg New York
2. Hotz J (1990) Die Historie der Wismutbehandlung. In: Malfertheiner P, Holz J, Ditschuneit H (eds) Wismut: Therapiekonzept bei Helicobacter pylori, Gastritis und Ulkuskrankheit. Zuckschwerdt, Munich
3. Morrow AW (1973) Request for reports: adverse reactions with bismuth subgallate. Med J Aust 60: 912
4. Burns R, Thomas DW, Barron VJ (1974) Reversible encephalopathy possible associated with bismuth subgallate ingestion. BMJ 1: 220–223
5. Buge A, Rancurel G, Poisson M, Dechy H (1974) Encephalopathies aigues au cours des traitements oraux par les sels de bismuth. Nouv Presse Med 3: 2315–2320
6. Bader JP (1987) The safety profile of De-Nol. Digestion 37 [Suppl 2]: 53–59
7. Greenwood NN, Earnshaw A (1984) Chemistry of the elements. Pergamon, Oxford
8. Marshall BJ (1991) The use of bismuth in gastroenterology. Am J Gastroenterol 86: 16–25
9. Herrmann WA, Herdtweck E, Pajdla L (1991) Colloidal bisuth subcitrate (CBS) isolation and structural characterization of the active substance against Helicobacter pylori, a causal factor of gastric diseases. Inorg Chem 30: 2579–2581
10. Pearson RG (1986) Acids and bases. J Am Chem Soc 85: 3563
11. Konturek SJ, Radecki T, Piastucki I, Drozdowicz D (1986) Advances in the understanding of the mechanism of cytoroprotective action by colloidal bismuth subcitrate. Scand J Gastroenterol 21 [Suppl]: 6–10
12. Coghill SB, Hopwood D, McPherson S, Hislop S (1983) The ultrastructural localisation of De-Nol (colloidal tripotassium dicitrate bismuthate TDB) in the upper gstrointestinal track of man and rodents following oral and instrumental administration. J Pathol 139: 105–114
13.. Nwokolo CU, Gavey CJ, Smith JTL, Pounder RE (1989) The absorption of bismuth from oral doses of tripotassium dicitrato bismuthate. Aliment Pharmacol Therap 3: 29–39
14. Slomiany BL, Nishikawa H, Bilski J, Slomiany A (1990) Colloidal bismuth subcitrate inhibits peptic degradation of gastric mucus and epidermal growth factor in vitro. Am J Gastroenterol 390–393
15. Shorrock CJ, Crampton JR, Gibbons LC, Rees WDW (1989) Effect of bismuth subcitrate on amphibian gastroduodenal bicarbonate secretion. Gut 30: 917–921
16. Nilius M, Schieffer S, Malfertheiner P (1991) Inhibition of H. pylori adhesion to human SMC by CBS and different proteases. Irish J Med Sci 161 [Suppl 10]: 10
17. Alstead S (1941) Action of bismth carbonate in gastric disease. Lancet II: 420–423
18. Bateson PR (1958) A comparative in vitro evaluation of a new bismuth salt bismuth aluminate. J Pharm Pharmacol 10: 123–131
19. Matts SGF, Swan CHJ, Kelleher J (1965) Double blind trial of bismuth aluminate and magnesium trisilicate in peptic ulceration with simultaneous gastric analysis. BMJ 1: 753–756
20. Marshall BJ, Armstrong JA, Francis GJ, Noke NT, Wee SH (1987) Antibacterial action of bismuth in relation to Campylobacter pyloridis colonization and gastritis. Digestion 27 [Suppl 2]: 16–30
21. Vogt K, Warrelmann M, Hahn H (1989) The minimum inhibitory concentrations of various bismuth salts against Campylobacter pylori. Zbl Bakt 271: 304–310
22. Goodwin CS, Blake P, Blincow E (1986) The minimum inhibitory and bactericidal concentrations of antibiotics and antiulcer agents against Campylobacter pyloridis. J Antimicrob Chemother 17: 309–314
23. Nilius M, Ströhle A, Espenhain E, Bode G, Malfertheiner P (1990) Coccoid like forms (CLF) of Helicobacter pylori – enzyme activity and antigenicity. Rev Esp Enf Digest 78[Suppl 1]: 28

24. Nilius M, Pugliese M, Malfertheiner P (1992) Electrophoretic characterization and inhibition of H. pylori catalase. Irish J Med Sci 161 [Suppl 10]: 51
25. Roine et al (1992) Colloidal bismuth subcitrate is a potent inhibitor of Helicobacter pylori associated alcohol dehydrogenase activity. Irish J Med Sci 161 [Suppl 10]: 47
26. Slomiany BL, Nishikawa H, Bilski J, Slomiany A (1990) Colloidal bismuth subcitrate inhibits peptic degradation of gastric mucus and epidermal growth factor in vitro. Am J Gastroenterol 85: 390–393
27. Sox T, Olson CHA (1989) Binding and killing of bacteria by bismuth subsalicylate. Antimicrob Agents Chemother 33: 2075–2082
28. Goodwin CS, Armstrong JA, Cooper M (1991) Colloidal bismuth subcitrate inhibits the adherence of H. pylori to epithelial cells. Ital J Gastroenterol 23 [Suppl 2]: 40
29. Van Caekenberghe DL, Breyssens J (1987) In vitro synergistic activity between bismuth subcitrate and various antimicrobial agents against Campylobacter pyloridis (C. pylori). Antimicrob Agents Chemother 31: 1429–1430
30. McNulty CAM, Gearty JC, Crump B, Davis M, Donovan IA, Melikian V, Lister DM, Wise R (1987) Campylobacter pyloridis and associated gastritis: investigator blind, placebo controlled trial of bismuth salicylate and erythromycin ethylsuccinate. BMJ 293: 645
31. Tytgat GN, Rauws JE, Langenberg W (1986) The role of colloidal bismuth subcitrate in gastric ulcr and gastritis. Scand J Gastroenterol 21 [Suppl 122]: 22
32. Marshall BJ, Armstrong JA, Graham J, Francis GJ, Nokes NT, Wee SH (1987) Antibacterial Action of bismuth in relation to Campylobacter pyloridis colonization and gastritis. Digestion 37 [Suppl 2]: 1630
33. Stanescu A, Malfertheiner P, Mayer D, Baczako K, Ditschuneit H (1989) Wismutsubnitrat – Therapie der Campylobacter-pylori-positiven chronischen erosiven Gastritis. Gastro-Entero-Hepatol 7:3
34. Stanescu A, Malfertheiner P, Mayer d, Baczako K, Ditschuneit H (1989) Wismutaluminat in der Gastroenterologie. Therapieeffekte bei chronischer erosiver Campylobacter-pylori-assoziierter Gastritis. Fortschr Med 107:623
35. McNulty CAM, Dent J, Wise R (1985) Susceptibility of clinical isolates of Campylobacter pyloridis to 11 antimicrobial agents. Antimicrob Agents Chemother 28: 837–838
36. Glupczynski Y, Thibaumont F (1989) Comparative in vitro susceptibility of Campylobacter pylori to different bismuth salts (abstract). Klin Wochenschr 67 [Suppl 18]: 24
37. Martin DF, Hollanders D, May SJ, Tweedle DEF, Ravenscroft MM, Miller JP (1981) Lancet I: 7–10
38. Tytgat GNJ (1987) Colloidal bismuth subcitrate in peptic ulcer – a review. Digestion 37 [Suppl 2]: 31–41
39. Bianchi-Porro B, Lazzaroni M, Parente F, Peprillo M (1986) The influence of colloidal bismuth subcitrate on duodenal ulcer relapse. Scand J Gastroenterol 21 [Suppl 122]: 36–38
40. Dobrilla G, Vallaperta P, Amplatz S (1988) Influence of ulcer healing agents on ulcer relapse after discontinuation of acute treatment; a pooled estimate of controlled clinical trials. Gut 29: 181–187
41. Coghlan IG, Tobin A, O'Morain C (1989) Campylobacter pylori and ulcer treatment. In: Rathbone BJ, Heathley RV (eds) C. pylori and gastroduodenal disease. Blackwell Scientific Publications, Oxford, pp 232–245
42. Rauws EA, Tytgat GNJ (1990) Cure of duodenal ulcer associated with eradication of Helicobacter pylori. Lancet 335: 1233–1235
43. Marshall BJ, Warren JR, Blincow ED, Phillips M, Goodwin CS, Murray R, Blackbourn SJ, Waters TE, Sanderson CR (1988) Prospective double-blind trial of duodenal ulcer relapse after eradication of Campylobacter pylori. Lancet II: 1437–1442
44. Axon ATR (1991) Helicobacter pylori therapy: effect on peptic ulcer disease. J Gastroent Hepatol 6: 131–132
45. Borody T, Cole P, Noonan S et al. (1988) Long-term Campylobacter pylori recurrence post-eradication. Gastroenterology 94: A43
46. McNulty CAM, Gearty JC, Crump B, Davis M, Donovan IA, Melikian V et al. (1986) Campylobacter pyloridis and associated gastritis: investigator blind, placebo controlled trial of bismuth salicylate and erythromycin ethylsuccinate. BJM 293: 645–649
47. Malfertheiner P, Stanescu A, Baczako K, Bode G, Ditschuneit H (1988) Chronic erosive gastritis – a therapeutic approach with bismuth. Scand J Gastroenterol 23 [Suppl 142]: 87–92

48. Marshall BJ, Dye KR, Plankey M, Frierson HF, Hoffman SR, Guerrant RL, McCallum RW (1988) Eradication of Campylobacter pylori infection with bismuth subsalicylate and antibiotic combinations. Am J Gastroenterol 83: 1035
49. Malfertheiner P, Stanescu A, Lehnhardt G, Bode G, Kemmer TP, Ditschuneit H (1990) In vivo and in vitro susceptibility of Helicobacter pylori. Gastroenterology 98: A82
50. Lechat P, Kisch R (1986) Bismuth induced encephalopathies: reappraisal of risks. Gastroenterol. Clinbiol 10: 562–569
51. Hasking GJ, Duggan JM (1982) Encephalopathy from bismuth subsalicylate. Med J Austr 2: 167
52. Martin-Bouyer G, Foulon B, Guerbois, H, Barrin C (1980) Aspects epidemiologiques des encephalopathies apres administration de bismuth par voie orale. Therapie 35: 307–313
53. Czerwinski AW, Ginn HE (1964) Bismuth nephrotoxity. Am J Med 37: 969–975
54. Winship KA (1983) Toxicity of bismuth salts. Adv Drug React Ac Pois Rev 2: 103–121
55. Urizar R, Vernier RL (1966) Bismuth nephropathy. JAMA 198: 207–209
56. Gaucher A, Netter P, Faure G, Hutin MF, Burnel D (1979) Bismuth-induced osteoarthropathies. Med J Aust 1: 129–130
57. Hudson M, Mowat NAG (1989) CBS (De-Nol) self-poisoning-reversible toxicity. BJ 299: 159
58. Karelitz S, Freedman AD (1951) Hepatitis and nephrosis due to soluble bismuth. Pediatrics 8: 772–777
59. Peters EE (1942) Bismuth stomatitis and albumin uria report of 6 cases. Am J Syph Gonnorhea Vener Dis 26: 84–95
60. Silverman SS (1944) Bismuth stomatitis during the treatment of syphilis in the axury. Mil Surg 95: 486–489
61. Goldman L, Clarke GE (1939) Erythema of ninth day syndrome associated with bismuth therapy. Am J Syph Gonorrhea Vener Dis 23: 224–227
62. Dobes WL, Alden HS (1949) Pityriasis rosea-like drug cruptions due to bismuth. South Med J 42: 572–579
63. Heyman A (1944) Systemic manifestations of bismuth toxicity observations on 4 patients with preexistent kidney disease. Am J Syph Gonorrhea Vener Dis 28: 721–732
64. Emile J de Bray JM, Vernat M, Morer T, Allain P (1979) Lc ostcopathies scapulaires et vertebrales des encephalophaties aigues myocloniques bismuthiques. A propos de 8 cas. Ann Med Intern 130: 75
65. Hillemand P, Palliere M, Laquais B, Bouvet P (1977) Traitement bismuthique et bismuthemie. Semaine des Hopiteaux de Paris 53: 1663–1669

Antibiotics in *Helicobacter pylori* Treatment

C.S. Goodwin

Introduction

The normal stomach is acid, and very few studies have been reported of the effect of antibiotics in acid media, especially on *Helicobacter pylori.* A few studies have compared the minimum inhibitory concentrations of antibiotics against *H. pylori* at a range of pH values. However, some of these have only been down to pH 5.5 [11], and virtually none have tested the effectiveness of antibiotics at the pH of the stomach, which is pH 2 or 3. It has been found that antibiotics are less active at pH 5.5 than at pH 7.5 [11]. Furthermore, the sensitivity of *H. pylori* to antibiotics should be assessed not only in cell-free liquid media, but in association with cells, and preferably in animal models of infection.

Tissue Culture Studies

At this conference, Boyanova et al. [11] reported using HEp-2 cells, to which *H. pylori* becomes adherent very quickly. In this model, antibiotics were added at different concentrations and removed after 1, 6, and 24 h. The viable bacteria were counted. Also synergy could be tesed by the addition of two antibiotics at once. By adding 1 mg/l metronidazole to 0.01 mg/l amoxicillin, the viable count of *H. pylori* decreased by 100 in comparison with amoxicillin alone. Lansoprazole 10 mg/l was bactericidal in this model, while 1 mg/l had no effect. This could be an extremely useful model, but does not operate at acid pH. However, when patients are treated with acid-reducing drugs, the pH of the stomach rises, and such a tissue culture model could be very useful to predict the effect of antibiotic treatment in this situation.

Goodwin et al. [2] have studied the action of colloidal bismuth subcitrate (CBS) against *H. pylori.* CBS 1 mg/ml was mixed with two strains of *H. pylori* for 30 min. The organisms were washed and then added to HEp-2 cell monolayers. CBS caused a 90% reduction in the number adhering to the cells.

Department of Medical Microbiology, Faculty of Medicine and Health Science, United Arab Emirates University, P. O. Box 17666, Al Ain, United Arab Emirates

Gasbarrini/Pretolani (Eds.)
Basic and Clinical Aspects of H. pylori Infection

Animal Models

Helicobacter felis can be transferred to the mouse stomach [10], so this site could be exposed to antibiotics in combination or singly to see whether the organism is eliminated. This may predict the response of antibiotic treatment against *H. pylori*. Other animals are more expensive and, therefore, less easy to use with multiple animals. Gnotobiotic piglets are infected by *H. pylori* and can be used to test antibiotic effectiveness. Ferrets cannot be infected with *H. pylori*, but *H. mustele* may be a useful model to test antibiotic treatment. Monkeys can be infected with *H. pylori*, but, again, they are very expensive for such experiments.

Antibiotics in Humans

An important bifurcation has occurred in the treatment of *H. pylori* infection. Up to now, therapy including bismuth has been the mainstay of eradication protocols, but recently reports have appeared on work with acid-reducing drugs and antibiotics without bismuth. Special attention should be paid to the gastric mucosal pharmacokinetics of bismuth compounds to ensure adequate delivery of bismuth [7]. The swallow tablet of colloidal bismuth subcitrate may give a low eradication rate when administered alone, in contrast to the chew tablet which has given a higher eradication rate on its own. Poor compliance of patients with treatment regimens may account for a significant proportion of failures, especially when prolonged treatment is given [3]. Triple therapy which includes metronidazole must only be used when one is sure that strains of *H. pylori* are metronidazole sensitive. Women may have a significantly higher rate of *H. pylori* strains resistant to metronidazole than males [12].

Recently, patients with duodenal ulcer have been treated for 12 days with amoxycillin (750 mg thrice daily) and metronidazole (500 mg three times daily); they also received cimetidine (800 mg at night for 4 weeks). This therapy achieved an eradication rate of 75%. Therapeutic failure was always associated with resistance to metronidazole [4]. Another treatment has been ranitidine plus oxacillin; 50% of patients remained free of *H. pylori* at 12 months [5]. A combination of ranitidine plus amoxicillin plus tinidazole was compared with omeprazole plus amoxicillin plus tinidazole. In the omeprazole group *H. pylori* was eradicated in 90% of patients, and in the ranitidine group in 80% of patients. These figures were obtained from endoscopies performed 1 month after the end of antibiotic treatment. The regimens were as follows: omeprazole, 20 mg/day for 4 weeks or ranitidine 300 mg/day for 6 weeks, plus amoxicillin 2 g/day for 15 days, and tinidazole 1 g/day for 10 days [8, 9]. A combination of CBS plus erythromycin plus omeprazole for 1 week, with endoscopy 5 weeks after treatment achieved eradication in 50% of patients. Side effects were rare [6]. These are very exciting and important developments in *H. pylori* treatment.

The scientific justification explaining the increased activity of antibiotics plus acid reducing drugs was shown by Westblom and Duriex, who administered clindamycin intramuscularly to guinea pigs and measured concentrations in serum and tissue. The luminal mucosa concentration of clindamycin at 1 h at pH 5.0 was fivefold greater than the concentrations seen under physiologic pH 2.0 conditions [13].

References

1. Boyanova L, Mégraud F, Lamouliatte H (1991) Application of a bactericidal assay using cell adherent bacteria to test drug combinations in vitro. Ital J Gastroenterol 23 [Suppl 2]: 36–37
2. Goodwin CS, Armstrong JA, Cooper M (1991) Colloidal bismuth subcitrate inhibits the adherence of *H. pylori* to epithelial cells. Ital J Gastroenterol 23 [Suppl 2]: 40
3. Glupczynski Y, Burette A (1990) Drug therapy for *Helicobacter pylori* infection: problems and pitfalls. Am J Gastroenterol 85: 1545–1551
4. Hirschl AM, Hentschel E, Berger J, Nemec H, Rotter ML (1991) Treatment of *Helicobacter pylori* infections with amoxycillin plus metronidazole: bacteriological, serological and histological results. Eur J Gastroenterol Hepatol 3: 3–7
5. Isakov VA, Grigoriev PY, Yakovenko EP (1990) Treatment of *Helicobacter pylori* positive duodenal ulcers (letter). Lancet 336: 755–756
6. Koster ED, Burette A, Nyst JF, Glupczynski Y, Deprez C, Jonas C, Otero J, DeReuck M, Deltenre M (1991) *Hp* treatment: bismith, omeprazole, antibiotics. Gastroenterology 100: A52
7. Lambert JR (1990) Safety profile of bismuth-containing medications. In: Malfertheiner P, Ditschuneit H (eds) *Helicobacter pylori*, gastritis and peptic ulcer. Springer, Berlin Heidelberg New York, pp 427–433
8. Lamouliatte H, Bernard PH, Boulard A, Cayla R, De Mascarel A, Megraud F, Quinton A (1991) *Helicobacter pylori* eradication prevents duodenal ulcer relapse. Gastroenterology 100: A104
9. Lamouliatte H, Bernard PH, Boulard A, Megraud F, De Mascarel A, Quinton A (1991) Controlled study of omeprazole-amoxicillin-tinidazole in *Helicobacter pylori* associated duodenal ulcers (abstract). Gastroenterology 100: A104
10. Lee A, Fox JG, Otto G, Murphy J (1990) A small animal model of human *Helicobacter pylori* active chronic gastritis. Gastroenterology 99: 1315–1323
11. McNulty Cam (1989) Bacteriological and pharmacological basis for the treatment of *Campylobacter pylori* infection. In: Rathbone BJ, Healthy RV (eds) *Campylobacter pylori* and gastroduodenal disease. Blackwell Scientific, Oxfort, pp 209–216
12. Weil J, Bell GD, Powell K, Jobson R, Trowell JE, Gant P, Jones PH (1990) *Helicobacter pylori* and metronidazole resistance. Lancet 336: 1445
13. Westblom TU, Duriex DE (1991) Enhancement of antibiotic concentrations in gastric mucosa by H_2-receptor antagonist: implication for treatment of *Helicobacter pylori* infections. Dig Dis Sci 36: 25–28

Clinical Application of Antibiotics in Eradicating *Helicobacter pylori*

C. O'Morain, H.X. Xia, and M.A. Daw

Introduction

Helicobacter pylori is sensitive to a wide spectrum of antibiotics in vitro but not in vivo. In vitro *H. pylori* is highly sensitive to β-lactam, macrolides, nitrofurantoin and quinilones. It is also sensitive to the ulcer-healing agents colloidal bismuth subcitrate and omeprazole but not to H_2 antagonists, sucralfate or prostaglandin analogues.

The striking discordance between in vitro and in vivo efficacy of antibiotics may be due to their inability to come into contact with the micro-organisms within the gastric mucous layer in sufficient concentration, either by diffusion from the lumen or from the lamina propria vessels after systemic absorption. In addition, some antibiotics are pH dependent for their activity. The organism is ideally adapted to the environment, being buried in the gastric pits and protected from the acid environment by the mucous layer. It is now accepted that at least 4 weeks should elapse before taking biopsies to determine eradication. The micro-organism can be suppressed temporarily at the end of treatment and re-emerge after 4 weeks.

Like other slowly growing micro-organisms, resistance against antibiotics can develop. Resistance can be induced in vitro by serial passage of the organism in culture media containing increasing concentration of the antibiotic. In the laboratory, another phenomenon is observed, that of synergism, antibiotics enhancing the activity of one another in the organism. This occurs in the case of metronidazole and tetracyline.

The ideal antibiotic treatment is one without side effects that can be given in a convenient dosage over a short period of time. This antibiotic should be able to find access to the organism and therefore diffuse across the cell membrane and be active at an acidic pH. It also may be effective by being secreted into the gastric juice.

Monotherapy with Antibiotics

Antibiotics on their own have been used in the eradication of *H. pylori*, and the best eradication rate achieved is about 50%. Glupczynski et al. [1] randomly assigned patients with gastritis to 1 g amoxicillin twice a day or placebo (Table 1).

Department of Gastroenterology, Meath/Adelaide Hospital, and Clinical Microbiology, St. James's Hospital, Dublin 8, Ireland, and Department of Medical Microbiology, Faculty of Medicine, Tripoli – Libya (GSPLAJ)

Gasbarrini/Pretolani (Eds.)
Basic and Clinical Aspects of H. pylori Infection

Table 1. Efficacy of monotherapy in clearing and eradicating *H. pylori*

Therapy	*n*	Dosage	Clearance	Eradication	Reference
CBS	30	2 tablets b.i.d, 4 weeks	32%	ND	Coghlan et al. [8]
		1 tablet q.i.d, 4 weeks	64%	ND	
BSS	17	3 tablets t.i.d, 8 weeks	47%	17	Borsch et al. [6]
Amoxicillin	22	2 × 1000 mg, 7 days	91%	ND	Glupczynski et al. [1]
	18	2 × 1000 mg, 14 days	72%	ND	Glupzynski et al. [1]
Ciprofloxacin	13	500 mg b.i.d, 14 days	0%	ND	Hirschl et al. [28]
Erythromycin	15	4 × 5000 mg, 14 days	7%	ND	McNulty et al. [4]
Metronidazole	5	2 × 5000 mg, 21 days	20%	ND	Hirschl et al. [28]

CBS, Colloidal bismuth subcitrate; BSS, bismuth subsalicylate; ND, not done.

Immediately after treatment 91% of the patients cleared the organism, compared to 16% of those on placebo. However, 2 weeks after treatment all the patients were culture positive. Oral ciprofloxacin 500 mg b.i.d. was unsuccessful in clearing the organism in 9 out of 14 patients evaluated [2]. Some of these patients with *H. pylori* acquired resistance. Similar disappointing results were observed when ranitidine was added to these antibiotics [3].

Erythromycin is effective in vitro against *H. pylori*. In a study of 15 patients with non-ulcer dyspepsia and *H. pylori*-associated gastritis treated with erythromycin ethylsuccinate (500 mg q.i.d.) only one was cleared of the micro-organism [4].

Morgan et al. conducted a double-blind placebo-controlled randomised trial in patients with *H. pylori*-associated gastritis using furazolidine (40 mg) and nitrofurantoin (400 mg) for 2 weeks. Of the patients treated with nitrofurantoin, 44% had *H. pylori* eradicated [5]. An appreciable number of patients experienced side effects to lead the author to conclude that this was not an appropriate treatment. Borsch [6] also reported poor results with nitrofurantoin a smaller dose of 100 mg for 10 days with only one of 13 patients having *H. pylori* eradicated.

Hollingsworth et al. measured ampicillin, erythromycin and metronidazole levels in gastric juice after intravenous administration of their antibiotics. The gastric juice contained no detectable ampicillin but had high levels of erythromycin. Erythromycin is excreted in the bile, and the high levels in the gastric juice might be due to duodenogastric reflux [7]. Metronidazole may be the antibiotic of choice as it is secreted into the gastric juice. However, resistance to it can present because of previous exposure (primary), or it can be acquired (secondary). Up to 20% of patients have primary resistance, and this figure is higher in underdeveloped countries. Acquired metronidazole resistance is as high as 50%–70% of cases if used as monotherapy. Bismuth salts have been used to eradicate *H. pylori*, and the low relapse rates of duodenal ulcer treated with bismuth may be due to the antibacterial properties of colloidal bismuth subcitrate [8–10]. The eradication rates in published data vary between 10% and 50%, with one dose of bismuth given four times a day showing superior results to two doses twice a day [11, 12].

Combined Therapy with Antibiotics

Synergism between antibiotics is observed in vitro and may prevent the development of resistance in vivo. The combination of amoxicillin and metronidazole seems to reduce, though not eliminate, the development of resistance [13]. A study of 23 patients with duodenal ulcer treated for 12 days with amoxicillin (250 mg b.i.d.) and metronidazole (500 mg b.i.d.) and also given cimetidine 500 mg at night for 4 weeks showed an eradication rate of 75% (Table 2). Therapeutic failure was due to either primary or acquired resistance. A similar eradication (83%) was reported by Oderda et al. for a course of amoxicillin plus tinidazole given for 6 weeks [14], and an eradication rate of 77% reported by Borsch et al. [15] with amoxicillin plus metronidazole given for 1 month. We achieved an eradication rate of only 56% for metronidazole 400 mg t.i.d. and amoxicillin 500 mg t.i.d. given for 1 week [16]. However, we found that the addition of amoxycillin to combined treatment of colloidal bismuth subcitrate and metronidazole did not improve eradication rates [17]. Furthermore, it did not prevent the development of resistance. Metronidazole and tetracycline are synergistic in vitro against *H. pylori* and may be the combination of choice. However, tetracycline given on its own is ineffective in eradicating *H. pylori* [18].

Combinations of bismuth salts and various antibiotics have been tried with the aim of improving the rate of long-term *H. pylori* eradication [19]. The results of this are superior to those when each drug is given alone. The success may be due to the local bactericidal effects of the bismuth compounds combined with the systemic effect of the antibiotics. The bismuth particles may be bound to the lipopolysaccharide layer of the bacterial outer membrane. An intact lipopolysaccharide-containing bacterial outer membrane is essential for bacterial survival so that bismuth might damage the outer membrane and then render the micro-organism relatively sensitive to antibiotics.

Rauws et al. treated 63 patients with non-ulcer dyspepsia with a combination of colloidal bismuth subcitrate (q.i.d. 4 weeks) and amoxicillin (375 mg t.i.d. for 4 weeks). Twenty-one patients remained culture negative 1 year after treatment [20]. Bayerdorffer et al. investigated the effect of a combination of ofloxacin (200 mg b.i.d.) and bismuth subsalicylate (600 mg t.i.d.) on 15 patients with duodenal ulcer. *H. pylori* was eradicated in only three out of nine patients

Table 2. Combination of antibacterial agents in eradicating *H. pylori*

Regimen	Dosage	*n*	Eradication rate	Reference
Metronidazole + amoxicillin	3 × 500 mg, 2 weeks 3 × 500 mg, 2 weeks	9	90%	Borsch et al. [6]
Amoxicillin + metronidazole	250 mg b.i.d, 4 weeks 500 mg b.i.d, 4 weeks	23	75%	Hirschl et al. [13]
Metronidazole + amoxicillin	400 mg t.i.d, 1 week 500 mg t.i.d, 1 week	90	56%	Patchett et al. [16]
CBS + amoxicillin	4 × 120 mg, 4 weeks 3 × 375 mg, 4 weeks	40		Rauws et al. [20]

CBS, Colloidal bismuth subcitrate.

evaluated 4 weeks after starting treatment. All strains were sensitive to ofloxacin before treatment but three acquired resistance after treatment [21]. Marshall found that the combination of colloidal bismuth and tinidazole eradicated *H. pylori* in 70% of patients [9].

Triple Therapy with Antibiotics

Borody et al. treated 10 dyspeptic patients with a combination of colloidal bismuth subcitrate (q.i.d.) tetracycline (500 mg q.i.d.) both for 4 weeks with metronidazole (200 mg q.i.d.) for the first 2 weeks. In eight patients tetracycline was replaced by amoxicillin (250 mg q.i.d.). The eradication rate of *H. pylori* evaluated after treatment was 94% (Table 3). However this regimen was associated with side effects, and two patients developed *Clostridium difficile*-associated colitis [22].

Rauws et al. found triple therapy with colloidal bismuth subcitrate, amoxicillin and metronidazole for 1 month to be effective in eradicating *H. pylori* in 39 out of 48 patients. However, three of the patients had to stop the treatment because of side effects. One of these patients developed an associated antibiotic diarrhoe [18]. Borsch et al. investigated the efficacy of a 14-day course of the combination of bismuth subsalicylate (600 mg t.i.d.), amoxicillin suspension (500 mg t.i.d) and metronidazole (500 mg t.i.d.) in treating patients with duodenal ulcer. Nine out of ten patients had *H. pylori* eradicated [6].

In a study we compared colloidal bismuth subcitrate with four antibiotic regimens. The antibiotic regimens were used for only 1 week, and we observed no side effects. Metronidazole (200 mg t.i.d.) or amoxicillin (500 mg t.i.d.) with colloidal bismuth subcitrate did not improve eradication rates, but metronidazole (400 mg t.i.d.) for 1 week significantly improved eradication rates (81%). The addition of amoxicillin did not improve eradication rates and did not prevent the development of resistance [17].

Bell et al. found a 2-week course of metronidazole (400 mg t.i.d.) to be more effective than a 1-week course in eradicating *H. pylori* when used in combination with colloidal bismuth subcitrate [23]. Triple therapy appears to be the most

Table 3. Effect of combined triple therapy treatment on *H. pylori*

Regimen	Dosage	*n*	Eradication rate	Reference
CBS	4 × 120 mg, 4 weeks	100	94%	Borody et al. [22]
+ tetracycline	4 × 500 mg, 4 weeks			
+ metronidazole	4 × 200 mg, 2 weeks			
CBS	1 tablet q.i.d, 4 weeks	48	81%	Rauws and Tytgat [18]
+ amoxycillin	375 mg t.i.d, 4 weeks			
+ metronidazole	500 mg t.i.d, 18–28 days			
BSS	600 mg t.i.d, 2 weeks	10	90%	Borsch et al. [6]
+ amoxycillin	500 mg t.i.d, 2 weeks			
+ metronidazole	500 mg t.i.d, 2 weeks			

CBS, Colloidal bismuth subcitrate; BSS, bismuth subsalicylate.

effective treatment, but it is complex as it requires the patient to take 10–12 tablets per day.

Compliance as well as resistance must be a factor in the failure to achieve eradication. Treatment of resistant *H. pylori* strains is still problematic. It is not clear whether the addition of tetracycline prevents the development of resistance or eradicates organisms that have primary resistance when used as triple therapy. Regimens without metronidazole have been advocated which include pivampicillin 500 mg b.i.d. for 2 weeks in conjunction with liquid colloidal bismuth subcitrate [24].

Our treatment of choice is triple therapy with colloidal bismuth subcitrate q.i.d. for 4 weeks with tetracycline 500 mg t.i.d. and metronidazole 400 mg t.i.d. for 1 week. This regimen is free of side effects; so far we have not observed any acquired resistance, and it has been effective in eradicating resistant strains [25]. The main disadvantage is that it requires patients to take multiple tablets. Logan et al. reported a 78% eradication rate with a 1-week treatment regimen of colloidal bismuth subcitrate 120 mg q.i.d. and amoxicillin 500 mg q.i.d. for 1 week and metronidazole 400 mg t.i.d. for 3 days (days 5–7) in patients with non-ulcer dyspepsia and peptic ulcer. The major cause of non-eradication was metronidazole resistance. Only 4 of the 21 resistant strains were cleared with this regimen. The authors proposed that biopsies be taken to test for metronidazole sensitivity before instituting treatment [26]. What is required is a simple, safe, non-toxic regimen to overcome the problem of *H. pylori* resistance. Regimens without metronidazole have been advocated for resistant strains.

Omeprazole

Omeprazole (a proton pump inhibitor) has antibacterial properties in vitro, but it is formulated in an acid-resistant capsule and is unlikely to have a direct effect on gastric *H. pylori* in vivo. However, omeprazole does have a suppressive effect on *H. pylori* [27].

The achlorhydric conditions probably render the *H. pylori* biologically inactive as it is not required to secrete urease and may adapt a cocoid form. However, achlorhydric conditions may allow antibiotics to be more active. Preliminary studies suggest that the combination of antibiotics can eradicate *H. pylori* in about 60% of cases.

However, we have found the combination of omeprazole and amoxicillin not to be successful in eradicating *H. pylori*. We have found that triple therapy with omeprazole 20 mg for 1 week and tetracycline 500 mg t.i.d. and metronidazole 400 mg t.i.d. to be effective in eradicating *H. pylori* in 60% of patients.

Conclusion

Eradication of *H. pylori* is one of the greatest challenges in medicine today even after successful eradication, as recrudescence or reinfection can occur. This has implications in terms of treatment because patients may relapse following successful eradication. It may be justifiable to treat asymptomatic relatives of patients with *H. pylori*. This is more feasible now as non-invasive techniques become available to detect the presence of *H. pylori*, for example, the ^{13}C-urea breath test and serology. Controlled trials are necessary in this area.

The ideal treatment of *H. pylori* is not yet available. This would need to be simple, safe and free of side effects. An antibiotic that has the desired profile against *H. pylori* has not yet been found.

References

1. Glupczynski Y, Burette A, Labbe M, Deprez C, De Reuck M, Delterne M (1988) *Campylobacter pylori* associated gastritis, a double-blind placebo controlled trial with amoxycillin. Am J Gastroenterol 83: 365–372
2. Stone JW, Wise R, Donovan IA, Gearty JC (1988) Failure of ciprofloxacin to eradicate *Campylobacter pylori* from the stomach. J Antimicrob Chemotherap 22: 92–93
3. Glupczynski Y, Labbe M, Burette A, Delmee M, Avesni V, Bruck C (1987) Treatment failure of ofloxacin in *Campylobacter pylori* infection. Lancet i: 1096
4. McNulty CAM, Gearty JC, Grump B et al. (1986) *Campylobacter pyloridis* and associated gastritis: investigator blind, placebo controlled trial of bismuth salicylate and erythromgen ethylsuccimate. Br Med J 293: 645–649
5. Morgan D, Kraft WC, Bender M, Pearson A (1988) Nitrofurans in the treatment of gastritis associated with *Campylobacter pylori*. Gastroenterology 95: 1178–1184
6. Borsch G, Mai U, Muller KM (1988) Monotherapy or polychemotherapy in the treatment of *Campylobacter pylori* related gastroduodenal disease. Scand J Gastroenterol 23 [Suppl 142]: 101–106
7. Hollingsworth JA, Goldie J, Siletti CF et al. (1988) Does gastric secretions of antibodies explain differential eradication rates of *Campylobacter pyloridis*? Workshop C. pylori Colorado (Keystone) 1988 (Abstract)
8. Coghlan JG, Gilligan D, Humphries H, McKenna D, Dooley C, Sweeney E, Keane C, O'Morain C (1987) *Campylobacter pylori* and recurrence of duodenal ulcers: a 12 month follow-up study. Lancet ii: 1109–1111
9. Marshall BJ, Goodwin CS, Warren JR, Murray R, Blincow ED, Blackbourn SJ, Phillips M, Waters TE, Sanderson CR (1988) Prospective double blind trial of duodenal ulcer relapse after eradication of *Campylobacter pylori*. Lancet ii: 1437–1442
10. Rauws EA, Tytgat GNJ (1990) Cure of duodenal ulcer associated with eradication of *Helicobacter pylori*. Lancet i: 1233–1235
11. Coghlan JG, Gilligan D, Humphries H et al. (1990) Efficacy of different dosage regimes in duodenal ulcer healing and eradication of *Helicobacter pylori*. Aliment Pharmacol Ther 4: 449–450
12. Lambert JR, Borromeo M, Eaves EA, Hanskey J, Korman M (1988) Efficacy of different dosage regimes of bismuth in eradicating *Campylobacter pylori*. Gastroenterology 94: A248 (abstract)
13. Hirschl AM, Hentschel E, Berger J, Nemec H, Rotter ML (1991) Treatment of *Helicobacter pylori* infection with amoxycillin plus metronidazole, bacteriological, serological and histological results. Eur J Gastroenterol Hepatol 3: 3–7
14. Oderda G, Vaira D, Holton J, Ainley C, Altare F, Ansaldi N (1989) Amoxycillin plus tinidazole for *Campylobacter pylori* gastritis in children: assessment by serum IgG antibody by G antibody, pepsinogen and gastrin levels. Lancet ii: 690–692
15. Borsch G, Mai U, Opferkuck W (1988) Oral triple therapy may effectively eradicate *Campylobacter pylori* in man. Gastroenterology 94: A44 (abstract)
16. Patchett S, Beattie S, Leen E, Keane C, O'Morain C (1991) Eradicating *Helicobacter pylori* and symptoms of non-ulcer dyspepsia. Br Med J 303: 1238–1240
17. O'Riordan T, Mathai E, Tobin A, McKenna D, Keane C, Sweeney E, O'Morain A (1990)

Adjuvant antibiotic therapy in duodenal ulcers treated with colloidal bismuth subcitrate. Gut 31: 999–1002
18. Rauws EAJ, Tytgat GN (1989) *Campylobacter pylori.* Den Ouden, Amsterdam
19. Rauws EAJ (1989) Therapeutic attempts at eradication of *Campylobacter pyloridis.* Eur J Gastroenterol Hepatol 1: 34–41
20. Rauws EAJ, Langenberg W, Hauthoff HJ, Zanen HC, Tytgat GNJ (1988) *Campylobacter pyloridis* associated with chronic antral gastritis. Gastroenterology 94: 33–40
21. Bayerdorffer E, Simon TH, Bastlein CL, Alenjann R, Kasper G (1987) Bismuth/ofloxacin combination for duodenal ulcer. Lancet ii: 1467–1468
22. Borody T, Code P, Noonan S, Eaves ER, Jansky J (1988) Longterm *Campylobacter pylori* recurrence post eradication. Gastroenterology 94: A43 (abstract)
23. Bell GD, Weil J, Powell K, Jobson R et al. (1991) *Helicobacter pylori* treated with combination of tripotassium dicitrato and metronidazole; efficacy of different treatment regimens and some observations on the emergence of metronidazole resistance. Eur J Gastroenterol Hepatol 3: 319–322
24. Weil J, Bell GD, Powell K, Morden A, Harrison G, Gant PW, Trowell JE (1991) *Helicobacter pylori*; treatment with combinations of pivampicillin and tripotassium dicitrato bismuthate. Aliment Pharmacol Ther 5: 543–548
25. Patchett S, Beattie S, Keane C, O'Morain (1992) Short-term triple therapy for H. pylori-associated duodenal ulcer disease. Aliment Pharmacol Ther 6: 113–117
26. Logan RPH, Gummett PA, Misiewicz JJ, Karim QN, Walker MM, Baron JH (1991) One week eradication regimen for *Helicobacter pylori.* Lancet ii: 1249–1252
27. Weill J, Bell GD, Powell K, Morden A, Harrison G, Gant PW, Jones PH, Trowell PE (1991) Omeprazole and *Helicobacter pylori*: temporary suppression rather than true eradication. Aliment Pharmacol Ther 5: 309–314
28. Hirschl AM, Hentschel E, Schutze K, Nemec H, Potzi R, Gangl A et al. (1988) The efficacy of antimicrobial treatment in *Campylobacter pylori*-associated gastritis and duodenal ulcer. Scand J Gastroenterol 23 [Suppl 142]: 76–81

Cytoprotective Drugs and *Helicobacter pylori* Infection

M. Del Tacca, G. Natale, and C. Blandizzi

Introduction

Cytoprotection has been defined as the ability of pharmacological agents, originally prostaglandins (PGs), to prevent or reduce gastric or intestinal mucosal injury produced by a variety of ulcerogenic and necrotizing agents, including ethanol, nonsteroidal anti inflammatory drugs (NSAIDs), steroids, bile and *Helicobacter pylori* (HP; Fig. 1). Gastric mucus plays an important role in maintaining or restoring gastroduodenal mucosal integrity because, other than acting as a physical barrier, mucus may create an unstirred layer of secreted bicarbonate and hence help to neutralize hydrogen ions.

The role of HP micro-organisms in gastric pathology is under active investigation at the present time. These bacteria are within mucosal layer and are associated with epithelial cells. Chen et al. [6] have provided histological evidence of the association between the presence of HP and the occurrence of gastric mucosa lesions.

Biochemical studies have indicated that HP markedly affects gastric mucus integrity by producing specific enzymes such as glycosyl hydrolase, protease and urease. A marked breakdown of gastric mucus by glycosyl hydrolase has been demonstrated by Nakajima et al. [16] on human gastric mucus from healthy volunteers (Fig. 2). Slomiany et al. [20] have shown that HP filtrate also contains proteases capable of rapid mucus degradation leading to disintegration of its polymeric structure.

Cave and Vargas [5] demonstrated that HP as a whole organism or as a sonicate can profoundly inhibit histamine-stimulated acid secretion from rabbit parietal cells. The extent of acid secretion inhibition corresponded to that of cimetidine $10^{-4} M$. Pronase completely eliminates the effect of HP, suggesting that the inhibitor factor is at least in part comprised of a protein. Presumably, the reduction in acid secretion helps HP to colonize the stomach.

Experiments in which human gastric mucus was incubated with urea in the presence of HP urease have revealed structural changes of mucus glycoproteins. On this basis, Sidebotham and Baron [19] have postulated that HP urease catalizes the transformation into ammonia of plasma urea transuded toward gastric surface. This urea metabolite would cause a rearrangement of mucus glycoproteins from a normal structure (spherical micellae) to a less viscous one

Institute of Medical Pharmacology, University of Pisa, Via Roma 55, 56126 Pisa, Italy

Gasbarrini/Pretolani (Eds.)
Basic and Clinical Aspects of H. pylori Infection

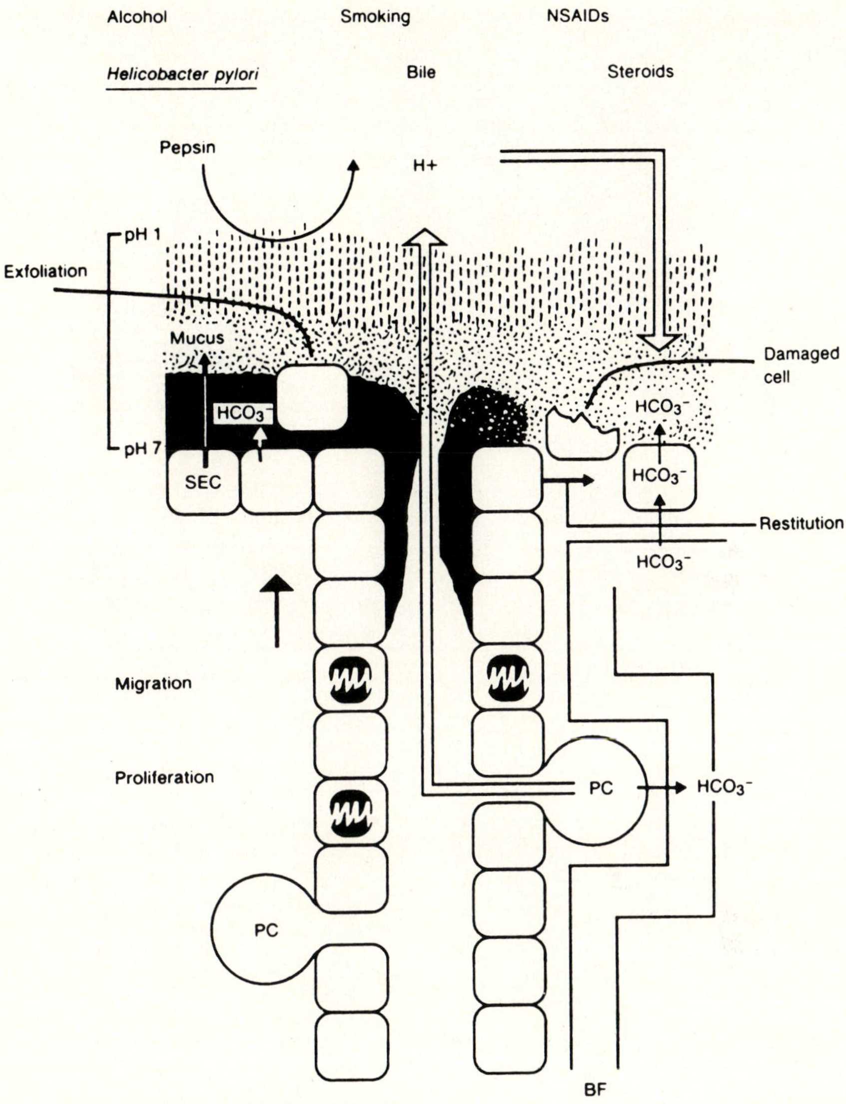

Fig. 1. Schematic representation of epithelial renewal in gastric mucosal protection. *BF*, Blood flow; *PC*, parietal cell; *SEC*, surface epithelial cell [12]

(lamellar micellae), thus favoring HP motility and colonization of gastric mucosa.

Taha et al. [23] used histopathological methods to assess the microstructure of human antral mucosa incubated with HP culture filtrate alone or in the presence of indomethacin. When administered alone, the filtrate or indomethacin did not affect the structure of the mucosa, whereas the combined treatment with filtrate plus indomethacin reduced the mass of viable cells, suggesting cytotoxic activity of HP filtrate. The precise structure of the toxic factor in the HP culture

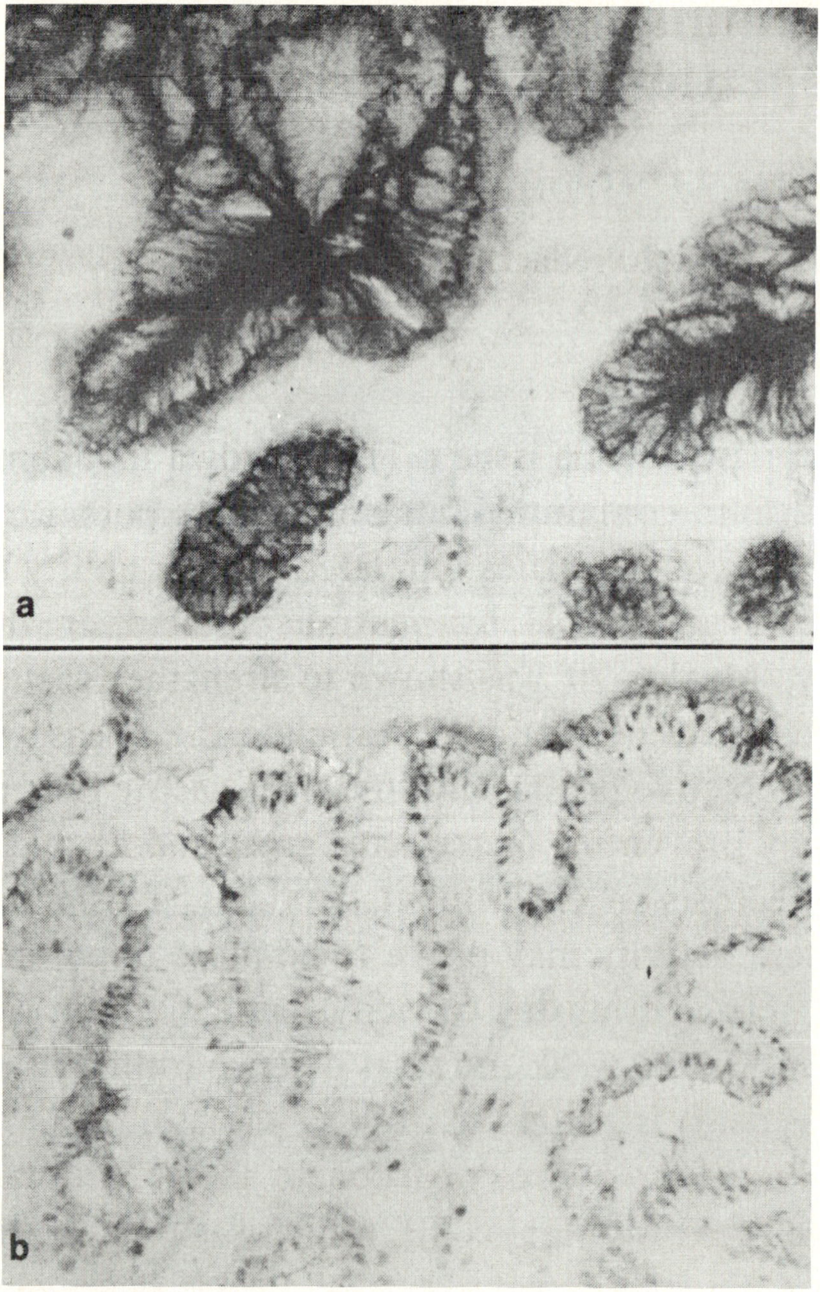

Fig. 2a, b. Breakdown of gastric mucus by enzymes derived from HP. Shown are sections of human gastric mucosa following incubation with saline (**a**) or enzyme preparation (**b**) and staining by means of the periodic acid–Schiff reaction [16]

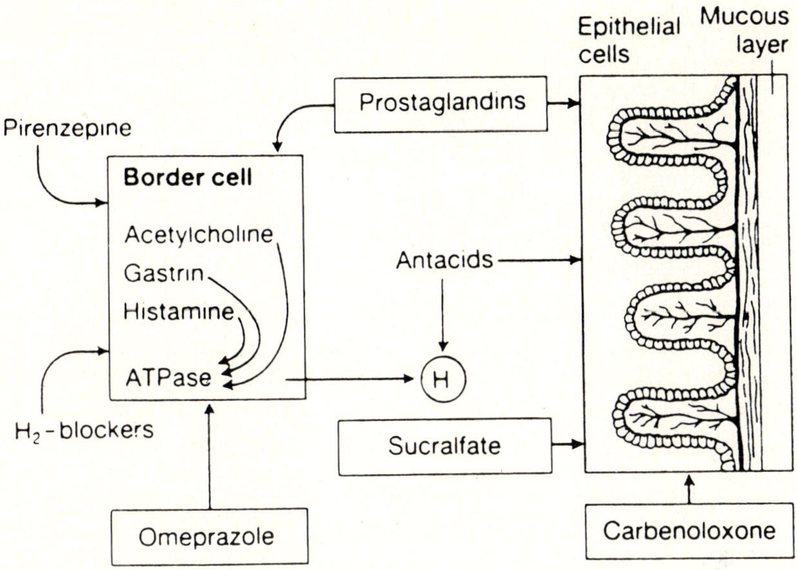

Fig. 3. Diagram showing the proposed sites of action of several gastroprotective drugs [26]

filtrate is not known, although it might be a protein, as suggested by Cave and Vargas [5]. Cytotoxic activity of culture filtrate of HP against in vitro human and animal cell lines has also been observed by Leunk et al. [14].

The cytoprotective drugs include well-documented agents such as PGs, sucralfate, bismuth salts, antacids, carbenoxolone and putative drugs, such as epidermal growth factor (EGF) or omeprazole (Fig. 3).

The most common mechanisms of the pharmacological activity of sucralfate, carbenoxolone, and bismuth derivatives involve PG and/or mucus production. In particular, the proposed mechanisms of sucralfate include formation of a barrier consisting of stable complexes of drug molecules and mucosal proteins on the eroded or ulcerated mucosa, deactivation of pepsin, and binding of both pepsin and bile acids [13]. Moreover, the basis of the protective and therapeutic activity of sucralfate seems to consist of stimulation of PG production and mucus release, as well as mucosal cell renewal [24]. Pirenzepine appears to cytoprotect by increasing mucosal blood flow [2]. Growth factors, such as EGF, might cytoprotect through preservation of cellular DNA synthesis [13]. The cytoprotective activity of omeprazole is still under investigation [4].

Both natural and synthetic PGs represent active cytoprotective agents with beneficial effects on inflamed or ulcerated gastrointestinal mucosa [21]. The pharmacological mechanisms mediating cytoprotective effects of PGs include: stimulation of mucus secretion, stabilization of cell membranes, increase in gastric mucosal blood flow, stimulation of bicarbonate secretion [21], trophic action, and strengthening of the phospholipid layer [10]. On the isolated surface epithelial cells from rat gastric mucosa Kobayashi et al. [10] found that PGs were the most active cytoprotective drugs. Among them the most potent were dimethyl-dinoprostone and misoprostol (Fig. 4). In a classic rat model of acute

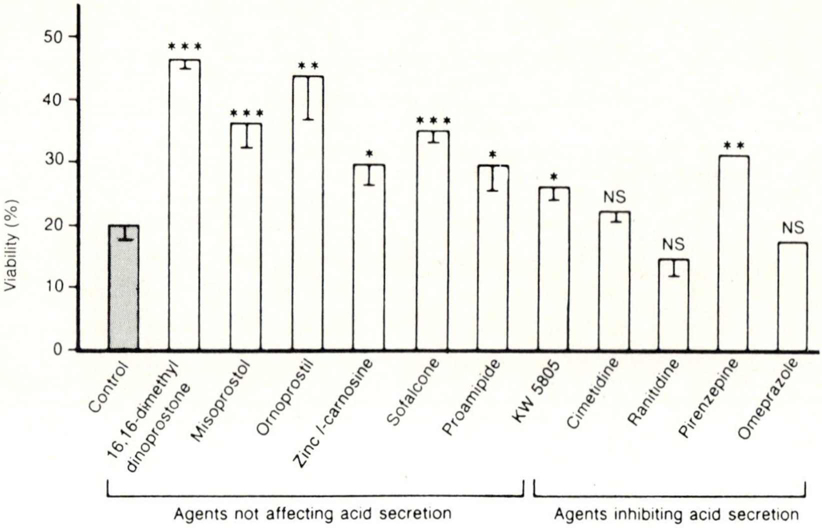

Fig. 4. Isolated surface epithelial cells of rat stomach. Effect of antiulcer drugs on 15% ethanol-induced damage (percentage of viable cells in the total cell counter). *$p < 0.05$; **$p < 0.02$; ***$p < 0.001$; *NS*, not significant [10]

gastric mucosal injury caused by absolute ethanol, Tarnawski et al. [25] demonstrated the higher protection rate displayed by 16-16-dimethyl-PGE_2. No data are at present available about the effects of PGs on HP-induced digestive lesions.

Berstad et al. [3] first demonstrated that aluminum-magnesium antacids given to patients with nonulcer dyspepsia and erosive prepyloric changes, with or without associated HP infection, decreased the density of HP without any improvement of the inflammatory reaction. Thus, suppressing HP infection by antacids may not benefit digestive pathology.

The effects of sucralfate and sulglycotide were examined on active gastritis and HP colonization of the gastric mucosa in nonulcer dyspepsia patients [1]. Although both treatments induced a marked regression of active gastritis, HP colonization remained unchanged at the end of the treatment, suggesting that remission of active gastritis may be independent of HP clearance (Table 1).

Colloidal bismuth subcitrate (CBS) is classified as a mucosal-protecting agent, but it also shows antibacterial action which may be useful for treating peptic diseases associated with HP infection [8]. Following a 6-week treatment with CBS, the incidence of HP decreases significantly, and this is accompanied by diminished severity of histological gastritis. By eradicating HP, CBS alters the natural history of the disease, and this may explain the lower incidence of peptic ulcer relapse after CBS [8].

As far as the relationship between HP infection and endogenous PGs is concerned, an increase in PG production could be expected as a response of neutrophils and macrophages to the infection with enhanced levels of both PGs and leukotrienes (LTs) [17]. Fukuda et al. [7] have demonstrated a significant enhancement of tissue concentration of LTB_4 in patients affected by gastritis

Table 1. Patients with nonulcer dyspepsia: evaluation of gastritis severity and HP density (both expressed as scores) at baseline and after treatment with sucralfate or sulglycotide (from [1])

Treatment	Before treatment	After treatment	p^a
Sucralfate ($n = 39$)			
Body			
Gastritis	2.82 ± 0.38	1.69 ± 0.36	< 0.05
HP density	1.76 ± 0.14	1.45 ± 0.13	NS
Antrum			
Gastritis	4.51 ± 0.21	2.10 ± 0.37	< 0.0001
HP density	1.89 ± 0.15	2.03 ± 0.13	NS
Sulglycotide ($n = 50$)			
Body			
Gastritis	3.68 ± 0.31	2.22 ± 0.32	< 0.01
HP density	1.59 ± 0.13	1.45 ± 0.13	NS
Antrum			
Gastritis	4.12 ± 0.23	2.62 ± 0.34	< 0.001
HP density	1.88 ± 0.14	1.82 ± 0.14	NS

[a] Wilcoxon's rank sum test.

associated with HP infection, which suggests a possible pathogenetic role of LTs in HP digestive disease. However, Taha et al. [23] demonstrated that PGE_2 production by tissue specimens of human gastric antral mucosa exposed to HP culture filtrate plus indomethacin was more markedly inhibited compared with indomethacin alone. This inhibition may be due to a combination of cyclooxygenase blockade and a reduction of viable cells induced by HP [23]. The relationship between bacterial toxins and PG synthesis is still unclear; however, other bacterial toxins such as lipopolysaccharides increase intestinal PG synthesis in the laboratory animals [18].

Understanding of the interaction between HP culture filtrate and indomethacin might have therapeutic implications if confirmed by in vivo studies. It could explain at least in part the higher incidence of complications related to NSAIDs in elderly patients who have a higher prevalence of HP colonization [9].

Other studies confirm that PG synthesis is increased in the presence of gastritis and gastric ulcer regardless of HP status [22]. The total amount of PGs produced under these conditions could result mainly from PGs produced by inflammatory cells, since both human neutrophils and macrophages have the capacity to synthesize PGs [15]. The lack of difference between PG values in patients with or without HP infection might depend on the density of the organisms [22].

Considering the possible interaction between HP and endogenous production of PGE_2 [23] or LTB_4 [7] and the fact that the cytoprotective effects of sucralfate, sulglycotide, or CBS are mediated by stimulation of endogenous PG production [1, 11], thus exogenous PGs may be beneficial for the restoration of mucosal integrity in the presence of HP infection.

In conclusion, although substantial evidence supports a critical role of HP participation in the multifactorial pathogenesis of peptic disease, the pharmacological effects of cytoprotective drugs in the treatment of HP infection are still unclear. No significant relationship has been found between cytoprotection by antacids, sucralfate, or sulglycotide and HP infection. In the case of bismuth derivatives, their efficacy against HP may be ascribed mainly to their antibacterial activity. The putative protective effect of PGs against HP mucosal lesions remains to be established.

References

1. Barbara L, Biasco G, Capurso L, Dobrilla G, Lalli A, Paganelli GM, Pallone F, Torsoli A (1990) Effects of sucralfate and sulglycotide treatment on active gastritis and *Helicobacter pylori* colonization of the gastric mucosa in non-ulcer dyspepsia patients. Am J Gastroenterol 85: 1109–1113
2. Bernardini MC, Blandizzi C, Morini G, Chiavarini M, Impicciatore M, Del Tacca M (1989) Pirenzepine prevents cysteamine-induced formation of gastroduodenal ulcers and reduction of mesenteric circulation. Arch Int Pharmacodyn Ther 302: 242–254
3. Berstad A, Alexander B, Weberg R, Serck-Hanssen A, Holland S, Hirschowitz BI (1988) Antacids reduce *Campylobacter pylori* colonization without healing the gastritis in patients with nonulcer dyspepsia and erosive prepyloric changes. Gastroenterology 95: 619–624
4. Blandizzi C, Gherardi G, Marveggio C, Del Tacca M (1991) Omeprazole-induced protection against experimental gastric ulceration is mediated by an increase in mucus secretion. Digestion 49(Sl): 14
5. Cave DR, Vargas M (1989) Effect of a *Campylobacter pylori* protein on acid secretion by parietal cells. Lancet ii: 187–189
6. Chen XG, Correa P, Offerhaus J, Rodriguez E, Janney F, Hoffmann E, Fox J, Hunter F, Diavolitsis S (1986) Ultrastructure of the gastric mucosa harboring *Campylobacter*-like organisms. Am J Clin Pathol 86: 575–582
7. Fukuda T, Kimura S, Arakawa T (1990) Possible role of leukotrienes in gastritis associated with *Campylobacter pylori*. J Clin Gastroenterol 12: S131–S134
8. Humphreys H, Bourke S, Dooley C, McKenna D, Power B, Keane CT, Sweeney EC, O'Morain C (1988) Effect of treatment on *Campylobacter pylori* in peptic disease: a randomised prospective trial. Gut 29: 279–283
9. Jones DM, Eldridge JA, Sethi P, Whorrell PJ (1986) Antibody to the gastric *Campylobacter*-like organisms "*Campylobacter pyloridis*" clinical correlation and distribution in the normal population. J Med Microbiol 22: 57–66
10. Kobayashi K, Arakawa T, Nakamura H (1990) An experimental model for evaluating the protective effects of antiulcer drugs. Drug Invest 2(1): 10–12
11. Konturek SJ, Bilski J, Kwiecien N, Obtulowicz W, Kopp B, Oleksy J (1987) De-Nol stimulates gastric and duodenal alkaline secretion through prostaglandin-dependent mechanism. Gut 28: 1557–1563
12. Kuwayama H, Matsuo Y, Eastwood GL (1990) Gastroduodenal mucosal injury by nonsteroidal anti-inflammatory drugs. Drug Invest 2(1): 22–26
13. Lambert JR (1990) Effect of antiulcer drugs on *Helicobacter pylori*. Drug Invest 2(1): 52–55
14. Leunk RD, Johnson PT, David BC, Kraft WG, Morgan DR (1988) Cytotoxic activity in broth-culture filtrates of *Campylobacter pylori*. J Med Microbiol 26: 93–99
15. Morley J, Bray MA, Jones RW (1979) Prostaglandin and thromboxane production by human and guinea pig macrophages and leucocytes. Prostaglandins 17: 730–736
16. Nakajima M, Tanaka N, Kuwayama H (1990) Digestion of human gastric mucus by extracellular enzymes of *Helicobacter pylori*. Drug Invest 2(1): 60–62
17. Parodi MC, Marugo M, Ciancamerla G, Santucci R, Fazzuoli L (1990) Prostaglandin E_2 and $F_{2\alpha}$ levels in the duodenal and antral mucosa of non-ulcer dyspeptic and duodenal ulcer patients. Hepatogastroenterology 37: 208–211

18. Peskar BM, Weiler H, Kroner EE, Peskar BA (1981) Release of prostaglandins by small intestine tissue of man and rat in vitro and the effect of endotoxin in the rat in vivo. Prostaglandins 21:9–14
19. Sidebotham RL, Baron JH (1990) Hypothesis: *Helicobacter pylori*, urease, mucus, and gastric ulcer. Lancet 335:193–195
20. Slomiany BL, Bilski J, Sarosiek J, Murty VLN, Dworkin B, VanHorn K, Zielenski J, Slomiany A (1987) *Campylobacter pyloridis* degrades mucin and undermines gastric mucosal integrity. Biochem Biophys Res Commun 144:307–314
21. Sontag SJ (1986) Prostaglandins in peptic ulcer disease: an overview of current status and future directions. Drugs 32:445–457
22. Taha AS, Boothman P, Holland P, McKinlay A, Upadhyay R, Kelly RW, Lee F, Russell RI (1990) Gastric mucosal prostaglandin synthesis in the presence of *Campylobacter pylori* in patients with gastric ulcers and non-ulcer dyspepsia. Am J Gastroenterol 85:47–50
23. Taha AS, Kelly RW, Gemmell CG, Lees FD, Russell RI (1990) The interaction between *Helicobacter pylori* culture filtrate and indomethacin: effects on the integrity of human gastric antral mucosa and its prostaglandin E_2 production in vitro. Aliment Pharmacol Ther 4:265–273
24. Tarnawski A, Hollander D, Cummings D, Krause WJ, Gergely H, Zipser RD (1984) Are antacids acid neutralizers only? Histologic, ultrastructural and functional changes in normal gastric mucosa induced by antacids. Gastroenterology 86:1276
25. Tarnawski A, Hollander D, Stachura J, Krause WJ, Gergely H (1985) Prostaglandin protection of the gastric mucosa against alcohol injury – a dynamic time-related process. Gastroenterology 8:334–352
26. Zeidler H, Muenzel P (1989) NSAIDs: new approaches to limiting gastropathy. Scand J Rheumatol 78:18–23

Approaches to the Treatment of *Helicobacter pylori* Infection

G. Bianchi Porro and M. Lazzaroni

The role of *Helicobacter pylori* in gastritis of the gastric antrum and corpus and in some closely related clinical manifestations, namely dyspepsia and peptic ulcer, has shed new light on the pathogenesis of these forms and changed the current therapeutic approach. Despite the multitude of proposals available and the unquestionably encouraging results seen in the prophylaxis of recurrent duodenal ulcer, the question still remains as to the indications for anti-infective therapy, and particularly its place among the current therapeutic options for type B gastritis, dyspepsia, and peptic ulcer.

Functional Dyspepsia

Functional dyspepsia is not yet clearly defined as a clinical entity, although various classifications have been suggested depending on the pathogenic element held to be predominant. Some authors [1] have proposed a classification into refluxlike dyspepsia, ulcerlike dyspepsia, dismotilitylike dyspepsia, and essential dyspepsia, but this has recently been up-dated and simplified to ulcerlike functional dyspepsia, dismotilitylike, and unspecified functional dyspepsia [2].

The continuing lack of precise therapeutic indications is due to the uncertain pathogenesis [3] and the methodological shortcomings concerning the use of populations that are not homogeneous as regards subjective manifestations or endoscopic findings (presence or absence of erosions or hyperemia of the gastric mucosa) and the investigational methods and evaluation criteria employed [4]. Another factor adding to the confusion is the elevated response to placebo, ranging from 20% to 60% in patients with various forms of dyspepsia [3].

Therapeutic experience to data is based on the use of antacids, antisecretory agents, prokinetics, and mucosal-protecting agents, either singly or in combination. The use of antacids, though widespread, is essentially disappointing. Analysis of experience in controlled studies in patients with ulcerlike or refluxlike dyspepsia (with or without inflammatory manifestations in the gastric or duodenal mucosa) with doses high enough to neutralize up to 500 mmol HCl/day has revealed no significant advantage over placebo [5–8]. Only an antacid-alginate combination has proved of some value, at least in patients with predominantly gastroesophageal reflux [9].

Gastrointestinal Unit, L. Sacco Hospital, Milan, Italy

Gasbarrini/Pretolani (Eds.)
Basic and Clinical Aspects of H. pylori Infection

H_2 antagonists (especially cimetidine and, more rarely, ranitidine) have generally been effective, although some controlled studies in small populations have not revealed significant differences compared with placebo. Meta-analyses [10] have shown a therapeutic gain of 18% (range 12%–24%) compared with placebo, particularly in patients with ulcerlike dyspepsia and histological evidence of antral gastritis or endoscopic findings of antral or duodenal erosions [11–13].

The role of pirenzepine is controversial. In some studies (published in journals sponsored by the manufacturers) a therapeutic gain of 25% (14%–36%) compared with placebo has been reported [10]. However, besides causing unwanted effects, use of this drug seems to be restricted to subjects with ulcerlike dyspepsia. In controlled studies [11, 14] in patients with refluxlike dyspepsia this antimuscarinic agent was not superior to placebo.

Prokinetic drugs have provided very promising results in various forms of dyspepsia, both with and without disturbances of gastric emptying. The dopaminergic antagonists metoclopramide and domperidone, and cisapride, which has serotinin-4 receptor agonist activity and favors acetylcholine release from the myoenteric plexus, give a therapeutic gain compared with placebo of 56% and 39% respectively [10, 15].

The complex cyto-/site-protective activity of sucralfate has provided the rationale for its use in dyspeptic patients with chronic gastritis or erosions of the gastroduodenal mucosa. The results are controversial. Compared with placebo, sucralfate has shown significantly greater activity mainly in patients without inflammatory manifestations in the gastric or duodenal mucosa [16]. On the other hand, sucralfate has shown greater activity than ranitidine, antacids, or misoprostol [17, 18] in inducing remission of histological and endoscopic lesions but not of clinical manifestations.

Against the background of this variety of therapeutic options, the role of anti-infective treatment in the dyspeptic syndrome and in the forms of gastritis associated with this condition is still uncertain. Anti-infective therapy is certainly known to play a positive role in *H. pylori* associated gastritis [19]. The use of bismuth compounds (colloidal subcitrate and subsalicylate) and antibiotics (including amoxycillin, nitroimidazoles, tetracyclines) has resulted in eradication of the micro-organism and cure of the gastritis in 15%–20% of patients (in the case of bismuth compounds alone) and more than 90% with combined regimes (triple therapy). However, these positive results are offset by significant uncertainty as to the clinical significance of type B gastritis. There is still debate as to whether it has causal significance in well-drained subjective manifestations or is merely a casual finding. The high prevalence of gastritis B in asymptomatic subjects and the lack of any close correlation between cure of mucosal inflammatory status and relief of subjective disturbances suggests that the gastritis is in fact of limited clinical significance; thus the utility of any kind of treatment is questionable [20–22].

In contrast with these considerations are the preliminary observations in case-control studies which, though open to methodological criticism, raise a worrying question as to the relationship between chronic gastritis and some forms of gastric cancer [23–25]. If this were to be confirmed, the clinical role of gastritis would take on a quite different meaning, probably justifying long-term anti-infective treatment even in asymptomatic subjects.

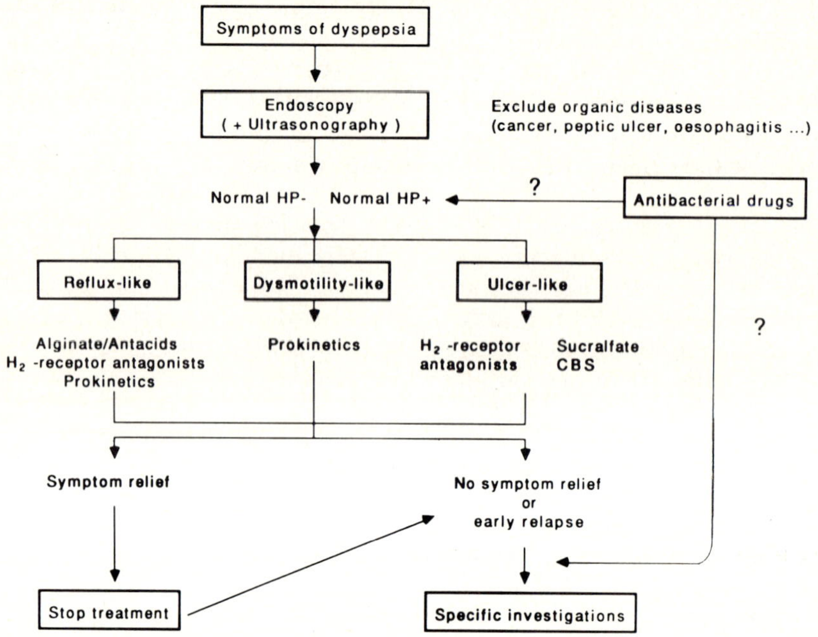

Fig. 1. Nonulcer dyspepsia and *H. pylori* (*HP*): which strategy? Some theoretical guidelines for the management of patients with dyspepsia with or without HP infection

Equally uncertain is the role of anti-infective therapy in functional dyspepsia [26] (Fig. 1). The available therapeutic studies provide conflicting findings and are not always acceptable from a methodological viewpoint [27]. A recent overview by Canadian authors [28] turned up some apparent methodological shortcomings both in the evaluation of the subjective symptomatology and in the design of the therapeutic protocols, which involved the use of antibiotics that can per se cause dyspeptic symptoms, thus altering the therapeutic conclusions, at least with the short observations times so far employed. In any case, as already mentioned, the results themselves are not in agreement [29–37] (Table 1).

Table 1. *Helicobacter pylori* and functional dyspepsia: clinical and histological outcome after antiinfective treatment

Reference	Gastritis score	HP prevalence	Symptoms	p^a
McNulty [33]	↓	↓	↓	NS
Borody [30]	↓	↓	↓	S
Lambert [31]	↓	↓	↓	S
Rokkas [29]	↓	↓	↓	S
Berstad [35]	↑	↓	=	
Loffeld [32]	↓	↓	=	
Kang [36]	↓	↓	↓	S
Holcombe [37]	ND	I	=	

↑, Worsening; ↓, improvement; =, no modifications.
[a] *p* values refer to symptom scores.

The significant correlation between eradication of *Helicobacter* and attenuation of inflammatory manifestations in the gastric mucosa has not been matched by relief of the clinical manifestations. In only four controlled studies was there a corresponding significant improvement in subjective symptoms, and this was in patients also treated with colloidal bismuth subcitrate, which has far more complex pharmacological properties than a simple antibacterial action.

Duodenal Ulcer

The role of anti-infective therapy in the short-term treatment of peptic ulcer in an attempt to improve the clinical results obtained with antisecretory agents, or with traditional mucosal protecting agents, is unconvincing at present. Contrary to expectations, isolated use of antibacterial drugs has not generally proved effective. The positive findings with metronidazole [38] and furazolidone [39, 40] warrant more rigorous confirmation in view of certain clear methodological shortcomings and because metronidazole can in any case exert indirect cytoprotective activity on the gastric mucosa independently of its antibacterial action [41].

The significant therapeutic results obtained with colloidal bismuth subcitrate (CBS), alone or in combination with one or two antibiotics, must be interpreted with caution in the light of the drug's intrinsic cytoprotective and antipeptic action and the fact that the bactericidal action is present in only about 50% of the patients achieving a cure.

The only indications as to the usefulness of *Helicobacter* eradication for accelerating and improving the cure rates in duodenal ulcer can be gleaned from two studies. On the basis of the experience of Bayerdorffer et al. [42] in an open pilot study, the combination of ofloxacin and ranitidine produced acceptable eradication (33%) but above all a significantly higher rate of ulcer healing than the H_2 antagonist alone: 93% versus 64% after four weeks of treatment.

Certainly more interesting but requiring confirmation is the controlled study by Graham et al. [43]. A triple therapy (CBS-metronidazole-tetracycline) combined with ranitidine 300 mg showed a therapeutic gain compared with the H_2 antagonist alone ranging from 19% to 14% over a period of 2–16 weeks.

On the other hand, short-term treatment with antibacterial drugs takes on an extremely interesting role in the prevention of ulcer recurrence [44, 45]. Their positive influence, at least in the medium term, on the natural history of the disease undoubtedly represents an important advance compared with traditional drugs, particularly antisecretory agents.

The trial results so far available [46–59] show that the risk of duodenal ulcer recurrence is closely correlated to the presence of *H. pylori* infection at the start of the observation period after healing, with recurrence rates after 12–18 months of observation ranging from 74% to 80% in HP-positive and 0% to 27% in HP-negative patients (Fig. 2).

These differences are certainly interesting and seem to provide ample justification for the claim [53] that eradication of the micro-organism cures duodenal

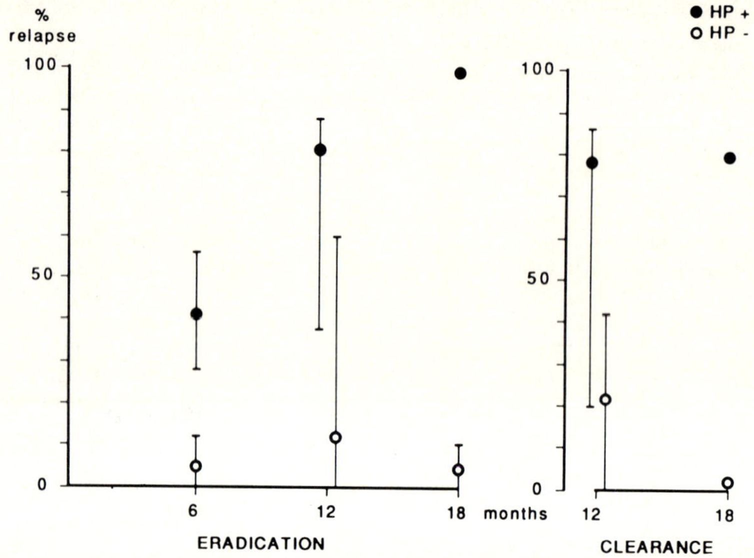

Fig. 2. Duodenal ulcer: long-term outcome after antibacterial treatment. Median values (and ranges) after eradication (*left*) or after clearance (*right*) of the micro-organism

ulcer and that anti-infective drugs are therefore an essential tool in the treatment of ulcer patients. However, objective analysis of the data available highlights a series of problems concerning the methods and interpretation of the results. The foundations of the theory of infection are seen to be fragile, and its therapeutic implications are not easy to put into clinical practice.

Methodological shortcomings include the following: trials not rigorously double-blinded, inadequate case lists, variability of criteria for judging success

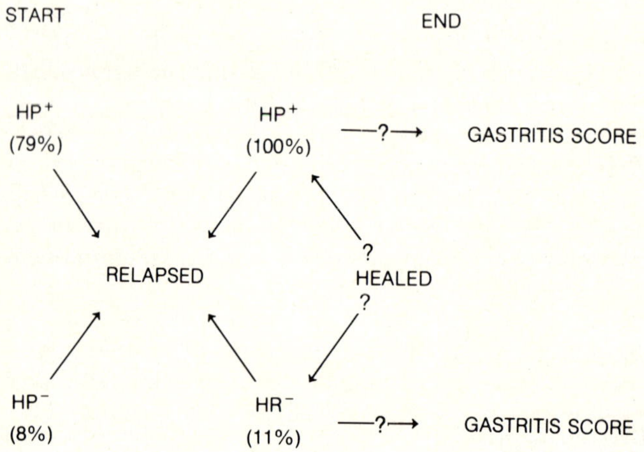

Fig. 3. Duodenal ulcer and *H. pylori* (*HP*) infection: Following after antibacterial treatment. Data concerning gastritis score and HP status in control patients are lacking

of the anti-infective therapy, lack of information about the course of inflammatory processes in the gastric and duodenal mucosa and on the prevalence of infection in the controls without recurrence (Fig. 3). Further problems still remain as regards:

- The type of patient to be treated with antibiotics. No specific group of ulcer patients has been identified as ideal candidates for anti-infective treatment. The best candidates – though this can be considered a subjective opinion – are probably young subjects with duodenal ulcer who do not agree to a long pharmacological follow-up, who have multiple recurrences, or who are resistant to treatment with H2 antagonists or (though highly improbably) to adequate treatment wth omeprazole. No precise indication emerges as to the usefulness of anti-infective treatment in gastric ulcer.
- The choice of treatment protocol. The plethora of current proposals, and the lack of a correct analysis of their risks and benefits and of patient compliance, certainly causes considerable perplexity as to the antibiotics to be used, with which drug(s): bismuth compounds? omeprazole?
- The duration of treatment, which, from the initial tests lasting 28 days, has been gradually reduced to 14 days, 1 week, and finally to only 1 day!
- The method of drug administration: in syrup or tablets (capsules), in single or divided doses, on an empty stomach or with meals.
- The modalities and timing of in vitro antibiotic susceptibility tests, particularly for metronidazole, to which *Helicobacter* has shown resistance in two or three out of ten patients.
- The approach of patients who are not cured after one cycle of combined treatment with antibiotics, or who present recurrence of infection but not of the ulcer.

Certainly these questions do not detract from the importance of the theory of infection in the etiopathogenesis of peptic ulcer, but they do show clearly that the attempt to translate their therapeutic implications into daily clinical practice is still in its infancy. State-of-the-art anti-infective treatment of peptic ulcer cannot be considered as replacing classical treatment with antisecretory drugs (H_2 antagonists or omeprazole) but may reasonably be a useful addition in well-defined patient groups under controlled clinical conditions.

References

1. Colin Jones DG (1988) Management of dyspepsia: report of a working party. Lancet 1: 576–579
2. Talley NJ, Colin Jones DG, Kock KL et al (1991) Functional dyspepsia: a classification with guidelines for diagnosis and management. Gastroenterol Int 4: 145–160
3. Talley NJ, Phillips SF (1988) Non ulcer dyspepsia: potential causes and pathophysiology. Ann Intern Med 108: 865–879
4. Petersen H, Loge I, Johannessen T et al. (1987) Dyspepsia: therapeutic response as a diagnostic tool. Scand J Gastroenterol 128: 108–113

5. Hyren O, Adami H, Bates S et al. (1986) Absence of therapeutic benefit from antacids or cimetidine in non ulcer dyspepsia. N Engl J Med 314: 339–343
6. Jonsson KA, Gotthard R, Bodemar G, Brodin U (1989) The clinical relevance of endoscopic and histological inflammation of gastroduodenal mucosa in dyspepsia of unknown origin. Scand J Gastroenterol 24: 385–395
7. Weberg R, Berstad A (1988) Low dose antacids and pirenzepine in the treatment of patients with non ulcer dyspepsia and erosive prepyloric changes. A randomized double blind placebo controlled trial. Scand J Gastroenterol 23: 237–243
8. Gottard R, Bodemar G, Brodin U, Johnsson KA (1988) Treatment with cimetidine, antacid or placebo in patients with dyspepsia of unknown origin, Scand J Gastroenterol 23: 7–18
9. McHardy G (1978) A multicentric randomized trial of Gaviscon in reflux esophagitis. South Med J 71:16
10. Dobrilla G, Comberlato M, Steele A, Vallaperta P (1989) Drug treatment of functional dyspepsia. A meta analysis of randomized controlled clinical trial. J Clin Gastroenterol 11: 169–177
11. Talley NJ, McNeil D, Hayden A, Piper DW (1986) Randomized, double blind, placebo controlled cross-over trial of cimetidine and pyrenzepine in non ulcer dyspepsia. Gastroenterology 91: 149–156
12. Johannessen T, Fjosne U, Kleveland PM et al. (1988) Cimetidine responders in non ulcer dyspepsia. Scand J Gastroenterol 23: 327–336
13. Nesland AA, Berstad A (1985) Effect of cimetidine in patients with non ulcer dyspepsia and erosive prepyloric changes. Scand J Gastroenterol 20: 629–635
14. Smith PM, Troughton AH, Gleeson F et al. (1990) Pirenzepine in non ulcer dyspepsia: a double blind multicentre trial. J Int Med Res 18: 16–20
15. Rosch W (1989) Efficacy of cisapride in the treatment of epigastric pain and concomitant symptoms in non ulcer dyspepsia. Scand J Gastroenterol 24 [Suppl 165]: 54–58
16. Kairaluoma MI, Hentilae R, Alavaikko M et al. (1987) Sucralfate versus placebo in treatment of non ulcer dyspepsia. Am J Med 83: 51–55
17. Guslandi M (1989) Comparison of sucralfate and ranitidine in the treatment of chronic non erosive gastritis. A randomized multicentre trial. Am J Med 86: 45–48
18. Safrany L, Schott B (1983) Vergleich von Sucralfat und Antazida in der Behandlung der unspezifischen Erosivhämorrhagischen duodenitis Therapiewoche 33: 5233–5236
19. Rauws EAJ, Tytgat GN (1989) *Campylobacter pylori*: treatment of gastritis. In: Rathbone BJ, Heatley RV (eds) *Campylobacter pylori* and gastroduodenal disease. Blackwell Scientific, Oxford, pp 225–231
20. Thalley NJ (1988) *Campylobacter pylori* associated gastritis. Is antibiotic therapy now justified? J Clin Gastroenterol 10: 10–12
21. Bartlett JG (1988) *Campylobacter pylori*: fact or fancy? Gastroenterology 94: 229–232
22. Sobala G, Dixon M, Axon ATR (1990) Symptomatology of *Helicobacter pylori* associated dyspepsia. Eur J Gastroenterol Hepatol 2: 445–449
23. Personnet J, Friedman GD, Vanderstreen DP et al. (1991) *Helicobacter pylori* infection and the risk of gastric cancer. N Engl J Med 325: 1127–1131
24. Nomura A, Stemmerman GN, Chyou PH et al. (1991) *Helicobacter pylori* infection and gastric carcinoma among Japanese Americans in Hawaii. N Engl J Med 325: 1132–1136
25. Forman D, Newell DG, Fullerton F et al (1991) Association between infection with *Helicobacter pylori* and risk of gastric cancer: evidence from a prospective investigation. Br Med J 302: 1302–1305
26. Shallcross TM, Rathbone, Heatley RV (1989) *Campylobacter pylori* and non ulcer dyspepsia. In: Rathbone BJ, Heatley RV (eds) Campylobacter pylori and gastroduodenal disease. Blackwell Scientific, Oxford, pp 115–166
27. Carrick 1988 Problems with clinical trials on *Campylobacter pylori*. J Clin Gastroenterol 10: 247–248
28. Veldhuizen van Zanten SJO, Tytgat KMAJ, Jalali S et al. (1989) Can gastritis symptoms be evaluated in clinical trials? An overview of treatment of gastritis, non ulcer dyspepsia and *Campylobacter pylori* associated gastritis. J Clin Gastroenterol 11: 496–501
29. Rokkas T, Pursey C, Uzeochina E et al. (1987) *Campylobacter pylori* and nonulcer dyspepsia. Am J Gastroenterol 11: 1149–1152
30. Borody T, Hennessy, Daskalopoulos G et al. (1987) Double blind trial of DeNol in non ulcer dyspepsia associated with *Campylobacter pylori* gastritis. Gastroenterology 92: 1324

31. Lambert JR, Borromeo M, Korman MG, Hansley J (1987) Role of *Campylobacter pylori* in non ulcer dyspepsia. A randomized controlled trial. Gastroenterology 92: 1488
32. Loffeld RJLF, Potters JVJP, Stobberingh E et al. (1989) *Campylobacter pylori* associated gastritis in patients with non ulcer dyspepsia: a double blind placebo controlled trial with colloidal bismuth subcitrate Gut 30: 1206–1212
33. McNulty CAM, Gearty JC, Crump B et al. (1986) *Campylobacter pyloridis* associated gastritis: investigator blind, placebo controlled trial of bismuth salicylate and erythromycin ethylsuccinate. Br Med J 293: 645–649
34. Rauws EAJ, Langerberg W, Houthoff HJ (1988) *Campylobacter pyloridis* associated chronic active antral gastritis, a prospective study of its prevalence and the effect of antibacterial and antiulcer therapy. Gastroenterology 94: 34–40
35. Berstad A, Alexander B, Weberg R, Serck-Hansen A, Holland S, Hirchowitz BJ (1988) Antacids reduce *Campylobacter pylori* colonisation without healing the gastritis in patients with non ulcer dyspepsia and erosive prepyloric changes Gastroenterology 95: 619–624
36. Kang JY, Tay HH, Wee A et al. (1990) Effect of colloidal bismuth subcitrate on symptoms and gastric histology in non ulcer dyspepsia. A double blind placebo controlled study. Gut 31: 476–480
37. Holcombe C, Thom C, Kaluba J, Lucas SB (1992) *Helicobacter pylori* clearance in the treatment of non ulcer dyspepsia Eur J Gastroenterol Hepatol ii: 87–92
38. Quintero-Diaz M, Sotto-Escobar A (1986) Metronidazole versus cimetidine in the treatment of gastroduodenal ulcer Lancet 1: 907
39. Zhao H, Li G, Guo J, Yan Z, Sun S, Li L, Duan Y, Yue F (1985) Furazolidone in peptic ulcer. Lancet 1: 907
40. Zheng Z, Wang Z, Chu Y, Li Y, Li Q, Lin S, Xu Z (1985) Double blind short term trial of furazolidone in peptic ulcer. Lancet 1: 1048–1049
41. Satoh H, Guth P, Grossman M (1983) Role of bacteria in gastric ulceration produced by indomethacin in the rat: cytoprotective action of antibiotics. Gastroenterology 84: 483–489
42. Bayerdorffer E, Pirlet TH, Sommer A, Kasper G, Ottenjann R (1988) Ofloxacin in der Therapie "resis tenter" Ulcera duodeni. Eine Pilot-Studie. Z Gastroenterol 2:155–159
43. Graham DY, Ginger M, Lew PAC (1991) Effect of triple therapy (antibiotics plus bismuth) on duodenal ulcer healing Ann Intern Med 115: 266–269
44. Coghlan JG, Tobin A, O'Morain C (1989) *Campylobacter pylori* and ulcer treatment. In: Rathbone J, Heatley RV (eds) Campylobacter pylori and Gastroduodenal disease. Blackwell, Oxford, pp 232–245
45. Axon ATR (1989) *Campylobacter pylori* – therapy review Scand J Gastroenterol 24 [Suppl 160]:35–38
46. Lambert JR, Borromeo M, Korman MG, Ansky J, Eaves ER (1987) Effect of colloidal bismuth (DeNol) on healing and subsequent relapse of duodenal ulcers. Role of *Campylobacter pyloridis* (abstract). Gastroenterology 92: 1489
47. Borody T, Cole P, Noonan S et al. (1988) Longterm *Campylobacter pylori* recurrence post eradication. Gastroenterology 94: A43
48. Coghlan JG, Gilligan Humphreis H et al. (1987) *Campylobacter pylori* and recurrence of duodenal ulcer. A 12 month follow up study. Lancet ii: 1109–1111
49. Marshall BJ, Goodwin CS, Warren JR et al. (1988) Prospective double blind trial of duodenal ulcer relapse after eradication of *Campylobacter pylori*. Lancet ii: 1437–1441
50. Smith AC, Price AB, Borriello P, Levi AJ. (1988) A comparison of ranitidine and tripotassium dicitrato bismuth (TDB) in relapse rate of duodenal ulcer. The role of *Campylobacter pylori*. Gastroenterology 94: A431
51. Borsch G, Wegener M, Reitemeyer E, Mai U, Opferkuch W (1989) Clinical results and medium term follow-up studies after eradication of *Campylobacter pylori*. In: Megraand F, Lamouliatte H (eds) Gastroduodenal pathology and *Campylobacter pylori*. Excerpta Medica, Amsterdam pp 599–603
52. Mannes GA, Bayerdorffer E, Hochter W et al. (1989) Early relapse after healing of *C. pylori* positive duodenal ulcers. Klin Wochenschr 67 [Suppl 13]: 44
53. Rauws EAJ, Tytgat GNJ (1990) Cure of duodenal ulcer associated with eradication of *Helicobacter pylori*. Lancet 335: 1233–1235
54. Patchett S, Beattie S, O'Riordan TO, Leen E, Keane C, O'Morain C (1990) Effect of eradication

of *Helicobacter pylori* on duodenal ulcer recurrence. The World Congress Gastroenterology, Sydney, 26–31 Aug 1990, abstract, p 953
55. Mannes GA, Bayerdorffer E, Hochter W et al. (1990) Relapse rate of *H. pylori* positive duodenal ulcers (DU) following antibacterial activity. Thc World Congress Gastroenterology, Sydney, 26–31 Aug 1990, abstract, p 955
56. Amstrong D, Blum AL, Damman H et al. (1990) The effect of *Helicobacter pylori* on the healing and relapse of duodenal ulcer. Rev Esp Enferm Dig 78 [Suppl 1]: 132
57. Bayerdorffer E, Mannes GA, Hochter W et al: (1990) Relapse rate of *H. pylori* (HP) positive duodenal ulcers (DU) following antibacterial therapy Rev Esp Enfern Dig 78 [Suppl 1]: 110
58. Coelho L, Passos MCF, Chausson Y, Castro LP (1990) *Helicobacter pylori* and duodenal ulcer relapse: effect of a bismuth free short term triple therapy. Rev Esp Enferm Dig 78 [Suppl 1]: 109
59. Pallen MJ, Clayton CL (1990) Vaccination against *H. pylori* urease. Lancet 336: 186 (letter)

Subject Index

Acid 4, 5, 74, 241, 243
– hypersecretion 52
– output 49, 52
– regurgitation 3
– secretion 4, 39, 48, 49, 122, 123, 241, 244, 252, 290
– – basal 5
– – peak 5
acridine orange stain 221
adherence 90, 260
– assays 228
– bacterial 91, 229
– properties 259
adhesins 85, 90, 91, 183, 192, 261
adhesion 65, 92, 260, 261
agglutinins 261
alcohol 5, 13, 24
– dehydrogenase 268
– use 12, 171, 173
ammonia 82, 261, 290
– toxic effects 262
amoxicillin 6, 12, 14, 30, 45, 237, 254, 255, 256, 275, 280, 281, 283, 285, 286, 287, 299
– suspension 286
ampicillin 244, 251, 259, 284
antacid-alginate 298
antacids 293, 294, 296, 298
antibiotic 42
– monotherapy 45
– therapy 101, 109
– – perioperative 44
– treatment 45
antibiotics 42, 45
antibodies
– *H. pylori* 19, 21, 30, 83, 84, 113, 124, 134, 136, 170
– – IgA 22, 159, 162, 163
– – IgG 20, 22, 171
– – neutralizing vacuplating activity
– – subclass IgG1, IgG2, IgG4, 159, 160, 163
antigen
– acid extract 155
– – glicin 19
– CAR5 109, CD20, 101, CD45RO 101, CD43 101, CD3, 114, CD4 114, CD8 114, HLA-DR 101, HM-CAP 155
antioxidants 110
antral cells 4
antritis 237
– endoscopic 13, 14
Archeabacteria 65
asialofetuin 94
autoradiography 67

Bacillus subtills 227
Bacillus thermoproteolyticus 93
belching 6
Beneckea spp 60
beta-lactams 241, 283
biopsies
– antral 21, 30, 74, 113, 145
– body 145
– duodenal 42
– from antrum 12, 42, 119, 125, 252
– from corpus 12, 42, 125
– from fundus 252
– gastric 12
bismuth 5, 6, 12, 41, 42, 237, 244, 248, 271, 281, 296
– aluminate 266, 271
– carboxylate 266
– colloidal subcitrate (CBS) 6, 29, 30, 258, 259, 260, 261, 262, 267, 268, 269, 272, 275, 280, 281, 283, 284, 285, 286, 287, 294, 295, 299, 301
– compounds 58, 266, 268, 269, 271, 272, 281, 285, 299, 303
– containing medicines (BCM) 258, 260, 261, 262, 263
– dialylacetate 276
– encephalopathy 276
– nefrotoxicity 276
– neuropathy 276
– osteoarthropathy 276
– salts 241, 259, 266, 272, 275, 276, 284, 285, 293
– subcarbonate 266, 271, 272, 276
– subcitrate 8, 26
– subgallate 266, 271, 272, 276
– – introxication 266
– subnitrate (BSN) 258, 259, 261, 271, 272, 276
– subsalicylate (BSS) 247, 258, 259, 260, 261, 262, 267, 275, 285, 286, 299

bismuth (*contd.*)
– therapy 238, 275
– thiolate 266
– trithioglycollamate 276
bloating 3, 13, 14
– postprandial 6
burping 13, 14, 15, 16
buspirone 5
broth
– coltures supernatants 82
– filtrates 80

CBS 12, 251, 254, 255, 258, 259, 260, 261, 262, 267, 268, 269, 272, 275, 280, 281, 283, 284, 285, 294, 295, 301
CLO-test 145
13 C-urea breath test 238, 252, 288
14 C-urea breath test 74, 78, 159
Campylobacter 61, 63, 185
– *coli* 61, 185
– *jejuni* 61, 63, 156, 227
– – flagellin mutant 187
cancer 4, 101
– development 101, 113
– gastric 35, 57, 136, 165, 175, 219, 238, 239, 256, 299
– – early 109
cancerogenesis 101, 110, 175
carbenoxolone 293
carcinoma
– gastric 52, 168, 169, 175, 176
catalase 157, 162, 223, 224, 268
– recombinant 225
cephalexin 244
cephalosporin 246
chemotaxis 63
– of *H. pylori* 63
chromatography
– affinity exchange 79
– anion exchange 66, 67, 93
– fast protein liquid (FPLC) 154
– ion exchange 79, 80
cimetidine 241, 242, 281, 285, 299
ciprofloxacin 45, 244, 254, 259, 284
cisapride 299
clarithromycin 254
clindamycin 245, 248, 259, 281, 282
Clostridium difficile
– associated colitis 286
Clostridium perfringens 85, 93, 95
coffee
– and nonulcer dyspepsia 5
– and ulcer recurrence 40
cohort effect 16, 175
collagens 227, 229, 231, 232
colonization 290
– antral 78
– gastric mucosal 74
– on gastric epithelial cells 195
cryofixation 66, 70
culture
– of antral biopsies 23, 74, 84, 113, 114, 119, 123, 139, 203
– of *H. pylori* 19, 23, 42, 45, 159, 206, 213
– – continuous 167
cyclooxygenase 295
cyprofloxacin 237
cytoprotection 290, 296
– impaired gastric 108
cytotoxicity 79, 80, 120
– bacterial 105
– – direct 102
– epithelial 108
cytotoxin 83, 84, 85, 156
– assay 82, 83
– production 82, 216
– test 84
cytotoxins 261

DNA
– cellular synthesis 293
– DNA solution hybridization 57
– endonuclease profiling 57
– fingerprints 209, 212
– fragments 190, 204, 214, 224
– homology 216
– pairs 210
– patterns 213
– restriction chromosomal 57, 184, 224
– sequences 213
DOC-PAGE 66
dental prostheses 173
dental therapy 173
diarrhea 19, 258
– antibiotic associated 280
diet 5
dietary practices 173
distress symptoms 9
diversity
– allelic 57
– chromosomal 58
– genetic 58
domperidone 299
duodenal ulcer 4, 39, 43, 46, 48, 50, 52, 57, 58, 82, 83, 86, 87, 101, 105, 108, 125, 237, 239, 241, 252, 275, 281, 284, 285, 286, 301
– disease 21, 49
– healing 238
– pathogenesis 41, 57
– recurrent 298
– relapse 238
– resistant 246
duodenitis 49, 237, 238, 243
dyspepsia 3, 5, 11, 12, 49, 101, 239, 298
– essential 298
– functional 11, 298, 300

-- dysmotility-like 298
-- ulcer-like 3, 11, 16, 298, 299
--- symptoms 7
-- unspecified 298
- motility-like 3
- nonspecific 3, 4
- nonulcer 3, 4, 5, 6, 8, 9, 11, 12, 13, 14, 15, 16, 26, 29, 30, 239, 252, 275, 284, 285, 287, 294
- reflux-like 3, 298
- ulcer-type 5

Elderly 125, 139, 165, 295
electron microscopy 61, 91, 185, 259, 262
electrotransformation
- of *H. pylori* 180
ELISA 23, 24, 25, 29, 114, 124, 131, 134, 147, 155, 157, 159, 166, 171, 196, 203, 225
emotional factors 8
emptying
- gastric 5, 122, 123
-- delayed 5, 124
- of the stomach 39
endoscopy 4, 19, 21, 24, 25, 30, 42, 84, 86, 113, 122, 125, 139, 143, 204
- resources 23
enzyme
- profile of *H. pylori* 58
epidermal growth factor (EGF) 268, 293
eradication 237, 252, 255, 277, 283, 287, 288,
- of *H. pylori* 301
-- rates 238, 254, 275, 285, 286
-- therapy 239
erythromycin 244, 248, 254, 259, 281, 284
Escherichia coli 167, 183, 193, 195, 197, 201, 268
- K38 190
esophagitis 21, 24
ethanol 290, 294
Eubacteria 65
extracellular matrix 227, 228, 231
- proteins 227

Famotidine 242
farm animals 173
ferrets 74, 281
fetuin 94
fibronectin 227, 229, 231
fingerprinting
- molecular of *H. pylori* 206, 212, 216
flagella 60, 156, 183, 185, 260
- sheated 60
flagellar sheath 60, 183, 187
flagellin 60, 156, 162, 183, 185, 223
- antigenicity 61
- genes 61, 183, 185
- sequences 61
flow cytometric analysis 114
flurofamide 75, 76, 77, 78

follicles
- lymphoid activated 102
food intolerance 5
fullness 3
- postprandial 3
furazolidone 284, 301

G cell
- mass 52
gastrectomy
- partial 35
- specimens 101
gastric juice 261, 267, 272, 283, 284
- aspirates 203, 204
gastrin 4
- secretion 39
gastritis 4, 16, 20, 21, 22, 24, 29, 30, 42, 48, 49, 51, 52, 57, 82, 101, 108, 109, 126, 169, 237, 283, 289, 295, 298, 299
- antral 49, 50, 51, 247, 254, 299
- asymptomatic 57, 58
- atrophic 39, 48, 50, 51, 52, 104, 136, 139,
-- fundic (FAG) 122, 124
- body 49, 50
- chronic 11, 16, 21, 30, 31, 83, 275
-- type B 29, 82, 113, 119, 168, 176, 219, 241, 298, 299
- endoscopic 26
- histological 12, 13, 14, 16, 49, 294
- interstitial 104
- scores 6
- superficial 39, 49, 50, 51, 52, 104
gastroscopy 74
Giemsa
- modified stain 12, 23, 125
glycocalyx 261
glycosylhydrolase 290
gnotobiotic piglets 183, 281
Gram stain 43
granulocytes
- eosinophilic 104
- intraepithelial 29
- neutrophilic 102

H2
- antagonists 5, 13, 16, 75, 244, 283, 299, 303
-- blocker 239
-- treatment 4, 12, 35, 36, 173
-- use 11, 170
- blockers 241, 244
- receptor antagonists 241, 243, 244, 248, 251, 275
- receptor blockers 41, 242
- receptors 241
H+
- backdiffusion 262
HML 1-cells 114, 116, 117
haemoagglutination 93, 131

haemoagglutinin
– activity 227, 232
haemoagglutinins 90, 91, 92, 95, 96
haemolysin 86
haemolysis 85, 86, 88
– heat shock proteins 157, 164
heartburn 3, 11, 13, 14, 15, 16
Helicobacter 78
– *felis* 281
– *mustelae* 74, 75, 76, 77, 78, 203, 281
– *pylori* 5, 6, 11, 12, 13, 14, 15, 16, 19, 21, 23, 26, 27, 28, 31, 35, 41, 42, 43, 45, 46, 48, 50, 51, 52, 57, 58, 60, 61, 62, 65, 69, 70, 82, 84, 85, 87, 88, 91, 92, 96, 113, 131, 134, 145, 154, 183, 189, 195, 206, 219, 223, 232, 237, 241, 258, 263, 269, 275, 280, 281, 283, 286, 287, 288, 290, 298
– – aflagellate variant 63
– – CCUG 17874 79, 80, 220
– – cells 67
– – colonization 11, 21, 43, 45, 108, 234, 244, 248, 294, 295
– – clearance 45, 105, 241, 244, 252, 294
– – cytotoxin 80
– – epidemiology 136, 168, 175
– – eradication 6, 16, 30, 105, 109, 134, 156, 162, 239, 241, 244, 255, 256, 275, 283, 285, 301
– – flagellin 163
– – gastritis 6, 11, 16, 101, 110 125, 299
– – identification 19
– – infection 4, 5, 12, 20, 21, 22, 25, 29, 31, 44, 45, 51, 78, 117, 124, 159, 164, 165, 167, 168, 171, 175, 203, 237, 251, 260, 262, 276, 295, 296, 301
– – intrafamilial clustering 168
– – isogenic mutants 179
– – isolates 57, 58, 79, 86, 179, 203, 213
– – – cytotoxic 79, 80
– – – non cytotoxic 79, 219
– – motility 63
– – species 74
– – strains 57, 82, 83, 91, 92, 119, 195, 206, 219, 227, 260, 269
– – – cytotoxic 79, 84, 119, 219
– – surface associated proteins 65
hydroxitryptamine (5-HT) 5
– blocker 5
– receptor 5
hyperacidity 4
hypergastrinemia 52
hypoachlorhydria 124
hypoacidity
– and intestinal metaplasia 51
hypomotility 5
– antral 5

IgA
– *H. pylori* specific 29, 30
– mucosal recognition 80
– plasma cells 102, 105
– seropositivity 29, 30
IgG
– amtibodies 104
– *H. pylori* specific 29, 30
– mucosal recognition 80
– plasma cells 102, 104
– seropositivity 29, 30
– serum antibodies 84
– subclasses 159
– – in monitoring treatment of *H. pylori* 163
IgE antibodies 104
immunoassay
– enzyme 19, 22
immunoblotting 60, 79, 119, 131, 157, 171, 187, 201
immunogold labelling 60
– electron microscopy 60
immunolabelling 201
indomethacin 291, 295
infiltration
– granulocytic 110
– mononuclear cell 29
– neutrophil 104
– polymorphonuclear leukocytes 42
inflammation
– gastric mucosal 42, 44, 82
– antral 108
injury
– gastric mucosal 294
intercellular junctions 63
interferon gamma (INF) 114, 117
interleukin 6 (IL-6) 114, 117
isoelectric focusing 94

Lactose
– intolerance 21
– malabsorption 20
laminin 227, 229, 231, 232
lansoprazole 251, 280
latex agglutination 131
– tests 166, 203
lectins 92
leukocytes
– polymorphonuclear 260
leukotrienes (LTs) 294
lipases 262
LTB4 294
lyfestyle habits 168
lymphocytes 42
– B 102, 105
– infiltrating gastric mucosa 113
– intraepithelial 114, 117
– T 102, 113, 114
lysolecithin 262

Macrolides 241, 283
macrophages 104
mast cells 104

metaplasia
– gastric 4, 108, 237, 243, 244, 248
– – in the dudenum 4, 41, 42, 44, 45, 243
– intestinal 39, 51, 101, 108, 109, 110, 136
metoclopramide 299
metronidazole 6, 12, 14, 26, 27, 28, 41, 45, 237, 244, 251, 259, 275, 280, 281, 283, 284, 285, 286, 287, 301
– resistance 237, 238, 284
– resistant organisms 238, 239, 281
mezlocillin 41, 45
misoprostol 293, 299
Morganella Morganii 203
motility
– of *Campylobacter* 61
– disorders 248
mucosa
– antral 87, 104, 105, 291
– corpus 104, 105
– duodenal 268
– – and inflammation 45, 243, 248
– fundic 48
– gastric 8, 21, 82, 168, 189, 242, 260, 268, 275, 295
– – antrum 39
– – body 49, 52
– – damage 119
– hydrophobicity 262
– pyloric 48
mucus
– gastric 244, 252, 262, 268, 283, 290
– glycoproteins 290
– layer 43, 244
multilocus enzyme electrophoresis 57, 58
mycobacterium
– *leprae* 157
– *tuberculosis* 227

Nausea 3, 11, 13, 19
necrotaxis 104
neutrophils 113
nitrofurantoin 244, 283, 284
nitroimidazole 45
nitroimidazoles 241, 299
NLHB of *H. pylori*
– adhesin subunit 189, 192
– antibody 189
– fibrillar structure 192
nonsteroidal antiinflammatory drugs (NSAIDs) 12, 125, 126, 127, 134, 170, 173, 238, 290, 295
nonulcer dyspepsia (NUD) 3, 4, 5, 6, 8, 9, 11, 12, 13, 14, 15, 16, 26, 29, 30, 101, 105, 108, 239, 252, 275, 284, 285, 287, 294

Oesophagitis 238
ofloxacin 246, 285, 286, 301
omeprazole 35, 41, 42, 237, 251, 252, 253, 254, 255, 256, 281, 283, 287, 293, 303
orosomucoid 94
oxacillin 246, 247, 281

Pain 4, 5
– abdominal 3, 21, 22, 30
– – upper 11
– – recurrent (RAP) 6, 19, 20, 29, 30
– – – in childhood 6
– epigastric 3, 13, 14
pantoprazole 251
parietal cell 4
– mass 38
penicillin 237, 244
pentagastrin 5
pepsinogen I and II
– serum basal concentrations 49
peptic ulcer 4, 12, 21, 26, 31, 82, 119, 125, 169, 219, 247, 258, 275, 287, 294, 298, 301
– active 12
– disease 5, 11, 29, 30, 82, 101, 108, 206, 241, 251, 258, 295
– healing 241
– inactive 12
– treatment 35
pernicious anemia 120
personality 5, 8
– traits 9
– variables 8, 9
phagocytosis 65
phospholipase 96
– activity 93, 262
– hydrolizing enzymes 85
– C 85, 188
– – production 86
phospholipases 262
phospholipids 88
Photobacterium fischeri 60
pirenzepine 293, 299
pivampicillin 287
placebo 9, 26, 78, 298, 299
– effect 9
– response 5, 6, 8
plasmid
– DNA 190
– pHL 319–24 184, 185
– pHPA 22 189
– pHPA 23 189
– pHPA 26 191
– pIC20R2 184
– pILL 753 197
– pRH 121 185
– vectors 224
polymerase chain reaction (PCR) 196, 199, 203
– nested 199
pool
– acidic storage 246

prokinetics 298
prolactin 5
– release 5
pronase 290
prostaglandin
– analogues 283
– E2 268
– synthesis 295
prostaglandins (PGs) 290, 293, 294, 295, 296
protease 96, 290
proteases 290
protein
– cytotoxin associated 79, 81
– 15 kDa 157, 162
– 48 kDa 195, 201
– – antibodies 119
– 50 kDa 223
– 54 kDa 60
– 55 kDa 66, 162
– 82 kDa 79
– 95 kDa 79
– 120 kDa 154, 156, 162, 167, 260
– 130 kDa 79, 119, 219, 220, 222
proteoglycans 227, 232
Proteus mirabilis 203
proton pump inhibitors (PPI) 251, 256, 275
Pseudomonas aeruginosa 62, 63, 91
psychotherapy 8

Quinolones 241, 283

Radicals
– free 110
ranitidine 241, 242, 247, 255, 281, 284, 299, 301
– bismuth citrate 77, 78
RAP 9, 19, 20, 21
– psychosomatic 21
recombinant phage 196
recrudescence 287
reflux
– bile 35
– duodenogastric 284
– esophagitis 251, 252
– gastroesophageal 7, 12, 298
– – disease 21
– symptoms
regurgitation 19, 31
relaxation response 8
resistance
– antimicrobial acquired 45
restriction endonuclease analysis
– of genomic DNA 206, 207, 212
– of PCR products 206, 207, 212
restriction endonucleases 214
ribopatterns
– of *H. pylori* 213, 215, 226
– – Hae III 216
– – Hind III 217
ribotyping
– of *H. pylori* 213
rifampin 259

Salmonella typhimurium 63, 185, 197, 201
SDS-PAGE 66, 68, 69, 70, 79, 93, 94, 96, 119, 159, 185, 190, 197, 201, 206, 207, 220
serodiagnosis
– of *H. pylori* 23, 131, 165, 166
seroepidemiological tests 165
serological tests 131, 164
serology 23, 31, 136, 143, 146, 159, 167, 239
– kit evaluation 139
seroprevalence 137
– of *H. pylori* antibodies 137, 168
serotonin-4 receptor 299
sewage plants 173
sialoproteins 90
Skirrow's medium 23, 43
S layers 65, 70
– of *H. pylori* 66
smoking 5, 12, 13, 24, 40, 171
solphomucins 261
southern hybridization
– *H. pylori* chromosome 184, 214
spectrometry
– atomic absorption 272
spiral bacteria 23
Staphylococcus aureus 201
steroids 290
Streptomyces presens 93
stress 8, 9
– psychological 5
sucralfate 26, 293, 294, 295, 296
sucralfates 283
sulglycotide 294, 295, 296
surface
– active phospholipids 262
– epithelium damage 104
– exposed proteins 195
– gastric epithelial 101, 104, 183
surgery
– gastrointestinal 12
– gastric 24
symptoms 3, 21, 29
– dyspeptic 15, 26
– gastrointestinal 129
– psychosomatic 9, 19
– scores 14, 16
– subjective 301
– ulcer-like 11, 16

– Tetracycline 237, 244, 275, 283, 285, 286, 287, 301
tetracyclines 241, 299
therapy
– autogenic 8
tight junctions 244

tinidazole 29, 237, 255, 281, 286
– resistant strains 255
– transformation mediated allelic exchange 185
transmission
– bacterial mode 136
transposon mutagenesis 179
Treponema pallidum 227
trimethoprim 251
tritirachium album 93
Tumor growth factor alpha (TGF) 104
Tumor necrosis factor alpha (TNF) 144, 117

Ulcer 4
– chronic benign 35
– complicated 35, 39
– disease 21, 23, 42, 256, 277
– gastric 35, 49, 50, 52, 57, 82, 83, 101, 105, 108, 113, 125, 126, 239, 295, 303
– – prepyloric 39
– gastroduodenal 35
– pathogenesis 35
– recurrent 35
– relapses 21
ulceration 24, 105
– mucosal 104
– peptic 24, 80, 125, 127, 260
– endoscopic 26
– – duodenal 26
– – gastric 26, 82
ulcerogenesis 101, 110
Ure A gene 203
urea 261, 290
– breath test 136, 203, 242
urease 82, 87, 163, 167
– activity 67, 82, 96, 179, 239, 262
– colonization factor 74, 78
– *H. pylori* 155, 223, 290
– – negative mutant 74, 75
– – – isogenic 181
– inhibition 74, 78
– inhibitor 74
– monoclonal antibody 62
– recombinant 62
– secretion 74
– test
– – CLO 26
– – microtiter 12
– – rapid 42, 43

Vacuolating activity 79, 80, 82
vacuolating toxin 119, 122
vacuolization intracytoplasmic 119, 219
vagotomy 39
– proximal (PGV) 41, 42, 43, 44, 45
– selective 35
– – highly (HSV) 35, 36, 243
– truncal 35
variation
– allelic 57
Vibrio cholerae 60, 93, 227
– mutants 162
Vibrio parahaemolyticus 60
virulence 183
– factors 65, 85, 223, 260
– of *H. pylori* 79, 119
visual analogue scale (VAS) 12, 16
vomiting 3, 11, 13, 19, 31

Warthin-Starry 42
Western blotting 120, 160, 222, 223
– techniques 159, 225

Yersinosis 20

Zollinger-Ellison syndrome 243

Printing: Saladruck, Berlin
Binding: Buchbinderei Lüderitz & Bauer, Berlin